Hormone Analysis: Methodology and Clinical Interpretation

Volume II

Editors

George W. Pennington, M.D., F.R.C. Path.
Director, Sheffield and Region
Endocrine Investigation Centre
Jessop Hospital for Women
Sheffield, England

Sandra Naik, M.B., Ch.B., D.A.
Medical Assistant in Endocrinology
Sheffield and Region Endocrine
Investigation Centre
Jessop Hospital for Women
Sheffield, England

CRC Press, Inc.
Boca Raton, Florida

Library of Congress Cataloging in Publication Data

Main entry under title:

Hormone analysis.

Bibliography: v. p.
Includes index.
1. Hormones—Analysis. 2. Endocrine glands—
Diseases—Diagnosis. I. Pennington, George W.
II. Naik, Sandra, CDNLM: 1. Hormones—Analysis.
QY330 H8115
RB48.5.H67 616.4'0756 80-13417
ISBN 0-8493-5539-7 (v. 1)
ISBN 0-8493-5540-0 (v. 2)

Direct all inquiries to CRC Press, Inc., 2000 N.W. 24th Street, Boca Raton, Florida 33431.

International Standard Book Number 0-8493- 5539-7 (Volume I)
International Standard Book Number 0-8493-5540-0 (Volume II)
Library of Congress Card Number 80-13417
Printed in the United States

PREFACE

The aim of this book is to provide an easily accessable framework of knowledge in the field of endocrinology for both the clinician and the laboratory-oriented worker. Methods of analysis are described which are known to work, while the references provide a continuing source of additional material. The clinical interpretation of results is important if disease entities are to be recognized. This usually demands a knowledge of the physiological activity of individual glands, and this is discussed in most of the chapters. Among the biomedical fields, endocrinology has been a massive growing point in recent years and it is no longer possible for single individuals to have an intimate knowledge of all aspects of the subject. It was our intention, therefore, to identify contributing authors, and within a broad framework to request that they write chapters within their own areas of competence.

As editors we have not attempted to impose conditions as to the precise way in which the contents of chapters should be written. It is our hope that this freedom has led to a freshness of approach that would appeal to the individual reader. In addition to a survey of each of the endocrine glands, additional chapters have been written dealing with quality control, and the cellular action and chemistry of hormones, while the relationship of hormones to genetics and sexual differentiation and their usefulness as tumor markers are also discussed. These are likely areas of considerable advancement of knowledge in the immediate future. Our task as editors has been greatly facilitated by the help and cooperation of the contributing authors. We also wish to express our appreciation to Dr. B. Bevan and Mr. R. Hall for their unfailing assistance in times of stress. We are greatful also for the forbearance shown by the staff of our publishers CRC Press. If this book assists the clinical and laboratory worker and teaches the students of medicine, science, and laboratory technology it will have served its purpose.

G. W. Pennington
Sandra Naik

THE EDITORS

George W. Pennington, M.D., F.R.C.Path., is a Consultant Chemical Pathologist specializing in Endocrinology for the Sheffield Area Health Authority, Sheffield, England. He is Director of the Sheffield and Region Endocrine Investigation Centre based at the Jessop Hospital for Women. Incorporated within the work of this Unit is a Supra Regional Assay Service for the whole of Great Britain for certain steroid and polypeptide hormones. The Centre is one of three providing a follow-up service for all reported cases of hydatidiform mole and choriocarcinoma.

Dr. Pennington graduated M.B., Ch.B. in 1956 from the University of Liverpool, England, and also M.R.C.S., L.R.C.P. (London) the same year. He subsequently obtained the degrees of M.D. (Liverpool) 1959, M.S. (California) 1961, and M.A. (Dublin) 1962, and proceeded from membership (M.R.C.Path., 1963) to Fellowship (F.R.C.Path., 1973) of the Royal College of Pathologists.

He was formerly Professor of Pharmacology at Trinity College, University of Dublin, and Consultant Endocrine/Pharmacologist to the Dublin Federated Hospitals, and has acted as an external examiner in the National University of Ireland, and the Universities of Liverpool and Edinburgh.

Dr. Pennington is a member of the Society for Endocrinology, and has held various offices in the Association of Clinical Pathologists. He was the official analyst to the Irish Turf Club and has carried out similar work on behalf of the English, Belgian, and Cyprus Turf Clubs. He is currently an Honorary Member of the Association of Official Racing Chemists.

He has been a member of national, regional, and local committees, and chairman of a number of them. He has lectured widely both within the United Kingdom and by invitation on a number of occasions in the U.S. He had the honor to give the first ''Dyke'' Memorial Lecture, and has been a recipient of the British Medical Association ''Walter Dixon Memorial Scholarship''.

Dr. Pennington has published over 70 research papers, mainly in the field of reproductive endocrinology, and has either written or contributed to six books.

Sandra Naik, M.B., Ch.B., D.A. (RCSI), is a Medical Assistant specializing in Endocrinology at the Jessop Hospital for Women, Sheffield, England. She is an Honorary Clinical Tutor in Chemical Pathology at the University of Sheffield.

After graduation, she worked in East Africa and India. On returning to the U.K. she worked as an anesthetist for six years. Dr. Naik has worked for ten years in the fields of male and female infertility and took part in setting up an A.I.D. service. She has also studied and researched various biochemical methods of monitoring normal and abnormal pregnancy. She has contributed to scientific papers in the fields of reproductive endocrinology.

CONTRIBUTORS

Kenneth D. Bagshawe, M.D., F.R.C.P., F.R.C.O.G
Professor of Medical Oncology
Charing Cross Hospital Medical School
London, England

Brian R. Bevan, Ph.D
Principal Biochemist
Sheffield Area Health Authority
Jessop Hospital for Women
Sheffield, England

Charles E. Blank, M.B., B.Ch., Ph.D.
Reader in Medical Genetics
Sub-Department of Medical Genetics
University of Sheffield
Sheffield, England

Raymond Hall, L.R.I.C., Fi.M.L.T
Senior Chief Medical Laboratory Scientific Officer
Sheffield and Region Endocrine Investigation Centre
Jessop Hospital for Women
Sheffield, England

N. H. Hunt, Ph.D.
Research Fellow
Department of Experimental Pathology
John Curtin School of Medical Research
Australian National University
Canberra City, Australia

V. H. T. James, D.Sc.
Professor of Chemical Pathology
St. Mary's Hospital Medical School
University of London
London, England

Norman R. Lazarus, Ph.D
Head, Biochemical Research Department
Wellcome Foundation Ltd.
Dartford, England

Patricia W. Major, Ph.D.
Lecturer in Pharmacology
Academic Division of Medicine
University of Sheffield
Sheffield, England

Vincent Marks, D.M., F.R.C.P., F.R.C. Path.
Professor of Clinical Biochemistry
University of Surrey
Guildford
England

T. J. Martin, M.D., F.R.A.C.P.
Professor of Medicine
University of Melbourne and
Repatriation General Hospital
West Heidelberg
Victoria, Australia

Linda M. Morgan, Ph.D.
Senior Biochemist
Department of Clinical Biochemistry
University of Surrey
Guildford, England

James Mosley, D.Phil.
Senior Scientific Officer
Sheffield Area Health Authority
Jessop Hospital for Women
Sheffield, England

Sandra Naik, D.A.
Medical Assistant in Endocrinology
Sheffield and Region Endocrine Investigation Centre
Jessop Hospital for Women,
Sheffield, England

Kevin J. O'Connor, Ph.D.
Scientist, Biochemical Research Department
Wellcome Foundation Ltd.
Dartford, England

George W. Pennington, M.D., F.R.C. Path.
Director Sheffield and Region Endocrine Investigation Centre
Jessop Hospital for Women
Sheffield, England

Ronald Robinson, Ph.D., F.R.I.C.
Consultant Biochemist, Pathology Laboratory
Warwickshire Area Health Authority
Warwick, England

James S. Scott, M.D., F.R.S.C.E., F.R.C.O.G.
Professor of Obstetrics and Gynaecology
Leeds Maternity Hospital and
University of Leeds
Leeds, England

Stephen Tomlinson, M.D., M.R.C.P.
Wellcome Senior Research Fellow in Clinical Science
Department of Human Metabolism and Clinical Biochemistry
University of Sheffield Medical School
Sheffield, England

TABLE OF CONTENTS

Volume I

Volume II

CHAPTER 1

MALE GONADAL FUNCTION

Sandra Naik

TABLE OF CONTENTS

I. ANATOMY AND PHYSIOLOGY

A. Anatomy of the Genital Tract

The adult testis measures approximately 2.5 cm from side to side, 3 cm from back to front, and is 4 cm in length. It is covered by a tough dense capsule called the tunica albuginea. The veins of the testis lie close to the subcutaneous tissues of the scrotum and the returning venous blood is close to scrotal temperature,[1] which is about 2.2°C cooler than body temperature. Within the testis there are approximately 200 pyramidal lobules, each of which contains one or more coiled seminiferous tubules. These convoluted tubules converge at the hilar region of the testis where they become straight and anastomose to form the 9 to 15 collecting tubules of the rete testis. The tubules of the rete testis unite to form the epididymis, a tube 5 to 7 m long, the head of which is attached to the superior pole of the testis and the tail of which leads into the vas deferens. This is a thick muscular tube which, on leaving the scrotum, enters the inguinal canal penetrating the internal inguinal ring to travel in the pelvis behind the bladder. It then passes over the ureter and enlarges into the ampullary portion which penetrates the prostate and opens into the prostatic urethra as the ejaculatory duct.

The seminal vesicles arise as outbuddings from the vas at the ampullary portion. They provide a source of nutrient fructose and a proteinaceous material that contains a substrate for the enzymatic processes of seminal coagulation. Cowper's glands empty into the bulbous urethra and Littre's glands empty into the urethra. The prostatic ducts empty into the prostatic urethra along with the ejaculatory ducts (see Figure 1).

B. Histology of the Testis

Histological examination of a normal testicular biopsy is shown in Figure 2.

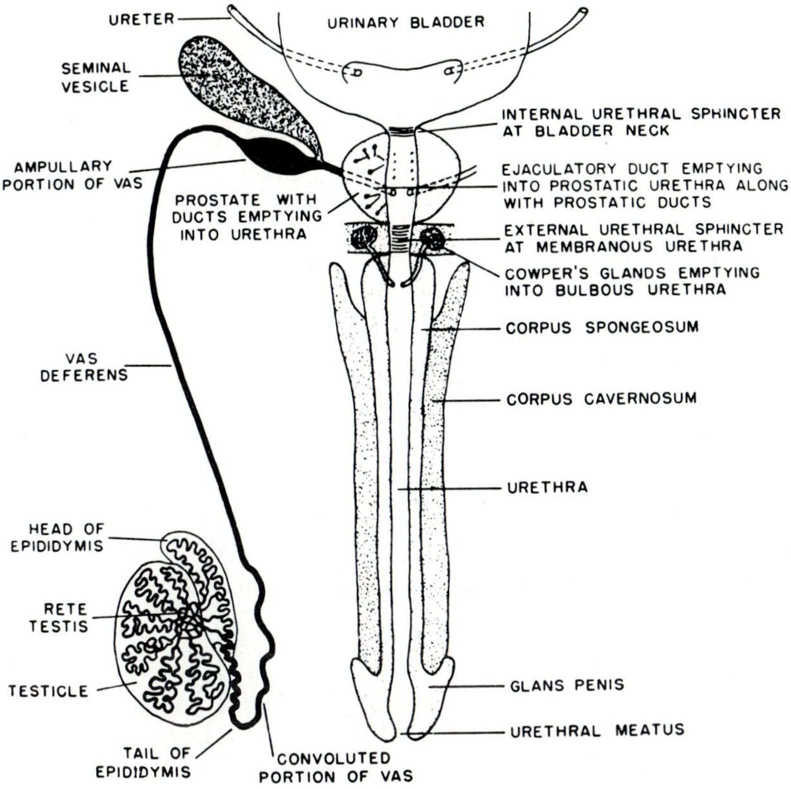

FIGURE 1. The male reproductive tract.

Seminiferous tubules are seen in cross section. They are rounded with a diameter of 170 to 250 μm with a thin basement membrane. Lying on this membrane are 0 to 12 Sertoli cells and resting and dividing spermatogonia. Close to the lumen, other cells of the spermatogenic series are seen in a sequential orderly arrangement.

The interstitial tissue consists of loose connective tissue situated between the seminiferous tubules. Small collections of Leydig cells are present in this stroma. These cells secrete testosterone which passes by the capillary venous or lymphatic route or by traversing the myoid cell layer to enter the seminiferous tubules.[2]

C. Spermatogenesis

Spermatogenesis is the process of development and maturation of the sperm cells. The basement membrane at the periphery of the tubules is lined by spermatogonia. The spermatogenic cells are arranged in an orderly manner from the basement membrane to the lumen. The spermatogonia proliferate to produce the primary spermatocytes, which undergo a long prophase. This is followed by the first maturation division that yields secondary spermatocytes. After a short interphase these cells undergo a second maturation division that results in the formation of spermatids that metamorphose without further division to form spermatozoa. Within these broad groups at least 13 germ cell types have been identified. The process of spermatogenesis, from pale type A spermatogonia to spermatozoa, takes 74 days[3] (Figure 3).

D. Transport of Spermatozoa

Testicular spermatozoa are transported to the epididymis by secretions from the

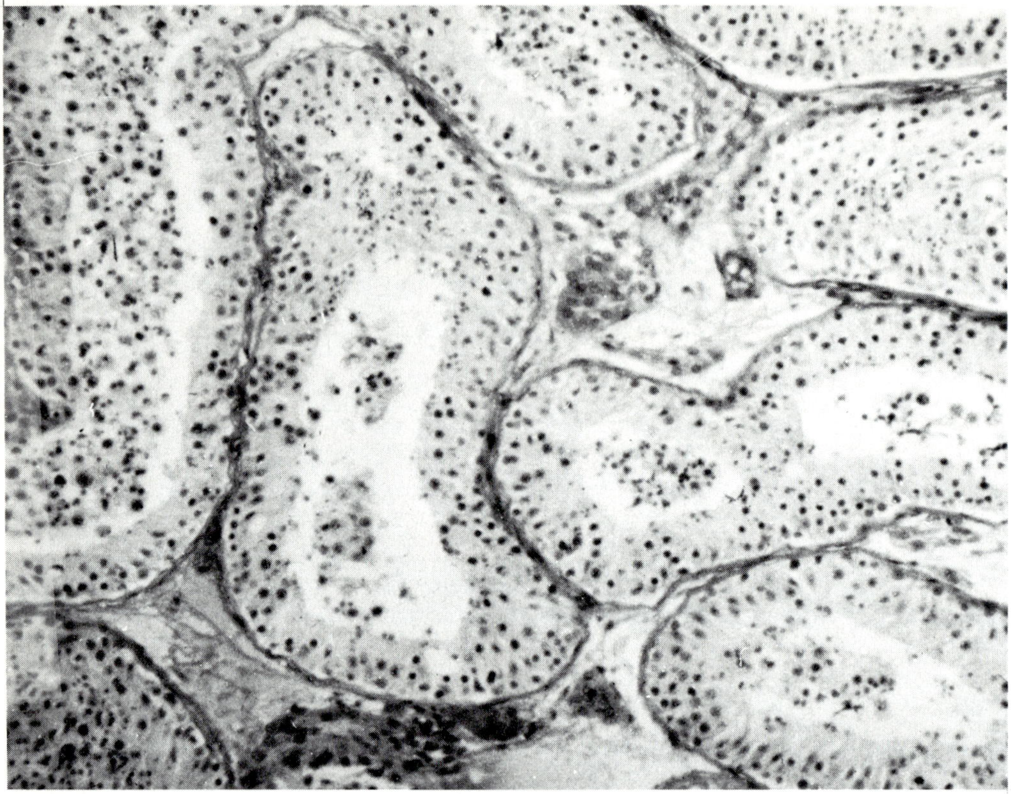

FIGURE 2. Human testis. The transections of the tubules show various stages of spermatogenesis. Leydig cells are visible in the interstitium.

testis and by ciliary and contractile activity of the luminal wall of the ductules. During their passage through the epididymis, spermatozoa undergo maturation with respect to motility and fertility. This includes development of the capacity for progressive motility, alteration of the plasma membrane, modification of the structural state of some of the tail organelles, and loss of the cytoplasmic droplet; the sperm nuclear chromatin and acrosome are also modified.[4]

The maintenance of the epididymis is under androgenic control. Testosterone is transported, bound to the high-affinity androgen-binding protein, from the seminiferous tubules into the epididymis.[5] In the epididymis, the androgen-binding protein disappears and testosterone is taken up by the cells and converted to 5α-dihydrotestosterone and 5α-androstane-3α,17β-diol. These androgens are necessary for the development of fertilizing capacity in the spermatozoa.[6]

It takes about 12 days for the sperm to reach the ampullary portion of the duct.[7] Phagocytosis of sperm occurs if they are not ejaculated at regular intervals.

The characteristic secretory product of the epididymis is glycerylphosphoryl-choline. It has not been established which epididymal secretions depend on androgens.[8]

E. The Spermatozoon

Under the light microscope, the structure of the sperm shows a head, middle piece, tail, and tail-end. The heads are oval in shape, the mean length is 4.4 μm and the width is about 3.0 μm. The midpiece has a length of approximately 3.0 μm and the tail is

Duration of Stage	Stage
	↓
	Spermatogonia
26 days	↓
	Primary Spermatocytes
16 days	↓
	Secondary Spermatocytes
16 days	↓
	Spermatids
16 days	↓
	Immature Spermatozoa

FIGURE 3. Spermatogenesis in the human testis.

about 50 μm in length. Under the electron microscope the head shape is oval, when viewed from the front. The nucleus extends throughout the length of the sperm head and is covered anteriorly by the thin acrosomal cap. The neck of the sperm connects the head to the midpiece and contains two centrioles. The midpiece, containing the axial bundle of fibrils and the surrounding mitochondrial sheath, is in turn joined to the tail section of the sperm.

The size distribution of human sperm is markedly positively skewed.[9] However sperm from one man tends to vary less in morphology than in count and motility.[10]

F. The Control of Testicular Function

The process of sperm formation within the testis is under endocrine control. The mechanisms regulating the testis are complex and involve the hypothalamus, the anterior pituitary, and the testis (Figure 4).

The hypothalamus produces releasing hormones which stimulate production of pituitary gonadotropin from the anterior pituitary gland. It has been suggested that gonadotropin releasing hormone can affect its own secretion by an ultrashort loop feedback mechanism.[11] Excess releasing factor production would prevent the hypothalamus from producing further factor. The short loop feedback of gonadrotropins on the hypothalamus may operate via peptidases which inactivate gonadotropin releasing factor.[12]

Gonadotropin releasing factor stimulates the anterior pituitary gland to secrete follicle stimulating hormone (FSH) and luteinizing hormone (LH), which are secreted in a pulsatile manner throughout the 24-hour period.[13] These pulses are superimposed on a basal secretion rate, and occur at intervals of 30 to 300 min. FSH is the hormone which controls spermatogenesis. However it is unable to initiate or maintain the process without the aid of other hormones.[14] LH and testosterone are also necessary. The precise target cells for FSH and the biochemical sequence of events initiated by this hormone have not been fully established. LH affects spermatogenesis by way of stimulating testosterone synthesis and release from the Leydig cells.[15] The site of action of LH is at the stage of conversion of cholesterol to pregnenolone and uses cyclic AMP as a second messenger. The biochemical steps mediating the secretion of testosterone have been described.[16]

The testis is able to control its own central control mechanisms by feedback regulatory systems which act on the hypothalamus and pituitary. There is a clear negative feedback role of testosterone on LH production.[17] It is only the free, unbound circulating testosterone which exerts this control.[18] Control may be effected by other steroids to which testosterone is converted such as dihydrotestosterone or the 3α and 3β

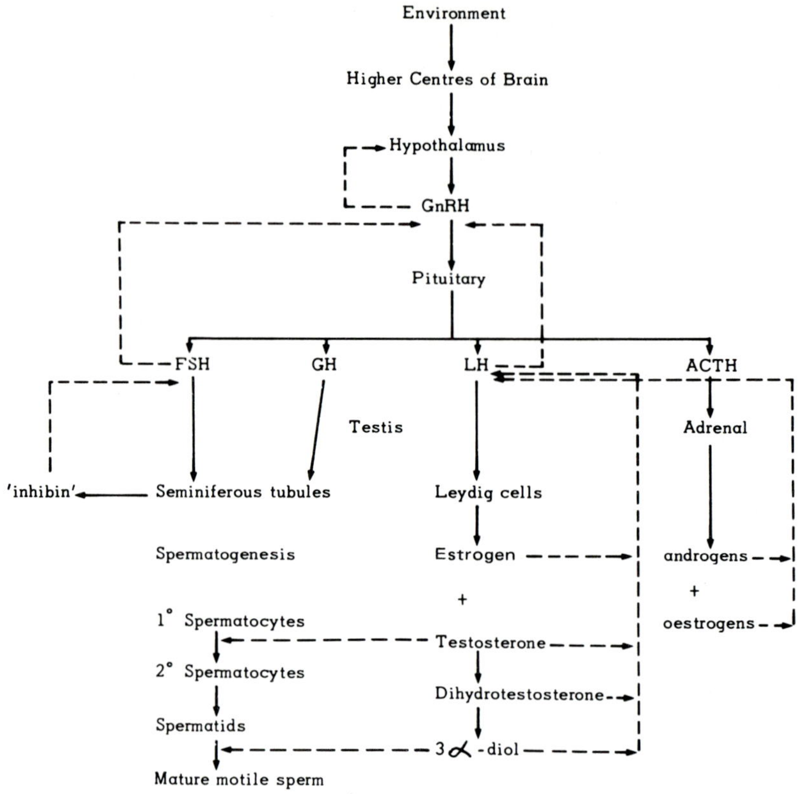

FIGURE 4. Integrated scheme of testicular control mechanisms in man: Gonadotropin releasing hormone (Gn-RH); follicle stimulating hormone (FSH); luteinizing hormone (LH); growth hormone (GH); 3 α-androstanediol (3α-diol) adrenocorticotropic hormone (ACTH).

isomers of 5α-androstanediol or by estradiol. The effect of androgens and estrogens on FSH secretion is disputed. FSH is less easily suppressed by testosterone and only large nonphysiological doses of estradiol can suppress FSH secretion in men. FSH acts on the seminiferous tubules and a feedback mechanism between tubular function and FSH secretion involving a nonsteroidal substance called inhibin as has been postulated; certainly extensive tubular damage is associated with a selective increase in FSH levels.[19] Recent evidence suggests that the cell involved in the regulation of FSH must be either type A spermatogonia or the Sertoli cell itself.[20] Other evidence indicates that the inhibitory substance is a water-soluble nonsteroidal compound.[21]

The adrenal gland produces small amounts of androgens and estrogens. It is not known whether these take part in the physiological feedback control of the testis. Prostaglandins have a direct effect on the testis. PGE_1 causes an increase in cAMP levels,[22] while PGE_1, PGE_2, and $PGF_{2}\alpha$ cause an increase in the affinity of human prostatic tissue for testosterone.[23]

G. Hormones of the Testis

The androgens secreted by the testis, as shown by an excess in testicular vein blood, are testosterone, androstenediol, 5-androstene-3β,17β-diol, androstenedione, dehydroepiandrosterone, pregnenolone, 17α-hydroxypregnenolone, and 17α-hydroxyprogesterone.[24] There is indirect evidence for the secretion of small amounts of dihydrotestosterones.[25] There is also direct secretion of very small amounts of the estrogens, estrone, and estradiol.[26]

1. Testosterone

The most important androgen secreted by the Leydig cells is testosterone. Testosterone may also be synthesized in the Sertoli cells of the seminiferous tubules.[27] In normal men, 60% of the testosterone is bound to sex hormone-binding globulin, 38% is bound to albumin, and 2% is free.[28] Variation in the concentration of sex hormone-binding globulin results in a large alteration in unbound testosterone. Only the unbound fraction of the steroid hormone is freely exchangeable and biologically active.

Mean plasma testosterone levels remain within the same range from the age of 20 years until they start to fall at the age of 50 to 60 years.[29] Reference values are shown in Table 1. A diurnal variation has been noted, the lowest levels being found between 20.00 and 22.00 hours and the highest levels being found in the early morning.[30] It should be noted that testosterone is secreted episodically, in addition to exhibiting ciradian rhythym.

Both the free and albumin-bound testosterone are available for metabolism in the liver. About half the testosterone is excreted as androsterone and etiocholanolone. A third isomer epidandrosterone is produced in very small quantities. The isomeric 5α- and 5β-androstane-$3\alpha,17\beta$-diols and estradiol are also minor metabolites of testosterone. Steroids are excreted in the urine conjugated with glucuronic or sulfuric acid (Figure 5).

2. Dihydrotestosterone

Dihydrotestosterone appears to be the active androgen at the target organ level. The majority of the circulating dihydrotestosterone comes from peripheral conversion of plasma precursors.[31] The conversion of testosterone takes place under the influence of an NADPH-dependent 5α-reductase enzyme in androgen-dependent tissues, which also contain a 5α-dihydrotestosterone receptor.

3. 17-Oxosteroids

The major portion of the 17-oxosteroids is androsterone and etiocholanolone, which are the major metabolites of testosterone. Nevertheless, estimation of the 17-oxosteroids does not provide a reliable guide to the secretion of testosterone, because the weaker androgens, androstenedione and dehydroepiandrosterone, secreted by the adrenal cortex, are also metabolized and excreted as 17-oxosteroids.

H. Physiological Effects of the Androgens

The androgens have widespread effects on the sexual and nonsexual organs of the body. They stimulate growth of the genital tract and the processes of spermatogenesis together with seminal fluid formation. Testosterone stimulates growth in general and particularly muscle, bone, kidney, and larynx growth.

Androgens have specific effects on hair growth and are responsible for the transformation of the vellus hair into terminal hair. They stimulate the secretion of the sebaceous glands and they affect the concentrations of many enzymes in the kidney, increasing the concentrations of acid phosphatase, arginase and β-glucuronidase. Erythropoiesis is stimulated by androgens.

II. TESTICULAR FUNCTION

Testicular function may be altered by inherited or acquired factors. Patients with testicular disease may present with androgen deficiency, infertility, or a combination of both disorders.

Table 1
VARIATION OF PLASMA TESTOSTERONE LEVELS WITH AGE

Age in years	Plasma level nmol/ℓ
20—30	9.7—41.7
30—40	12.1—35.0
40—50	8.8—35.5
50—60	8.8—32.9
60—70	4.2—30.1
70 +	1.0—29.0

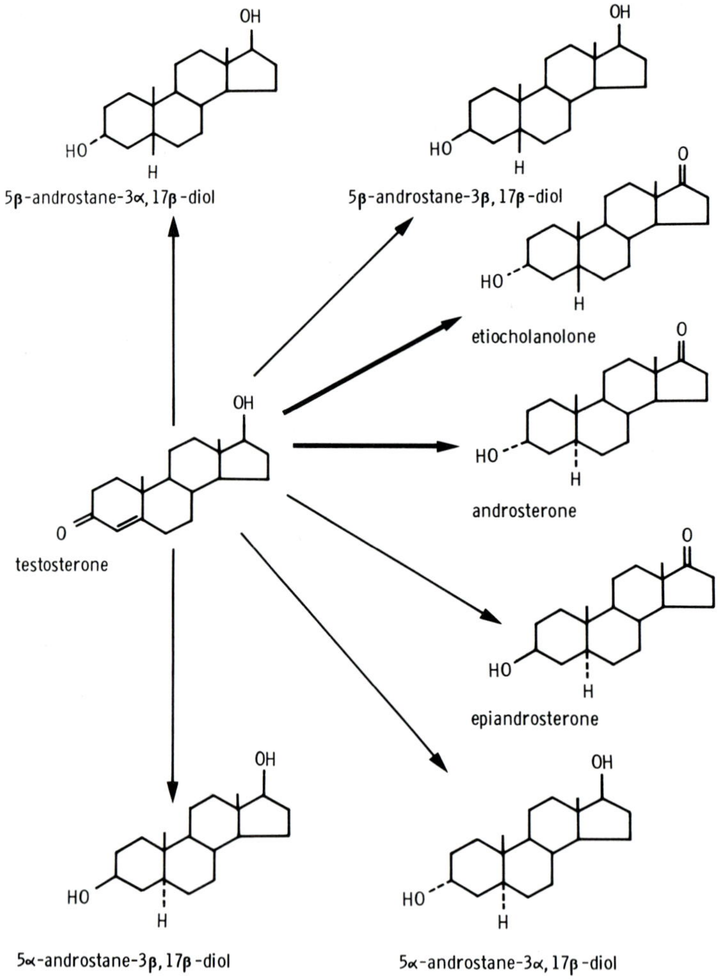

FIGURE 5. Metabolites of testosterone.

A. Infertility

It has been estimated that 10 to 15% of marriages in this country are infertile and in half of these a male factor has been identified.

1. Semen Analysis

The most important investigation in the evaluation of male infertility is the semen analysis (Figure 6). When considering the results of the analysis it should be remembered that large fluctuations in sperm density and in motility may occur under standard conditions from week to week. Wherever possible, judgment should be based on a series of specimens before and during treatment. The conditions under which the specimen is collected must be carefully controlled; the patient is asked to produce the specimen into a clean plastic container by masturbation after 3 days' continence The specimen should be examined as soon as liquefaction has occurred and certainly within 2 hours of production.

The semen is ejaculated in a liquid form and becomes a coagulum immediately after ejaculation, then liquefies again within 20 min and remains in a viscous state, allowing the spermatozoa to gain full motility. The cause of abnormally high residual viscosity of semen after it has coagulated and liquefied is not known.

After a period of 3 days' abstinence the volume of semen fluid is between 2.0 and 5.0 $m\ell$. A low semen volume may be associated with infertility as adequate access of spermatozoa to the cervical mucus may not be possible. The pH of freshly ejaculated semen is around 7.5 which is optimal for the survival of spermatozoa. In cases of prostatic disease the pH rises to above 8.0.

The sperm cell count method is similar to the laboratory method of performing blood cell counts, the red blood cell field of the standard Neubauer counting chamber being used. The sperm count is measured in millions/$m\ell$. In men of proven fertility the logarithmic mean is 65 million/$m\ell$[32]. A high proportion of infertile men have counts under 20 million/$m\ell$ and counts below this level are considered to represent oligospermia. Nevertheless, so long as any normal motile sperm are present, no figure can be set below which pregnancy cannot be achieved. It has been suggested that unless other parameters are abnormal, sperm counts of 10 million/$m\ell$ and above cannot be considered as major factors in infertility.[33]

Poor sperm morphology may be found in the presence of good sperm counts. In a fertile specimen, at least 60% of the sperm present should be morphologically normal. The persistent presence of more than 40% of abnormal forms is associated with a high incidence of infertility. The presence of more than 3% of immature sperm indicates that the testes are under stress. This occurs after illness and during treatment for infertility. Figure 7 shows a photomicrograph of stained spermatozoa.

The motility of the sperm is a very important factor in determining male fertility. A direct linear relationship between conception rate and percentage of motility has been demonstrated. Poor sperm motility may be found in normal men after a long period of continence; this may be caused by deterioration of sperm stored for a time in the duct system.

2. The Seminal Plasma

Seminal plasma represents the combined secretions of the epididymis, vas deferens, ampulla, seminal vesicles, prostate, and the glands of Cowper and Littre. Among its components are nitrogenous bases such as choline, spermine, and spermidine, many specific proteolytic enzymes which are associated with the processes of semen coagulation and liquefaction, and oxidative and hydrolytic enzymes including acid phosphatases and 5-nucleotidase. At least 14 prostaglandins have been identified in the seminal plasma. The two most prominent ones are prostaglandins E_1 and E_2. The carbohydrates found in the plasma are partly free and partly bound to proteins. The principal free sugar is fructose but in addition, sorbital, innosital, glucose, ribose, and fucose are present. Most of the bound carbohydrate is in the form of glycoprotein. Among

1. Volume 2 - 4 ml
2. pH 8
3. Viscosity liquefaction complete within 20 minutes
4. Motility at 2 hr - 60%
5. Count over 20 M/ml
6. Morphology 60% normal
7. Fructose 91 - 520 mg / 100 ml.

FIGURE 6. The semen analysis — normal findings.

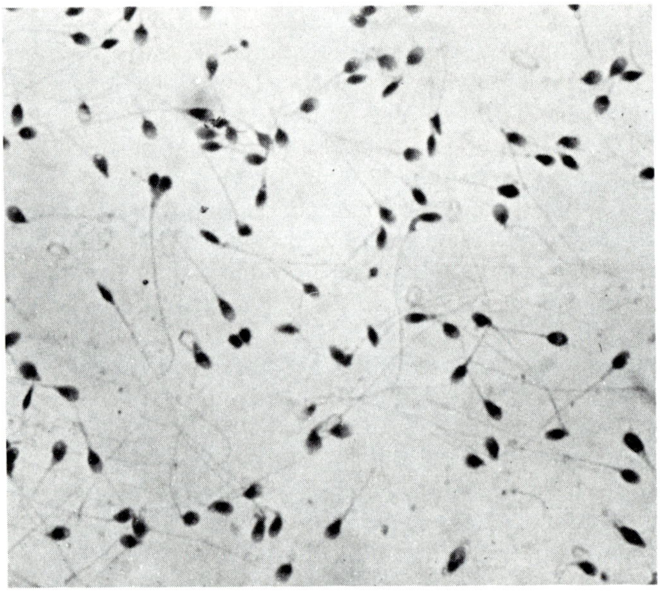

FIGURE 7. Photomicrograph of stained spermatozoa.

the organic acids secreted, citric acid is present in very high concentrations. An index of prostatic function may be determined by measuring the concentrations of citric acid and acid phosphatase. Estimations of fructose and ascorbic acid demonstrate the activity of the ampulla and seminal vesicle. The full value of measuring compounds in seminal plasma has not been fully assessed.

3. Factors Affecting Testicular Function.

Temperature — The testes, situated in the scrotum, are at a temperature of about 2°C cooler than the intra-abdominal temperature. If they are exposed to temperatures higher than that of the body for a sufficient length of time, cessation of maturation of sperms at the secondary spermatocyte stage occurs.

Radiation — Unshielded exposure to excessive radiation can produce permanent destruction of spermatogenic epithelium. If reconstruction of the germinal epithelium does occur, several years may be required before the processes are complete.

General health — Recent febrile illnesses and allergic phenomena may produce temporary oligospermia, reduction of motility, and structural changes in the spermatozoa. The semen picture may be depressed for several months after a serious illness.

Past infections — Postpubertal mumps orchitis may cause some degree of atrophy of the involved testis. When atrophy does not occur, fertility is not impaired. Tuberculosis and venereal disease may give rise to epididymitis and consequent obstructive azoospermia.

Cryptorchism — If both testes remain undescended by the time puberty is reached the chances of germinal cell damage and subsequent infertility are high. About 7% of cryptorchid testes are abnormal.[34] The incidence of testicular tumors in the undescended testis is 20 to 50 times greater than in the normally situated testis.[35] High levels of pituitary FSH are a consequence of defective spermatogenesis and may be found after operation when the prognosis regarding fertility is poor.

Trauma — Interference with the testicular blood supply in hernia repairs and in late correction of torsion of the testis will cause permanent testicular destruction. Previous traumatic conditions such as rupture of the tunica albuginea may cause permanent impairment of testicular function.

Drugs — Several drugs are known to cause depression of spermatogenesis. These interfere with the development of spermatozoa and cause azoospermia, oligospermia, or the production of mature spermatozoa which are biologically incompetent to fertilize. Among these drugs are nitrofurantoin, monoamine oxidase inhibitors, antimalarials, and antimetabolites. Prior treatment with estrogens or androgens in large doses may permanently inhibit spermatogenesis.

B. Androgen Deficiency

Eunuchoidism arises from dysfunction of the Leydig cells. Infertility and eunuchoidism may coexist as testosterone is necessary for the normal processes of spermatogenesis. The severity of eunuchoidism depends on the degree of androgen deficiency and the time of onset. The clinical features may demonstrate small infantile genitalia; lack of facial, pubic, and axillary hair; long limbs with muscle hypotonia; and an infantile larynx.

1. Klinefelter's Syndrome

This syndrome occurs in two per 1000 live male births. The clinical and endocrinological picture is variable. Usually, levels of pituitary follicle stimulating hormone are elevated. Levels of testosterone are usually reduced but may be in the normal range. The diagnosis is confirmed by finding Barr bodies in the buccal smear and detecting a 47 XXY chromosome karyotype. The testis is grossly affected, showing varying degrees of abnormality of the seminiferous tubules. The Leydig cells also show varying abnormalities.

2. Ullrich-Turner's Syndrome

This syndrome consists of hypogonadism accompanied by somatic abnormalities. The endocrine picture is of low testosterone levels together with elevated levels of pituitary FSH and LH.

3. Anorchia

In this condition the testes are absent. Levels of testosterone are low and do not respond to the HCG stimulation test. Levels of pituitary FSH and LH are invariably high.

4. Incomplete Male Pseudohermaphrodism

a. Androgen Receptor Defect[36]

The clinical picture includes infertility, gynecomastia, hypospadias, a urogenital sinus, scrotal malfusion, and eunuchoidism. The endocrine picture depends on the

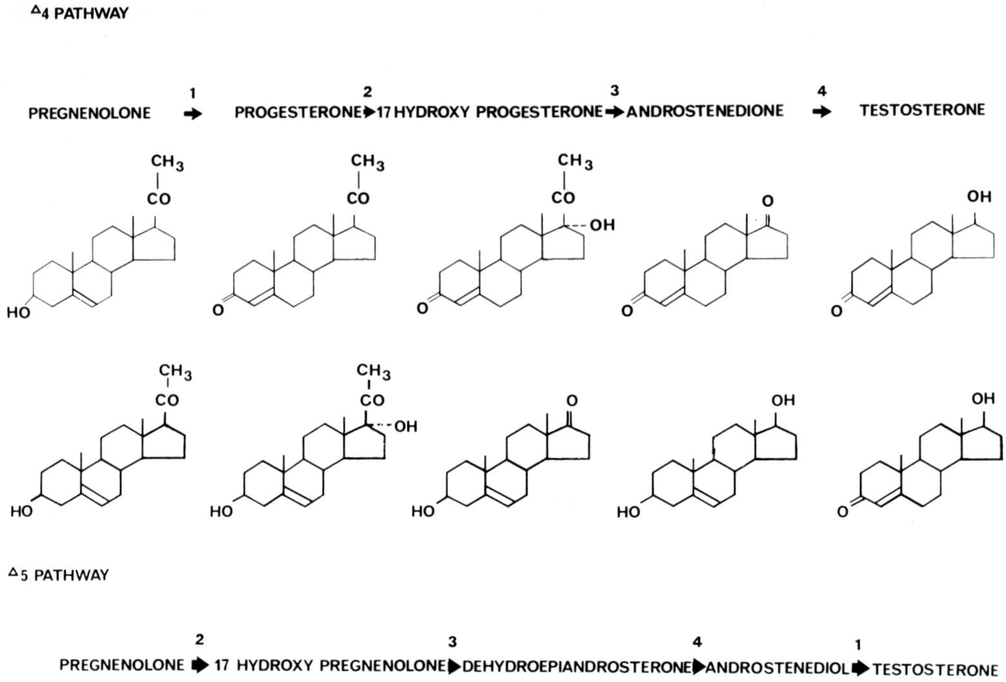

FIGURE 8. Defects in testosterone biosynthesis. The biosynthetic pathways from pregnenolone to testosterone are shown, the enzymes being indicated by numerals. The table shows the steroids which may be estimated to identify the enzyme defect. In all cases, the level of testosterone is reduced.

Enzymes indicated by numerals	Increased output of steroid
1. 3β-hydroxysteroid dehydrogenase	dehydroepiandrosterone
2. 17α-hydroxylase	corticosterone
3. 17—20 lyase	pregnanetriolone
4. 17-hydroxysteroid dehydrogenase	pregnanetriol

degree of Leydig cell hyperplasia which is present. Levels of LH and testosterone are usually raised, and there is an increased production rate of estrone and estradiol.

b. 5 α-Reductase Defect[37]

This condition presents as pseudovaginal perineoscrotal hypospadias. Testicular histology is normal in this condition, and testosterone and estrogen levels are normal. The lack of 5α-reductase prevents the conversion of testosterone to dihydrotestosterone in the peripheral tissues.

c. Testosterone Biosynthesis Defects

All the predictable defects have been described[38] and the measurement of various steroids may be used to identify the enzyme defect (Figure 8).

5. Hypopituitarism and Selective Gonadotropin Defect

Eunuchoidism may be the presenting symptom in hypopituitarism and it is important to consider the possibility of additional endocrine deficiencies. Hormonal defects in hypopituitarism include low serum testosterone levels and low output of FSH and LH.

6. Hyperprolactinemia

Elevated prolactin levels may be associated with the hypogonad state. The causal relationship between hyperprolactinemia and hypogonadism is not fully understood. About one third of men with hyperprolactinemia have galactorrhea, yet almost all are impotent, with loss of libido.[39] Diseases of the hypothalamus and pituitary gland may cause hyperprolactinemia, as may certain drugs including butyrophones, phenothiazines, some antihypertensives, estrogens, histamine-2 receptor antagonists, monoamine oxidase inhibitors, and centrally acting antiemetics.

7. Myotonic Dystrophy

The features of this condition are frontal balding, cataracts, and hypogonadism. Serum testosterone levels are low and levels of pituitary FSH and LH are elevated. The gonadal abnormality usually appears in adult life and presents as infertility due to progressive disorganization and fibrosis of the seminiferous tubules.[40]

8. Alcoholism

Alcoholism may produce impotence and testicular atrophy. Serum testosterone levels are usually low. When cirrhosis of the liver occurs, as well as low testosterone levels, elevated serum estradiol levels are present. Pituitary gonadotropin secretion remains normal.

C. Surgical Aspects of Infertility and Testicular Function

1. Varicocele

The precise role of a varicocele in causing impaired spermatogenesis is not known. Fertility is not always affected in the presence of a varicocele. Varicoceles usually occur on the left side; radiographic evidence has shown that there is an anastomosis of the venous circulation between the testes, and this accounts for the bilateral depressing effect of the toxic factors, produced in this condition, on normal sperm production. A consistent effect on the hypothalamic-pituitary-gonadal axis has not been observed. Levels of serum LH, FSH, testosterone, and estradiol show no significant differences from normal controls.[41] It has been reported[42] that after varicocelectomy, 71% of patients had a marked improvement in semen quality and that 55% of their wives became pregnant.

2. Epididymal Obstruction

This may be caused by congenital anomalies or by previous infection. When the semen is azoospermic but contains fructose, and the testicular biopsy shows normal spermatogenesis, epididymal obstruction may be suspected. Levels of pituitary FSH and LH and of testosterone are normal in these cases.

3. Previous Vasectomy

A vasovasostomy may be performed to restore potency. Autoimmunization occurs in some men who have ductal obstruction; therefore, testing for sperm-agglutinating and sperm-immobilizing antibodies in the seminal plasma and sera should be performed. No abnormalities of endocrine function are present in this condition.

D. Testicular Tumors

The incidence of testicular malignancies in the total male population is only 0.02%. However in men aged between 20 to 35 years, testicular tumors constitute one of the most common forms of malignancy.

1. Seminomas

Seminomas comprise 45% of all testicular tumors. Occasionally small occult foci of malignant teratoma, undetected in the primary tumor, may give rise to teratoma metastases. The assay of alpha-fetoprotein and of HCG may be of value in detecting this group.

2. Teratomas

Teratomas comprise 40% of testicular tumors. Plasma and urinary HCG levels are elevated in some patients and denote the presence of a trophoblastic component. A falling titer does not correlate well with the therapeutic response; however, a rising titer does indicate tumor recurrence.

3. Interstitial Cell Tumors

These tumors are very rare. Functionally they fall into two groups, those producing androgens and those producing estrogens. When the virilizing type develops in prepubertal boys, precocious sexual development occurs. Output of 17-oxosteroids and of testosterone is increased in this type. Tumors that produce estrogenic effects are found only in adult men, in whom gynecomastia, impotence, and decreased hair growth is found. Urinary estrogen excretion is elevated.

4. Sertoli Cell Tumors

The majority of these tumors are benign. No characteristic pattern of hormonal output has been observed.

III. INVESTIGATIVE PROCEDURES IN TESTICULAR FUNCTION

A. Hormone Measurement

1. Thyroid Function

Thyroid dysfunction is a rare cause of male infertility, being implicated in less than 1% of cases.[43] Function may be assessed by measuring total thyroxine, triiodothyronine uptake, the free thyroxine index, and if indicated, thyroid stimulating hormone levels in the plasma.

Hypothyroidism may be accompanied by impotence and oligospermia. The metabolism of androgens is altered in hypothyroidism; secretion of androgens is decreased; and the metabolic transformation of testosterone is shifted towards etiocholanolone rather than androsterone.[44] Hyperprolactinemia may be present in association with hypothyroid states.

Patients with hyperthyroidism have been found to have elevated levels of testosterone and luteinizing hormone in their serum.[45]

2. Adrenal Function

Congenital adrenal hyperplasia is the disorder of adrenal function that is responsible for abnormal spermatogenesis. If the patients are not treated during childhood, they have small stature and sterility. The hypogonadism in these patients is due to suppression of gonadotropins by the excess androgen of adrenal origin.[46] Treatment with cortisone in these cases will suppress androgen production and restore the pulsatile release of pituitary LH.

3. Gonadal Function

For spermatogenesis to progress, testosterone must be present in high concentrations within the seminiferous tubules. Any disorder leading to a defect in testosterone synthesis will inhibit spermatogenesis.

There are a variety of hereditary disorders in which defective testosterone synthesis occurs prenatally, giving rise to ambiguous genitalia in male infants. A defect in any one of the five enzymatic steps necessary for the conversion of cholesterol to testosterone may lead to incomplete virilization and ambiguous genitalia. Three of these hormones are common to the synthesis of adrenal hormones and deficiency causes congenital adrenal hyperplasia, as well as ambiguous genitalia in male infants.[47-49]

The hormones currently estimated as an index of testicular function are testosterone in the blood and the output of estrogen in the urine, or the estimation of 17β-estradiol in blood. 17-Hydroxyprogesterone in blood or pregnanetriol in the urine may also be estimated.

a. Method for Testosterone: Radioimmunoassay[50,51]

Reagents:

Phosphate buffered saline (PBS) — 0.05 *M* pH 7.4 containing sodium azide 0.1%.

0.1% gelatin in PBS — Freshly prepared each time.

Antisera to testosterone — For use the antisera are diluted in 0.1% gelatin PBS so as to give 30% binding in the zero standard.

Radioactive testosterone, (1,2,6,7,(n)-^{3}H) testosterone — The specific activity of this substance is approximately 85 Ci/mmol. For use a solution is prepared in 0.1% gelatin PBS to give 6 nCi/0.1 mℓ.

Diethylether — Freshly redistilled.

Dextran-coated charcoal — 500 mg charcoal (Norit A) and 50 mg Dextran T-70 are suspended in 100 mℓ 0.1% gelatin PBS.

Apparatus: Liquid scintillation counter, Packard 3380, using a PPO *bis*-MSB counting fluid.

Method:

Plasma 500 μℓ (female) or 100 μℓ plus 400 μℓ diluent (male) is extracted with diethylether (5.0 mℓ) by mechanical shaking for 20 min. The two layers are allowed to separate and then are placed in the deep freeze at −20°C for 30 min. The ether phase is transferred to clean tubes by decanting and evaporated to dryness under nitrogen at 40°C. The extract is taken up in 500 μℓ diluent.

Standard testosterone, in the range 5 to 60 nmol/ℓ is prepared in charcoal-treated plasma. This is then processed in the same way as male plasma. 100 μℓ extract is transferred to 75 × 12-mm glass tubes, in duplicate for samples and in triplicate for standards.

Addition of 100 μℓ antisera is made to all tubes except the nonspecific binding tubes, which receive 100 μℓ diluent. The tubes are incubated at 4°C for 30 min. Next 100 μℓ tritiated testosterone is added to all tubes which are then incubated at 4°C for 1 hr. The tubes are transferred to an ice bath and 500 μℓ of cold dextran-charcoal mixture is added and the tubes are rotex-mixed. They are replaced in the ice bath for 15 min after which they are centrifuged at 2000 r/min for 15 min at 4°C.

Of the supernatent 500 μℓ is pipetted into plastic mini-vials to which 4 mℓ of scintillation counting fluid is added and the vials are then counted.

Calculation:

The standard curve is calculated using the four parameter log-logit method of Hales. The concentration of testosterone in the unknown samples is calculated by reading from the graph. An appropriate factor is applied in the case of female plasma.

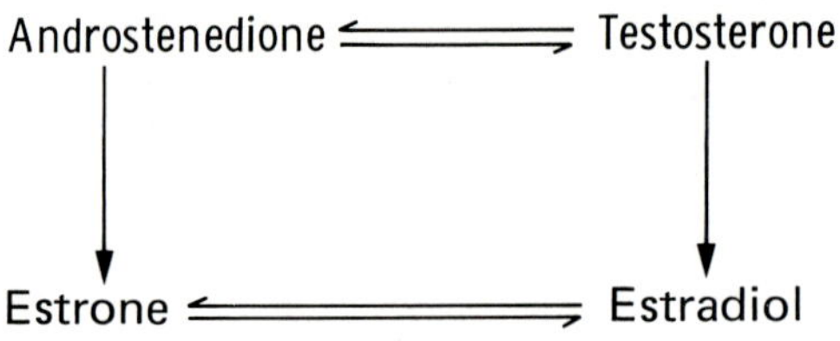

FIGURE 9. Interconversion of androgen and estrogen in normal man.

Precision: Coefficient of variation = 15%.

b. Estrogens

The most important blood estrogens in men are estrone and estradiol. Virtually all the estrone and estradiol are derived from androstenedione and testosterone. Only about 10% of these steroids are of gonadal origin (Figure 9). In men with gynecomastia the origin of the estrogens is very complex; in some instances the production of estrogen from all sources is normal and the only hormonal abnormality is decreased testosterone production, in which case the feminization relates to the increased amount of estrogen relative to androgen. In other cases there is an increased secretion of estrogens or of estrogen precursors such as androstenedione. In the majority of cases of gynecomastia not associated with hypogonadism, hormone measurements are within the normal range. On occasion however, the measurement of estrogen may be elevated and this may be the only manifestation of an adrenal or testicular tumor.

Estradiol 17β — This hormone may be estimated in cases of gynecomastia, hypogonadism, and in testicular tumors. Reference values in normal males: <174 pmol/ℓ.

Urinary estrogens — Reference values: 5 to 40 nmol/24 hr.

c. 17-Hydroxyprogesterone and Pregnanetriol

The secretion rate of 17-hydroxyprogesterone by the testis is one third that of testosterone.[52] The excretion of its metabolite, pregnanetriol, is a reasonable index of Leydig cell function. The hormones may be estimated in cases of male pseudohermaphrodism, where deficiency of 17-hydroxysteroid dehydrogenase is suspected. In this condition elevated levels will be found.

4. Pituitary Function

Luteinizing hormone and follicle stimulating hormone — Secretion of these hormones is an episodic process. Circulating levels vary from hour to hour. Therefore a 24-hr urine collection may give a more accurate assessment of pituitary status than a single venepuncture. Serum FSH and LH level reach adult ranges by the age of 16 years. Levels then plateau until the fifth decade when elevation in levels occurs, and increases again in the sixth and subsequent decades.[53]

Reference values in normal males — LH (24-hr urine), 4—45 IU/24 hr; LH (blood), 2—20 IU/ℓ; FSH (24-hr urine), 2—22 IU/24 hr; and FSH (blood), 4—30 IU/ℓ.

Prolactin — The secretion of prolactin is an episodic process and stress conditions will cause an increase in blood levels. Elevated levels may be the only evidence of a small pituitary adenoma and may be found in patients with hypogonadism due to a pituitary tumor or pituitary stalk lesion.[54] Reference values less than 600 mU/ℓ.

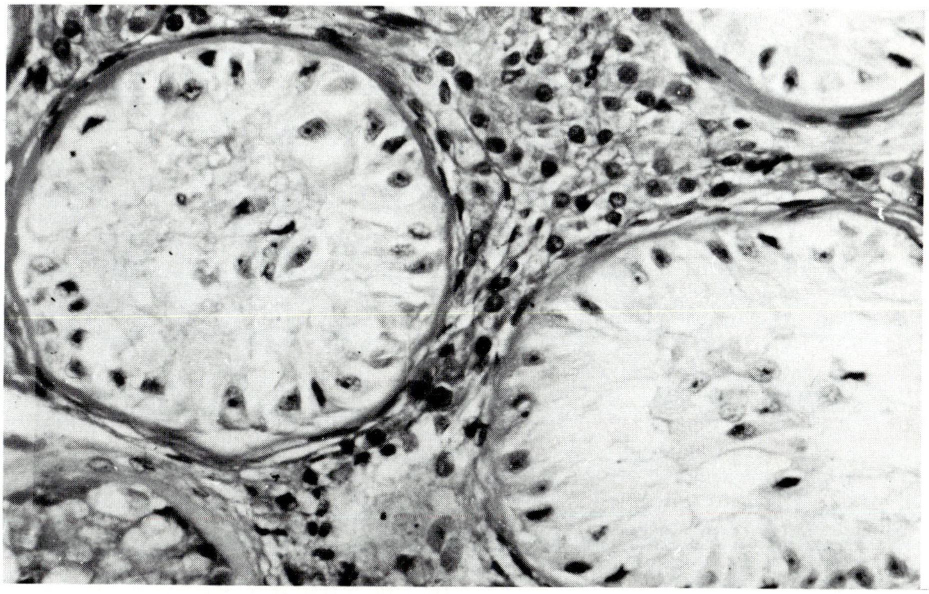

FIGURE 10. Histological section of testis showing complete lack of germinal cells. Sertoli-cell-only syndrome.

Human chorionic gonadotropin — Measurement of this hormone may be necessary in the investigation and treatment of testicular tumors.

Reference values — Less than 3 IU/ℓ.

IV. INTERPRETATION OF BASAL HORMONE MEASUREMENTS

A. Gonadal Defects

Oligospermia and azoospermia — Hormone levels are usually normal in these patients. No correlation has been found between sperm density and testosterone output. There is no relationship between FSH levels and the sperm count[55] but a relationship between serum FSH and testicular biopsy has been reported. FSH levels were elevated when spermatids were not visible on biopsy.[56] Other studies have not confirmed this.[57]

Primary testicular failure — In primary gonadal failure the main lesion is of the germinal epithelium, Leydig cell involvement being variable. FSH levels are always elevated, LH levels are usually raised, and testosterone output reduced. In Sertoli-cell-only syndrome (Figure 10) the FSH level is raised but as the Leydig cells are normal, testosterone and LH levels are normal. In the majority of cases, the cause is not known but similar findings occur in mumps and gonococcal orchitis, cryptorchidism, and irradiation damage. Elevated levels of FSH are present in seminiferous tubule hyalinization and in 50% of patients with germinal cell arrest. Azoospermic men in whom FSH levels are raised may be advised that the prognosis for fertility is poor because the number of germinal cells remaining in the testes is insufficient to restore fertility despite therapy.

B. Hypothalamic and Pituitary Disease

In hypothalamic and pituitary disease, low levels of all pituitary hormones are usually found. However some hormone levels may fall within the normal adult range.

Pituitary tumor — In tumors of the pituitary gland, FSH levels may be within the

Table 2
BASAL HORMONAL LEVELS IN DISORDERS OF THE HYPOTHALAMIC-PITUITARY-TESTICULAR AXIS IN MEN[a]

	Hormone levels			
Diagnosis	**LH**	**FSH**	**Prolactin**	**Testosterone**
Gonadal defects				
Oligospermia	N or E	N or E	N	N
1° testicular failure	E	E	N	D
Varicocele	N	N	N	N
Hypothalamic and pituitary defects				
Pituitary tumor	D or N	N	E or N	N
Hypogonadotropic eunuchoidism	D	D	N	D
Isolated LH defect	D	N	N	D
Gynecomastia	N	N	N or E	N or D

[a] N = Normal, D = decreased, E = elevated. The most common findings are indicated by the letters on the left hand side of each column.

normal range. LH secretion is often the first aspect of pituitary function to fail, so that low levels may be found in the presence of otherwise normal function. Elevated levels of prolactin may be demonstrated and may suggest the presence of a pituitary microadenoma. High quality radiographs of the skull and pituitary fossa should detect the presence of a tumor.

Hypogonadotropic eunuchoidism — In the classical form of this condition, FSH and LH levels are below the normal range and testosterone levels are within the female range. In Kallman's syndrome, in addition to hypogonadism, anosmia, color blindness, and midline facial deformities are present. The pathological basis for Kallman's syndrome lies in the hypothalamus, leading to the absence of gonadotropin releasing hormone. Like prepubertal boys, these patients show little or no response to stimulation with clomiphene citrate.[58] Secretion of thyroid stimulating hormone and adrenocorticotropic hormone is normal but deficient growth hormone secretion has been noted.[58]

Isolated LH Deficiency; "Fertile Eunuch" — These patients have variable degrees of spermatogenesis and sperm counts ranging from azoospermia to the normal range.[59] Serum testosterone and LH levels are low while FSH output is normal.[60]

The usual pattern of basal hormone levels is shown in Table 2.

V. DYNAMIC TESTS OF HYPOTHALAMIC-PITUITARY-TESTICULAR FUNCTION

It is frequently evident from measurement of basal levels of FSH, LH, and testosterone that there is a lesion in the hypothalamic-pituitary-testicular axis. In a number of patients borderline hormonal levels are found and in order to establish whether the axis is functioning normally, stimulation tests may be required.

A. Gonadotropin Releasing Hormone (Gn-RH)

This synthetic decapeptide releases LH and FSH in a dose-related manner. In the

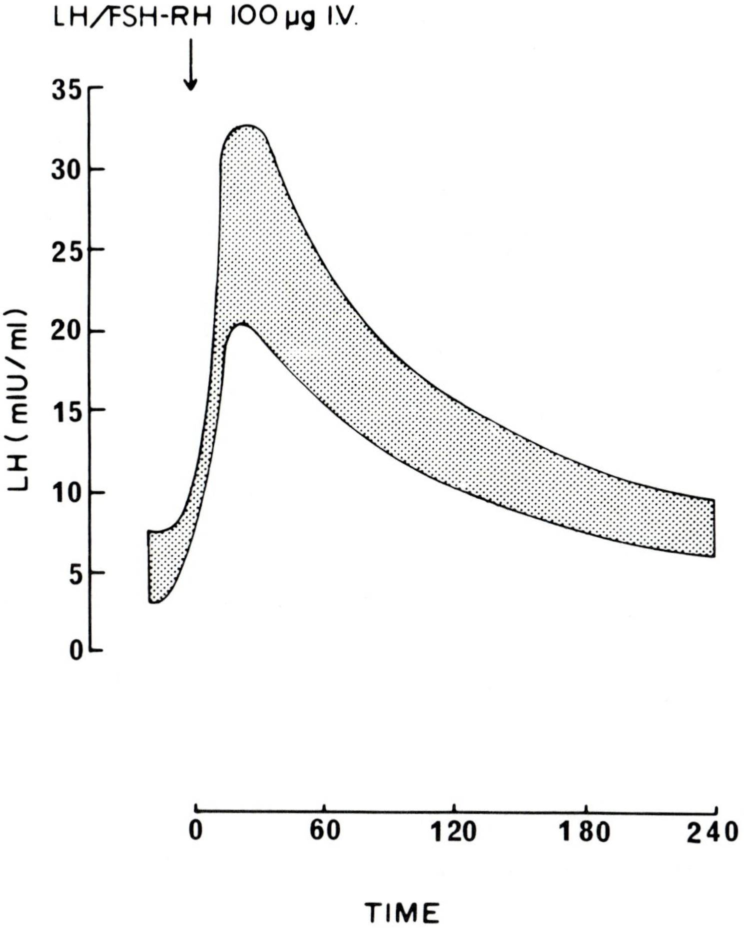

FIGURE 11. Serum LH response to Gn-RH (LH/FSH-RH). The shaded area indicates the range of response in normal men.

standard test serum LH and FSH levels are measured before and 20 and 60 min after the injection of 100 μg Gn-RH. Normal responses have been recorded in diseases of the hypothalamus and pituitary; therefore a normal response does not exclude hypothalamic or pituitary disease. An absent response or one which is impaired indicates the presence of dysfunction.

Normal males — Increases of serum LH are greater than those of FSH. Levels rise to a peak at 20 min and then decline (Figure 11). Larger increases are seen in men over 40 years of age.

Pituitary disease — In isolated gonadotropin defect most patients show an absent or subnormal response of LH; however the FSH response is often normal. In panhypopituitarism no rise in FSH or LH occurs. All patterns of response are to be found in patients with pituitary tumors. In the majority, however, the response is subnormal.

Gonadal disease — In primary gonadal failure there is a deficiency in the feedback mechanism of testosterone at the hypothalamic-pituitary level. Excessive responses to Gn-RH are found in these patients. In men with azoospermia or oligospermia, who have normal testosterone levels, there is a normal LH response to Gn-RH but an excessive FSH response indicating a diminished feedback effect of ''inhibin''.

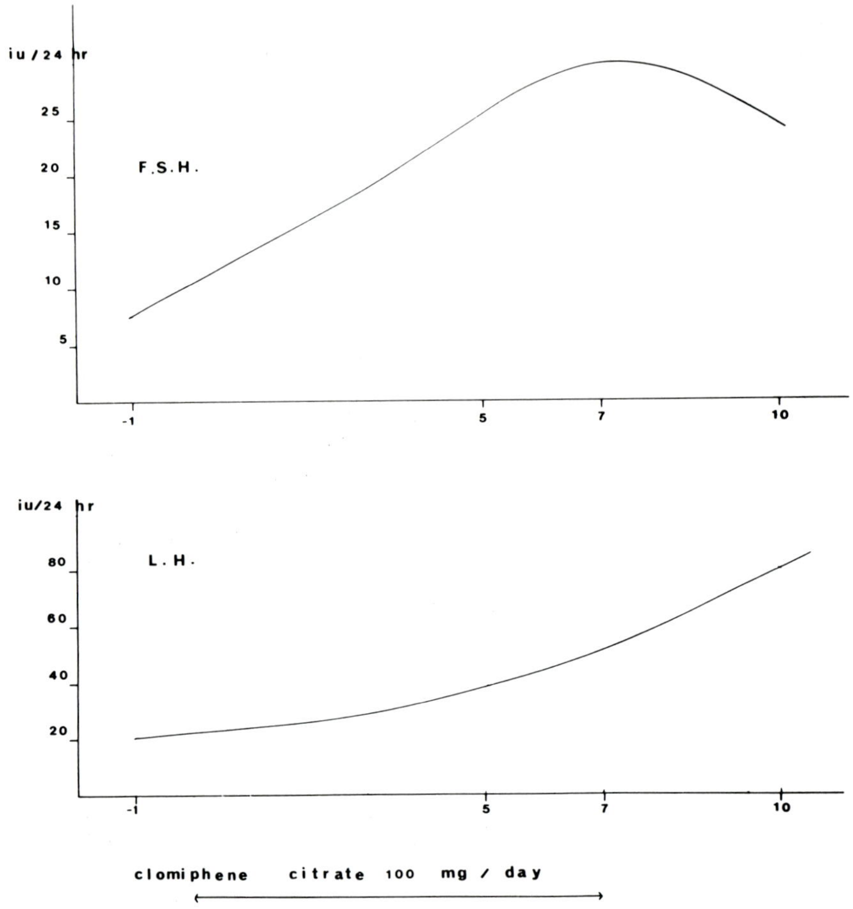

FIGURE 12. Urine FSH and LH responses in a normal man after administration of clomiphene citrate (100 mg) daily.

B. Clomiphene Stimulation Test

The effect of this tri-aryl ethylene compound, which acts on the hypothalamus,. is to elevate levels of FSH and LH. A normal response indicates a functioning hypothalamic-pituitary axis and a subsequent rise in testosterone output indicates that the testes can be stimulated by endogenous LH. The test is performed by giving 100 mg of clomiphene citrate orally daily for 7 days. On days 1, 5, 7, and 10, 24-hr specimens of urine or serum are assayed for FSH and LH (Figure 12). Serum testosterone may be assayed on the same days.

Normal males — The normal response shows a doubling in LH levels and a smaller rise in FSH. Testosterone responses are more variable than those of LH but normally there is a doubling in output. The increase in the levels of FSH and LH after clomiphene citrate may be prevented by the simultaneous administration of exogenous androgens.[61]

Pituitary disease — In isolated gonadotropin deficiency there is a lack of response to clomiphene citrate. In panhypopituitarism the low basal levels of FSH and LH do not increase after stimulation. There is a variable pattern of response in patients with pituitary tumors. This pattern depends on their basal hormone levels.

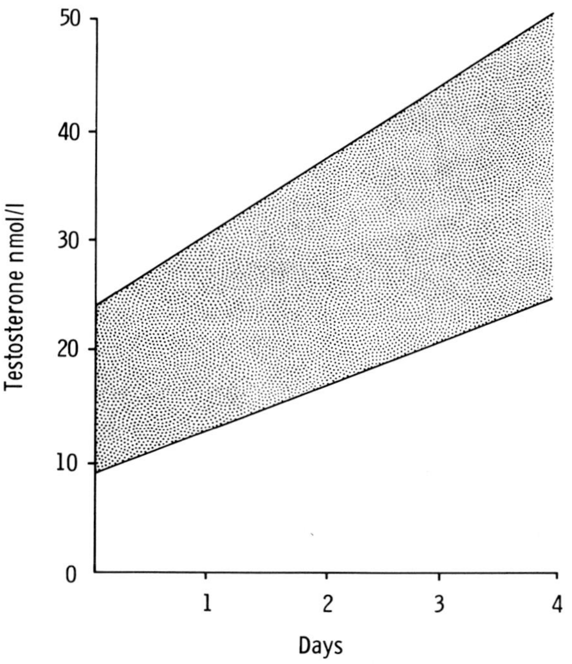

FIGURE 13. Serum testosterone response to administration of HCG (3000 IU daily) for 4 days. The shaded area indicates the range of response in normal men.

Gonadal disease — In primary gonadal failure the already elevated levels of FSH and LH do not rise further after stimulation. The majority of infertile men, with oligospermia or azoospermia, have a normal response to clomiphene.

C. Human Chorionic Gonadotropin (HCG) Stimulation

HCG may be used as a substitute for LH to stimulate testosterone secretion by the testes. HCG is given at a dose of 3000 IU daily by intramuscular injection, for 4 days. Serum testosterone levels are estimated prior to injection and on days 2 and 4.

Normal males — Serum testosterone levels usually double by day 4 of the test. The range of response is variable and the levels may rise 200% (Figure 13).

Pituitary disease — In isolated gonadotropin deficiency there is usually a small rise in testosterone output following HCG administration. In patients with panhypopituitarism of recent onset there is a marked testosterone rise which is slightly below that seen in normal men.[62] In patients with pituitary tumors the response depends on the basal levels of LH which are present.

Gonadal disease — In men with absent testes the low testosterone fails to respond. There are subnormal responses in cases of Sertoli-cell-only syndrome and germinal cell arrest.[63] In most men with azoospermia or oligospermia the response is normal.

VI. TESTICULAR BIOPSY

Testicular biopsy is indicated in patients with unexplained oligospermia or azoospermia, in whom the gonadotropin levels are normal, to distinguish between obstructive azoospermia and impaired spermatogenesis. The procedure should be performed bilaterally in order to detect any difference in the pathological process in each testis.

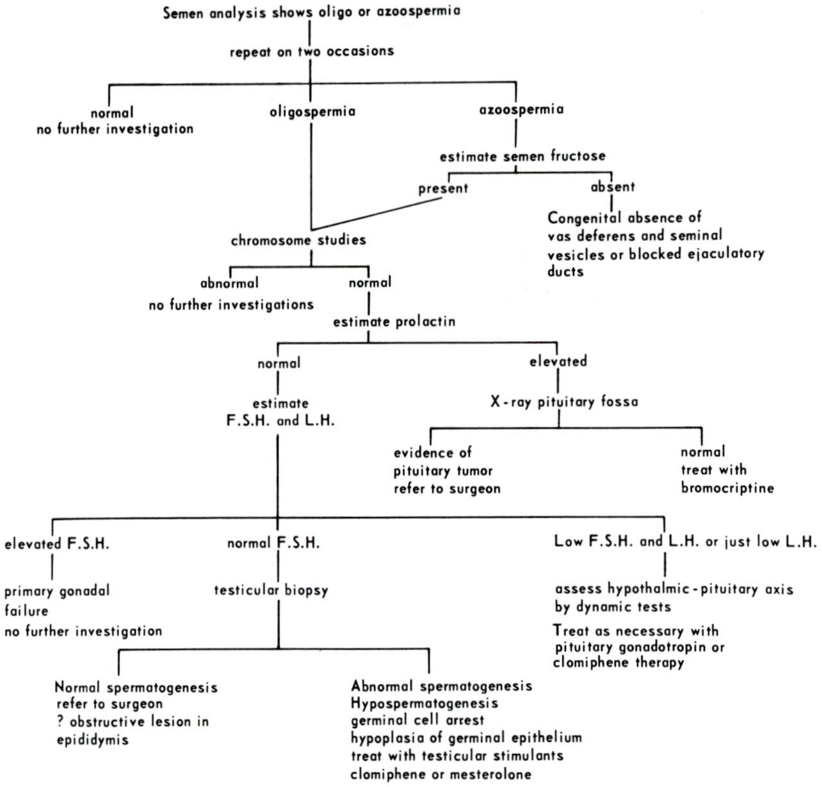

FIGURE 14. A flow diagram which indicates a possible method of investigating a man with oligospermia or azoospermia. Note that several stages may be combined; for example, a single blood sample at an early stage in investigation may be used for determination of FSH, LH, prolactin, thyroid function tests, and chromosome studies.

It has been found that neither semen analysis nor testicular size correlates with testicular biopsy findings.[64] In patients with chromosomal abnormalities or in whom the gonadotrophin levels are elevated, testicular biopsy is not indicated, as therapeutic measures will be ineffective.

Various scoring systems from testicular biopsy material have been devised, relating the proportions of each expected cell type with normal values.[65-67]

VII. KARYOTYPE

Chromosome abnormalities contribute significantly to the etiology of male infertility. Simple examination of cells from a buccal smear will indicate whether the male is chromatin negative. In a series of reports[68-71] various sex chromosome aberrations, structural autosomal rearrangements, and supernumerary marker chromosomes were found in about 6% of 1000 infertile men. An abnormal karyotype has been found in 20% of azoospermic men. On account of these findings, a karyotype should be performed on all azoospermic men.

A flow diagram for the investigation of men presenting with oligospermia or azoospermia is shown in Figure 14.

REFERENCES

1. **Gunn, S. A. and Gould, T. C.,** Vasculature of the testes and adnexa, in *Handbook of Physiology,* Vol. 5, Greep, R. O. and Astwood E. B., Eds., American Physiological Society, Washington, D.C. 1975, 117.
2. **Christensen, A.K.,** Leydig cells, in *Handbook of Physiology,* Vol. 5, Greep, R. O. and Astwood, E. B., Eds., American Physiological Society, Washington, D.C., 1975, 57.
3. **Heller, C. G. and Clermont, Y.,** Kinetics of the germinal epithelium in man, *Recent Progr. Horm. Res.,* 20, 545, 1964.
4. **Bedford, J. M.,** Maturation, transport and fate of spermatozoa in the epididymis, in *Handbook of Physiology,* Vol. 5, Greep, R. O. and Astwood, E. B., Eds., American Physiological Society, Washington, D.C., 1975, 303.
5. **Hansson, V., Ritzen, E. M., French, F. S., and Nayfeh, S. N.,** Androgen transport and receptor mechanisms in testis and epididymis, in *Handbook of Physiology,* Vol. 5, Greep, R. O. and Astwood, E. B., Eds., American Physiological Society, Washington, D.C., 1975, 173.
6. **Lubicz-Nawrocki, C. M.,** The effect of metabolites of testosterone on the viability of hamster epididymal spermatozoa, *J. Endocrinol.,* 58, 193, 1973.
7. **Rowley, M., Teshima, J. F., and Heller, C. G.,** Duration of transit of spermatozoa through the human male ductular system, *Fertil. Steril.,* 21, 390, 1970.
8. **Roy, S., Das, R. P., and Taneja, S. L.,** Effect of androgen on different biochemical constituents of human semen, *Andrologia,* 7, 195, 1975.
9. **Brotherton, J. and Barnard, G.,** Estimation of number, mean size and size distribution of human spermatozoa in oligospermia using a Coulter counter, *J. Reprod. Fert.,* 40, 341, 1974.
10. **Hartman, C. G., Schoenfield, C., and Copeland, E.,** Individualism in the picture of infertile men, *Fertil. Steril.,* 16, 632, 1965.
11. **Hyyppa, M., Motta, M., and Martini, L.,** "Ultrashort" feedback control of follicle-stimulating hormone-releasing factor secretion, *Neuroendocrinology,* 7, 227, 1971.
12. **Kuhl, H., and Taubert, H. D.,** Short-loop feedback mechanism of luteinising hormone: LH stimulates hypothalamic L-cystine arylamidase to inactivate LH-RH in the rat hypothalamus, *Acta Endocrinol. (Copenhagen),* 78, 649, 1975.
13. **McCann, S. M.,** Regulation of secretion of follicle-stimulating hormone and luteinizing hormone, in *Handbook of Physiology: 7. Endocrinology. Part IV. The Pituitary Gland,* Part 2, American Physiological Society, Washington, D.C., 1974, 489.
14. **Mancini, R. E., Vilar, D., Donini, P., and Lloret, A. P.,** Effect of human urinary FSH and LH on the recovery of spermatogenesis in hypophysectomised patients, *J. Clin. Endocrinol. Metab.,* 33, 888, 1971.
15. **van der Molen, H. J., de Bruijn, H. W. A., Cooke, B. A., de Jonge, F. H., and Rommerts, F. F. G.,** Regulation of the production of testicular steroids, in *The Endocrine Function of the Human Testis,* James, V. H. T., Serio, M., and Martini, L., Eds., Academic Press, New York, 1, 459, 1973.
16. **Catt, K. J. and Dufau, M. L.,** Basic concepts of the mechanism of action of peptide hormones, *Biol. Reprod.,* 14, 1, 1976.
17. **Stewart-Bentley, M., Odell, W., and Horton, R.,** The feedback control of luteinising hormone in normal men, *J. Clin. Endocrinol. Metab.,* 38, 545, 1974.
18. **Ruder, H., Corvol, P., Mahoudeau, J. A., Ross, G. T., and Lipsett, M. B.,** Effects of induced hyperthyroidism on steroid metabolism in man, *J. Clin. Endocrinol. Metab.,* 33, 382, 1971.
19. **Hunter, W. M. Edmond, P., Watson, G. S., and McLean, N.,** Plasma LH and FSH levels in subfertile men, *J. Clin. Endocrinol. Metab.,* 39, 740, 1974.
20. **Mecklenburg, R. S., Hetzel, W. D. Gulyas, B. J., and Lipsett, M. B.,** Regulation of FSH secretion: use of hydroxyurea to deplete germinal epithelium, *Endocrinology,* 96, 564, 1975.
21. **Baker, H. W. G.,** Testicular control of follicle stimulating hormone secretion, *Recent Progr. Horm. Res.,* 32, 429, 1976.
22. **Cooke, B. A., Rommerts, F. F. G., van der Kemp, J. W. C., and van der Molen, H. J.,** Effect of LH, FSH, prostaglandin E, and other hormones on cyclic AMP and testosterone production in rat testis tissues, *Mol. Cell. Endocrinol.,* 1, 99, 1974.
23. **Farnsworth, W. E. and Wilks, J. W.,** Prostaglandin F 2α and human prostatic affinity for testosterone, *Prostaglandins,* 9, 67, 1975.
24. **Laatkainen, T., Laitinen, E. A., and Vihko, R.,** Secretion of free and sulphate conjugated neutral steroids by the human testis. Effect of the administration of HCG, *J. Clin. Endocrinol. Metab.,* 32, 59, 1971.
25. **Saez, J. M., Forest, M. G., Morera, A. M., and Bertrand, J.,** Metabolic clearance rate and production rate of testosterone and dihydrotestosterone in normal subjects, during pregnancy and in hypothyroidism, *Jour. Clin. Invest.,* 51, 1226, 1972.

26. **Baird, D. T., Galbraith, A., Fraser, I. S., and Newsam, J. E.,** The concentration of oestrone and oestradiol-17β in spermatic venous blood in man, *J. Endocrinol.*, 57, 285, 1973.
27. **Lacy, D.,** Androgen dependency of spermatogenesis and the physiological significance of steroid metabolism in vitro by the seminiferous tubules, in *The Endocrine Function of the Human Testis,* Vol. 1, James, V. H. T., Serio, M., and Martini, L., Eds., Academic Press, London, 1973, 493.
28. **Vermeulen, A.,** The physical state of testosterone in the plasma, in *The Endocrine Function of the Human Testis,* Vol. 1, James, V. H. T., Serio, M., and Martini, L., Eds., Academic Press, London, 1973, 157.
29. **Vermeulen, A., Rubens, R., and Verdonck, L.,** Testosterone secretion and metabolism in male senescence, *J. Clin. Endocrinol. Metab.*, 34, 730, 1972.
30. **Rowe, P. H., Lincoln, G. A., Raley, P. H., Lehane, J., Stephenson, M. J., Shenton, J. C., and Glover, T. D.,** Temporal variations of testosterone levels in the peripheral blood plasma of men, *J. Endocrinol.*, 61, 63, 1974.
31. **Mahoudeau, J. A., Bardin, C. W., and Lipsett, M. B.,** The metabolic clearance rate and origin of plasma dihydrotestosterone in man and its conversion to the 5α-androstanediols, *J. Clin. Invest.*, 50, 1338, 1971.
32. **Naghma-E-Rehan, Sobrero, A. J. and Fertig, J. W.,** Semen of fertile men: statistical analysis of 1,300 men, *Fertil. Steril.*, 26, 492, 1975.
33. **Zucherman, Z., Rodriguez-Rigan, L. J., Smith K., and Steinberg, E.,** Frequency distribution of sperm counts in fertile and infertile males, *Fertil. Steril.*, 28, 1310, 1977.
34. **Gross, R. E., and Replogle, R. L.,** Treatment of undescended testis: opinions gained from 1767 operations, *Postgrad. Med.*, 34, 266, 1963.
35. **Hinman, F., Jr., Spence, H. F., Culp, O. S., Glenn, J. F., and Marshall, V. F.,** Panel discussion: anomalies of external genitalia in infancy and childhood, *J. Urol.*, 92, 1, 1965.
36. **Wilson, J. D., Harrod, M. J., Goldstein, J. L., Hemsell, D. L., and MacDonald, P. C.,** Familial incomplete male pseudohermaphrodism, Type 1. Evidence for androgen resistance and variable clinical manifestations in a family with the Reifenstein syndrome, *N. Engl. J. Med.*, 290, 1097, 1974.
37. **Walsh, P. C., Madden, J. D., Harrod, M. J., Goldstein, J. L., and MacDonald, P. C.,** Familial incomplete male pseudohermaphrodism, Type 2. Decreased dihydrotestosterone formation in pseudovaginal perineoscrotal hypospadias, *N. Engl. J. Med.*, 290, 944, 1974.
38. **Givens, J. R., Wiser, W. L., Summitt, R. L., Kerber, I. J., Anderson, R. N., Pittaway, A. B., and Fish, S. A.,** Familial male pseudohermaphrodism with gynecomastia due to deficient testicular 17-ketoreductase activity, *N. Engl. J. Med.*, 291, 938, 1974.
39. **Thorner, M.O.,** Prolactin, in *Clinics in Endocrinology and Metabolism. The Hypothalamus and Pituitary,* Vol. 6, Besser, G. M., Ed., W. B. Saunders, London, 1977, 201.
40. **Harper, P., Penny, R., Foley, T. P., Migeon, C. J., and Blizzard, R. M.,** Gonadal function in males with myotonic dystrophy, *J. Clin. Endocrinol.*, 35, 852, 1972.
41. **Swederloff, R. S. and Walsh, P. C.,** Pituitary and gonadal hormones in patients with varicocoele, *Fertil. Steril.*, 26, 1006, 1975.
42. **Dubin, L. and Amelar, R. D.,** Varicocelectomy as therapy in male infertility. A study of 504 cases, *J. Urol.*, 113, 640, 1975.
43. **Dubin, L. and Amelar, R. D.,** Etiologic factors in 1294 consecutive cases of male infertility, *Fertil. Steril.*, 22, 469, 1971.
44. **Hellman, L. and Bradlow, H. L.,** Recent advances in human steroid metabolism, *Adv. Clin. Chem.*, 13, 1, 1970.
45. **Clyde, H. R., Walsh, P. C., and English, R. W.,** Elevated plasma testosterone and gonadotropin levels in infertile males with hyperthyroidism, *Fertil. Steril.*, 27, 662, 1976.
46. **Molitor, J. T., Chertoio, B. S., and Fariss, B. L.,** Long-term follow-up of a patient with congenital adrenal hyperplasia and failure of testicular development, *Fertil. Steril.*, 24, 319, 1973.
47. **Kirkland, R. T., Kirkland, J. L., Johnson, C.M., Horning, M. G., Librik, L., and Clayton, G.W.,** Congenital lipoid adrenal hyperplasia in an 8-year-old phenotypic female, *J. Clin. Endocrinol. Metab.*, 36, 488, 1973.
48. **New, M. I.,** Male pseudohermaphroditism due to 17α-hydroxylase deficiency, *J. Clin. Invest.*, 49, 1930, 1970.
49. **Schneider, G., Genel, M., Bongiovanni, A. M., Goldman, A. S., and Rosenfield, R. L.,** Persistent testicular Δ^5= isomerase-3-hydroxysteroid dehydrogenase (^{5}-3-HSD) deficiency in the Δ^5-3-HSD form of congenital adrenal hyperplasia, *J. Clin. Invest.*, 55, 581, 1975.
50. **Hillier, S. G., Brownsey, G. G., and Cameron, E. H. D.,** Some observations on the determination of testosterone in human plasma by radioimmunoassay using antisera raised against testosterone-3-BSA and testoserone-11α-BSA, *Steroids*, 21, 735, 1973.
51. **Chen, J. C., Zorn, E. M., Hallberg, M. C., and Wieland, R. G.,** Antibodies to testosterone-3-bovine serum albumin applied to assay of serum 17β ol androgens, *Clin. Chem.*, 17, 581, 1971.

52. **Strott, C. A., Yoshimi, T., and Lipsett, M. B.,** Plasma progesterone and 17α hydroxyprogesterone in normal men and children with congenital adrenal hyperplasia, *J. Clin. Invest.,* 48, 930, 1969.
53. **Isurugi, K., Fukutani, K., Takayasu, H., Wakabayashi, K., and Tamaoki, B. I.,** Age-related changes in serum luteinizing hormone (LH) and follicle-stimulating hormone (FSH) levels in normal men. *J. Clin. Endocrinol. Metab.,* 39, 955, 1974.
54. **Child, D.F., Nader, S., Mashiter, K., Kjeld, M., Banks, L., and Fraser, T.R.,** Prolactin studies in functionless pituitary tumours, *Br. Med. J.,* 1, 604, 1975.
55. **Leonard, J. M., Leach, R. B., Couture, M., and Paulsen, C. A.,** Plasma and urinary follicle-stimulating hormone levels in oligospermia, *J. Clin. Endocrinol. Metab.,* 34, 209, 1972.
56. **Franchimont, P., Millett, O., Vendrely, E., Letawe, J., Legros, J. J., and Netter, A.,** Relationship between spermatogenesis and serum gonadotrophin levels in azoospermia and oligospermia, *J. Clin. Endocrinol. Metab.,* 34, 1003, 1972.
57. **De Kretser, D. M., Burger, H. G., and Hudson, B.,** The relationship between germinal cells and serum FSH levels in males with infertility, *J. Clin. Endocrinol. Metab.,* 38, 787, 1974.
58. **Boyar, R. M., Finkelstein, J. W., Witkin, M., Kapen, S., Weitzmann, E., and Hellman, L.,** Studies of endocrine function in isolated gonadotropin deficiency, *J. Clin. Endocrinol. Metab.,* 36, 64, 1973.
59. **Paulsen, C. A.,** The Testes, in *Textbook of Endocrinology,* Williams, R.H., Ed., W. B. Saunders, Philadelphia, 1974, 323.
60. **Santen, R.J. and Paulsen, C. A.,** Hypogonadotrophic eunuchoidism. 2. Gonadal responsiveness to exogenous gonadotrophins, *J. Clin. Endocrinol.,* 36, 55, 1973.
61. **Marshall, J. C., Anderson, D. C., Burke, C.W., Galvao-Teles, A., and Fraser, T. R.,** Clomiphene citrate in men: increase of cortisol, luteinising hormone, testosterone and steroid-binding globulins, *J. Endocrinol.,* 53, 261, 1972.
62. **Anderson, D. C., Marshall, J. C., Young, J. L., and Fraser, T. R.,** Stimulation tests of pituitary-Leydig cell function in normal male subjects and hypogonadal men, *Clin. Endocrinol.,* 1, 127, 1972.
63. **De Kretser, D. M., Burger, H. G., and Hudson, B.,** Diagnostic aspects of male infertility, in *Male Fertility and Sterility. Proc. Serono Symp.,* Vol. 5, Mancini, R. E., and Martini, L., Eds., Academic Press, New York, 1974, 337.
64. **Meinhard, E., McRae, C. U., and Chisholm, G. D.,** Testicular biopsy in evaluation of male infertility, *Br. Med. J.,* 3, 577, 1973.
65. **Hellinga, G., Swaen, G. J. V., and Van der Esch, E. P.,** Morphological semiquantitative scoring of testicular biopsy in infertility, *Andrologia,* 4, 55, 1972.
66. **Skakkebaek, N. E. and Heller, C.G.,** Quantification of human seminiferous epithelium. 1. Histological studies in twenty-one fertile men with normal chromosome complements, *J. Reprod. Fert.,* 32, 379, 1973.
67. **Skakkebaek, N. E., Hulten, M., Jacobsen, P., and Mikkelsen, M.,** Quantification of human seminiferous epithelium. 11. Histological studies in eight 47, XYY men, *J. Reprod. Fert.,* 32, 391, 1973.
68. **Kjessler, B.,** Meiosis in a man with a D/D translocation and clinical sterility, *Lancet,* 1, 1421, 1964.
69. **Kjessler, B.,** Karyotypes of 130 childless men, *Lancet,* 2, 493, 1965.
70. **Kjessler, B.,** Karyotype, meiosis, and spermatogenesis in a sample of men attending an infertility clinic, *Monogr. Hum. Genet.,* 2, 1, 1966.
71. **Kjessler, B.,** Chromosomal constitution and male reproductive failure, in *Male Fertility and Sterility, Proc. Serono Symp.,* Vol. 5, Mancini, R. E. and Martini, L., Eds., Academic Press, New York, 1974, 231.

Chapter 2

FEMALE GONADAL FUNCTION: THE OVARY

Sandra Naik and George W. Pennington

TABLE OF CONTENTS

I. ANATOMY AND PHYSIOLOGY

Reproductive processes result from a complex series of interactions between the hypothalamus, the pituitary, the ovaries, and the genital tract. The hypothalamus and pituitary gland are considered elsewhere.

The ovaries have two main functions: the production and release of secondary oocytes and the synthesis and secretion of the steroid hormones. These functions are carried out by the same ovarian organelles. Gametogenesis and the processes of ovulation and menstruation occur within the period of reproductive life. Gonadal steroids are secreted throughout life, being at their maximum levels during the reproductive years.

A. Basic Features of the Ovary

The ovaries are two nodular structures attached to the posterior surface of the broad ligament by a peritoneal fold of tissue called the mesovarium. The blood vessels, lymphatic ducts, and nerves traverse the mesovarium and penetrate the ovary at its hilum.

Microscopically the ovary consists of three distinct regions, an outer cortex, a central medulla, and an inner hilum. The ovary is covered by a layer of surface cells which are separated from the cortex by the tunica albuginea. The tunica albuginea increases in density with advancing age and may be thickened in pathological conditions, such as the Stein-Leventhal syndrome.

The appearance of the cortex is dependent on the age of the female. In the newborn it is packed with oocytes and primitive follicles. There is a growth phase between birth and puberty. This increase in weight of the ovary is due to an accumulation of stromal residue left after maturation and atresia of the follicles, and also to an increase in volume achieved by the maturing follicles. As the ovary matures, medullary tissue grows into the cortex, separating the individual primordial follicles. At adolescence the surface of the ovary is smooth and follicles are visible. At this time cyclic ovulation is initiated. The normal functioning adult ovary contains follicles and corpora lutea in various stages of maturation and regression, as well as corpora albicanta and corpora fibrosa. During the reproductive phase of life the ovarian surface becomes repeatedly scarred by ovulation. The stroma of the cortex is composed of a surface zone of compact fibrous tissue and a deeper area of looser, more cellular tissue. The ovarian stroma is responsible for the synthesis of ovarian androgens, while the follicles synthesize estrogens.[1] The postmenopausal ovary is gametogenically nonfunctioning and it declines in weight from about 14 g in the fourth decade to about 5 g in the sixth decade. The outer surface is wrinkled and without luster. At this time the cortical stroma becomes hyperplastic. As in the cortex, the stromal elements of the medulla become fibrotic and the blood vessels in this region become sclerotic.

The medulla represents the core of the organ and is formed by loose connective tissue. From the hilus the blood vessels enter or leave the medulla, where their branches run a spiral course. Well-developed perivascular networks of cholinergic and adrenergic nerves are found in the medulla. Hilus cells are present near the hilus of the ovary; these cells are very similar to the interstitial cells of the testis and they produce androgens. The hilus cells are sensitive to stimulation by gonadotropins[2] and tumors arising from them produce virilizing effects.

B. Ovarian Organelles

1. The Follicle

Follicles are scattered throughout the cortical zone. In the ovaries of children they are present in large numbers, mostly at the stage of primordial follicles. During reproductive life they decrease in number.

a. Primordial Follicle

The most immature form of follicle is known as the primordial follicle. This consists of a primary oocyte, which is blocked in the first prophase of meiosis, surrounded by a single layer of spindle-shaped cells.

b. Primary and Secondary Follicle

The flat spindle-shaped cells of the primordial follicle become cuboidal and the follicle is known as the primary follicle. Successive mitotic divisions of the cuboidal cells occur, giving rise to the zona granulosa and the zona pellucida, which derives from secretions of the endoplasmic reticulum of follicular cells. It is composed of mucopolysaccharide with a sialic acid component. The zona pellucida separates the cuboidal granulosa cells from the oocyte. This zone is surrounded by a pseudostratified layer of follicular cells called the corona radiata. Encircling the follicle is a differentiated cellular layer of stroma called the theca interna. The portion of theca merging with surrounding stroma is termed the theca externa.

c. Graafian Follicle

Epithelioid transformation of the theca interna occurs and the follicular cells secrete fluid. Steroid hormones have been identified in this fluid. It appears that there is a critical sequence of hormonal changes that take place within the follicular fluid before ovulation;[3] the endocrine events occurring prior to ovulation dictate the subsequent activity of the corpus luteum. This accumulation of fluid is followed by the appearance of cleft-like spaces among the granulosa cells; gradually a cavity, the antrum, is formed. The ovum surrounded by the follicle cells projects into the lumen of the cavity and this projection is called the cumulus oophorus.

d. Follicular Atresia

From fetal life until the menarche, maturation stops before the follicle reaches diameters equal to those required for ovulation and the follicle degenerates. This degenerative process is called atresia. The factor which determines atresia is not known. It is characterized by cessation of mitosis in the granulosa, the separation of granulosa cells from the basal lamina and by death of the oocyte. The nuclear fragments float in the follicular fluid and the cells of the cumulus oophorous slough off. The follicle collapses and is invaded by fibroblastic connective tissue. The structure is then known as the corpus fibrosum.

e. Ovulation

One of the maturing follicles enlarges and ruptures, extruding the oocyte surrounded by the cumulus oophorus. At the time of rupture the first meiotic division is resumed and completed with extrusion of the first polar body. This leaves the secondary oocyte surrounded by cumulus.

2. The Corpus Luteum

The life of this organ commences immediately following ovulation. After the ovum is extruded the wall of the follicle collapses and the site of ovulation becomes plugged by fibrin and then fibrous connective tissue. The granulosa cells proliferate and alter to lutein cells, which produce progesterone. This process is followed by vascularization. Vessels from the theca interna penetrate the basal lamina. The theca interna involutes except where it is incorporated into the septa which divide the corpus luteum into compartments. In these areas they remain as theca lutein cells and are known as paralutein cells which produce estrogens.

If fertilization and implantation do not occur, the corpus luteum starts to involute. This process is characterized by vacuoles forming in the luteal cells with progressive hyalinization. The structure is then known as the corpus albicans.

C. Menstrual Cycle

The reproductive period in women occupies about 30% of the life span, commencing at the menarche and ending at the menopause. The length of the cycle varies throughout life, tending to become more uniform with age.[4] The initial and last few years of menstrual life are often marked by a variation in pattern. The mean cycle length is 28 days, but regular cycle lengths of 23 to 35 days may be considered normal. In view of the varying lengths of normal regular menstrual cycles, a definite point in the cycle for plotting reference data has been established. This point is the LH (luteinizing hormone) peak.

For descriptive purposes the menstrual cycle may be divided into three parts, the follicular phase, the ovulatory phase, and the luteal phase. These phases are derived from the corresponding state of the ovary.

1. The Follicular Phase

This phase has a mean length of around 14 days. It starts on the first day of menstruation. During this time 10 to 20 follicles start to develop under the stimulus of follicle stimulating hormone and later of luteinizing hormone (Figure 1). It is probable that the follicle destined for ovulation begins to grow during the luteal phase of the preceding cycle. The theca interna secretes estrogens by approximately day 8 of the cycle and concentrations increase during this part of the cycle. During the last half of the follicular phase, the diameter of the largest follicle, which is destined to ovulate, increases rapidly. The remaining follicles become atretic. Coincident with the development of the largest follicle, the concentration of follicle stimulating hormone (FSH) declines and that of LH rises.

2. Ovulation

This extends over a period of about 60 hours. A surge of LH accompanied by a lesser surge of FSH begins 24 hr prior to ovulation. Associated with this, there is a sharp peak in estrogen output, which occurs before or coincident with the surge in gonadotropins.

3. Luteal Phase

During this secretory phase the Graafian follicle collapses and the corpus luteum is formed: this has a life span of about 14 days. The luteal cells produce progesterone and both the luteal and paraluteal cells produce estrogens. The abrupt termination of the release of progesterone from the corpus luteum determines the onset of menstruation. In vitro work has shown that the production of progesterone is correlated with the hormonal environment during the follicular phase of the cycle.[5]

4. Basal Body Temperature (BBT)

Progesterone is a thermogenic agent. Careful temperature measurements taken immediately on waking before rising, drinking, or smoking may be used as a rough assessment of ovulation. In a normal cycle the temperature remains fairly constant until ovulation, when there is a slight drop followed by a rise which should last for at least 10 days. The temperature falls prior to menstruation. In some cases the temperature chart shows no correlation with hormonal output.[6]

5. Effect of Stress

Stress may postpone or inhibit ovulation and menstruation if it occurs in the follicular phase of the cycle. When stress occurs in the luteal phase, the preovulatory phase of the subsequent cycle may be prolonged. This indicates that the ovulatory surge of LH is postponed or abolished but that the functioning life of the corpus luteum is not affected.

II. OVARIAN STEROID HORMONE SECRETION

A. Survey of Methods

Ovarian steroid secretion and metabolism may be studied by the following methods:

1. Measurement of steroid metabolites in urine. This method is widely used. Urinary

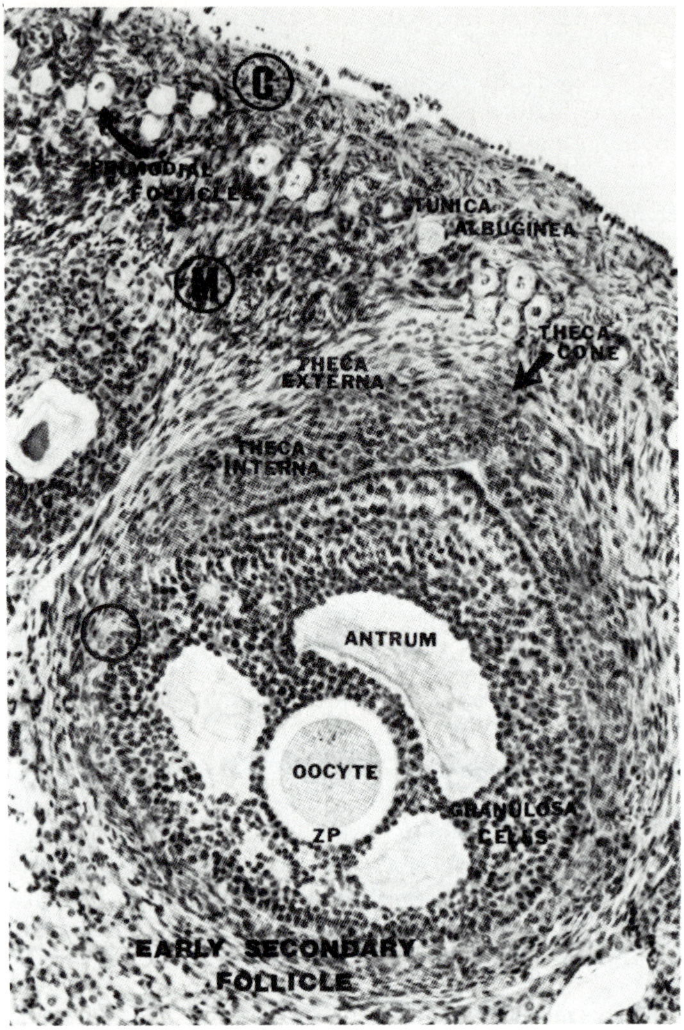

FIGURE 1. Light micrograph showing a follicle migrating (presumably by the theca cone) from the cortex (C) into the medulla (M). Once the follicle enters the medulla, it develops a theca interna and externa. The newly delivered plasma FSH stimulates antrum formation and reduces the aromatase enzyme activity and LH receptors in the granulosa cells. The primordial follicles form a thick band just beneath the tunica albuginea. Compare the size of the immature oocyte in the primordial follicle with that of the fully grown oocyte and its zona pellucida in the early secondary follicle. (From Erickson, G. F., *Clin. Obstet. Gynecol.*, 21, 31, 1978. With permission.)

excretion reflects ovarian secretion only if the steroid is secreted exclusively by the ovary and is metabolized to a unique metabolite. The accuracy of the 24-hr urine collection must be assured. This method of assessment will not reveal acute changes in ovarian activity but will reflect the overall pattern of steroid secretion and metabolism.

2. Measurement of hormones in peripheral venous blood. This method enables serial samples to be collected easily and rapid changes in secretion may be studied.

The way in which the concentration in plasma reflects ovarian secretion depends on its rate of metabolism and clearance.

3. Direct sampling of ovarian venous effluent. Direct proof of ovarian steroid secretion may be obtained by demonstrating that the concentration in ovarian venous effluent is higher than that in peripheral venous blood. This technique is performed by percutaneous catheterization via the femoral vein, thereby avoiding the stress of surgery.
4. Technique of isotope dilution. In this method a tracer amount of radioactively labeled steroid is introduced into the blood stream. Its fate is followed by the collection of serial samples of blood and/or urine. The rate of metabolism may then be expressed as the metabolic clearance rate.

B. Steroids Secreted by the Ovary

The secretion of steroid hormones is controlled by a negative feedback loop involving the hypothalamus and anterior pituitary. There may also be some degree of neural regulation governing the endocrine cells in the ovary. Isolated adrenergic fibers and possibly nerve terminals have been observed in the cortical stroma. These may have some physiological function regarding the changes which occur in stromal connective tissue.

The human ovary secretes progesterone, pregnenolone, 17α-hydroxyprogesterone, dehydroepiandrosterone, androstenedione, testosterone, estrone, and estradiol.[7]

1. Estrogens

a. General

The three classical estrogens are estrone, estradiol and estriol.

Estradiol. In the normal ovarian cycle, virtually all the estradiol is secreted by the ovary. By day 7 of the cycle the preovulatory follicle is secreting over 90% of the estradiol present. The concentration rises rapidly from day 5 to reach a peak either 1 day before or on the day of the LH peak. Following the midcycle elevation levels drop sharply after which there is a slow increase to plateau between day 4 and day 10 after the LH peak. In this luteal phase nearly all the estradiol originates from the corpus luteum. Following the plateau, levels fall to their nadir at the time of menstruation (Figure 2).

Estrone. Estrone is secreted in variable amounts by both the ovaries and adrenals. Most of the estrone in the cirulation is derived from peripheral metabolism of other precursors. A small contribution comes from estradiol but the majority is formed by the conversion of androstenedione.

The most abundant form of estrogen found in peripheral plasma is estrone sulfate.[8,9] At midcycle its concentration is approximately 5 times that of estradiol 17β and 15 times that of estrone.

Urinary Estrogens. The total excretion of the estrogen metabolites in urine is a reflection of the integrated secretion of the preceding 24 hours. Similar peaks of output to those of estradiol are shown in the urine sample. Urinary estrogens may also be estimated separately but the same two peaks are shown and individual breakdown is rarely required. The excretion of urinary total estrogens is shown in the diagram of composite levels during the menstrual cycle (Figure 5).

b. Radioimmunoassay of Estradiol in Plasma[10]*

Reagents

1. Add 1.0 mℓ distilled water to the standards ϕ-E and reference sera L & H. Let stand for 5 min and mix gently in order to obtain an homogenous solution.

* Kit Method of Nordiclab, Finland.

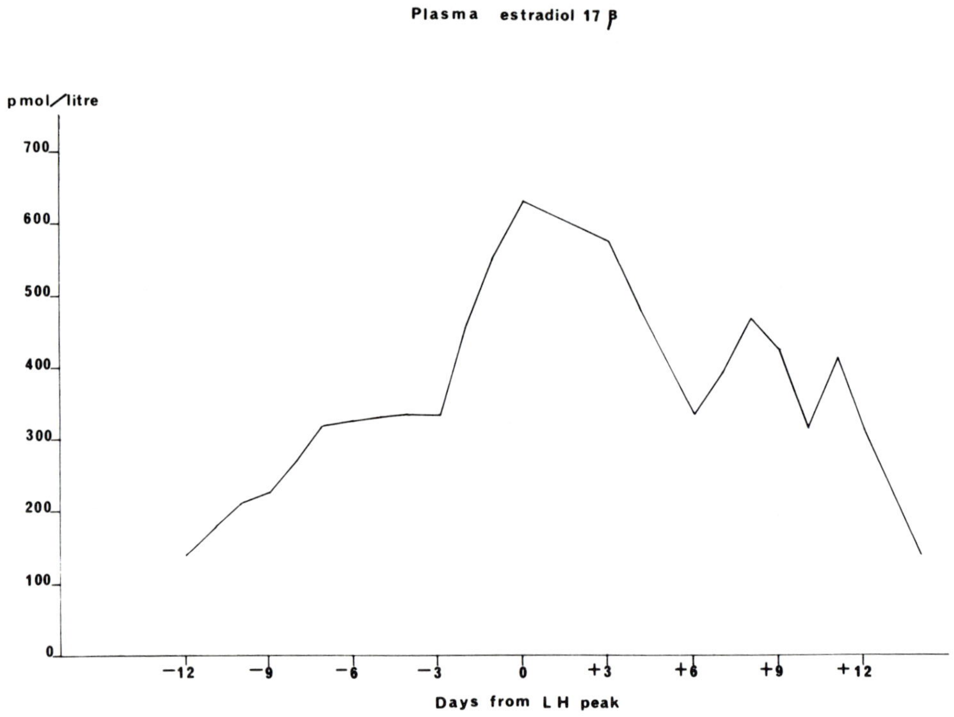

FIGURE 2. Concentration of estradiol 17β in the peripheral plasma. Day 0 in the graph is the day of maximum LH secretion.

2. Add 10.0 mℓ distilled water to the antiserum and ^{125}I tracer bottles (each for 50 tubes). Mix gently, avoid foaming.
3. Set up and mark glass tubes or high quality polypropylene tubes (available from Nordiclab) — four tubes for each standard ϕ-E, NSB, reference and patient sample, and two tubes for total.

Method

1. Pipette 0.20 mℓ of each standard ϕ-E, reference L & H, and patient sample in duplicate into the tubes above. Into NSB tubes add 0.20 mℓ of any patient serum in duplicate.
2. Dispense accurately 1.00 mℓ of distilled diethylether (calibrated glass dispenser) into all tubes to be extracted and stopper the tubes immediately and tightly (polyethylene caps) in order to prevent evaporation.
3. Shake vigorously for 15 min with a high efficiency horizontal shaker.
4. Let the phases separate and freeze the water phase (−40°C). Transfer the whole ether phase into the premarked assay tubes by decanting.
5. Evaporate to dryness under a stream of nitrogen or air at +37°C.
6. Pipette 0.2 mℓ of red tracer solution into all assay tubes and mix thoroughly in order to introduce dried residue into solution again.
7. Pipette 0.2 mℓ of blue antiserum solution into all tubes except NSB and total. Mix thoroughly.
8. Incubate for 60 min at 37°C; let cool to room temperature.
9. Mix polyethylene glycol solution by inverting a few times before dispensing and add 0.5 mℓ into all tubes except total. Mix thoroughly with a vortex.

10. After solution stands for a few min, centrifuge for 15 min at no less than 2000 g.
11. Aspirate the supernatant by a constant speed and manner using, e.g., Pasteur-pipette connected to a water suction. Check that there is no liquid phase left in the tubes after standing for a few minutes.

Counting

Count all the tubes for radioactivity for at least 60 sec in gamma counter.

Calculation

The standard curve is calculated using the four parameter log-logit method. The concentration of estrogen in the unknown samples is calculated by reading from the graph.

Factors affecting assay results

Drugs — Estrogen-containing therapy including oral contraceptives.

Interaction of sex hormone binding globulin — The steroid hormones in blood are bound to protein. A significant amount of estradiol binds to the hemoglobin of the erythrocytes. Estrogens are bound to sex hormone binding globulin (SHBG). It is known that the bound fraction is biologically inactive.[12] Only nonprotein-bound steroid can diffuse out of the plasma compartment into the interstitial space. SHBG levels are about twofold higher in adult women than in men. This difference is due to the sensitivity of SHBG production to estrogens and the antagonistic effect of androgens.

Factors causing altered levels of SHBG

Cirrhosis of liver — SHBG levels are elevated in men with cirrhosis of the liver. Estradiol levels have been shown to be little changed, but plasma levels of estrone and estriol are elevated. Accompanying these changes there is a fall in unbound testosterone.[13]

Thyrotoxicosis — SHBG levels are increased in this condition.[14]

Acromegaly — Low levels of SHBG are found. It has been shown that SHBG is inhibited by administration of growth hormone in growth hormone deficiency.[15]

Hirsutism — SHBG levels are reduced to half normal values in hirsute women. The low levels are secondary to excess androgens or to lack of estrogens.

c. Metabolism of Estrogens

The liver is responsible for the greater part of steroid hormone metabolism.[16] The hormones are partly excreted in the bile and reabsorbed from the gastrointestinal tract, the bulk of the metabolites appearing in the urine as sulfates or glucosiduronate conjugates. Double conjugates also occur. The metabolism of the estrogens is discussed elsewhere. For most clinical practice the estimation of total estrogens in the urine is adequate. Two methods are described.

d. Estimation of Total Estrogens in the Urine — Method 1[17]

Extraction procedure

Extraction is performed using the semiautomatic extractor.

Reagents

Kober reagent is prepared by dissolving 20 g quinol in 1 ℓ of 66% sulfuric acid (analytical grade).

Ittrich reagent is prepared by dissolving 10 g *para*-nitrophenol in 10 mℓ methanol.

It is made up to 500 mℓ with redistilled tetrachloroethane. This reagent is stored at 4°C.
Quinol — 1 g quinol is dissolved in 100 mℓ redistilled ethanol. This is stored at 4°C.
5 *M* sodium hydroxide
1 *M* sodium hydroxide
Concentrated hydrochloric acid (analytical grade)
Petroleum ether — bp 60 to 80°C, redistilled
Diethyl ether, peroxide-free
Sodium bicarbonate (8%)
Solid sodium chloride
Solid sodium bicarbonate
Carbonate buffer — pH 10.5, prepared by mixing 850 mℓ of 8% sodium bicarbonate and 130 mℓ of 5 *M* sodium hydroxide
Estriol standard — 150 nmol/ℓ of estriol in ethanol prepared from a stock solution containing 1.5 nmol/ℓ

Method

Hydrolize 1 mℓ urine, diluted with 5 mℓ distilled water and 0.9 mℓ concentrated hydrochloric acid, by heating in an autoclave at 120°C (15 lb/in^2) for 15 min. The sample is transferred to the semiautomatic extractor tube and 1 g sodium chloride is added to aid the extraction of estriol. When dissolved, 6 mℓ diethyl ether is dispensed into the tubes and shaken for 3 min. The lower aqueous layer is removed via the capillary end of the extraction tube. The extract is washed with 2 mℓ carbonate buffer for 3 min and 6 mℓ petroleum ether and 6 mℓ 1 *N* NaOH is added. The phenolic steroids are extracted into the alkali by shaking for 3 min. The upper organic layer containing the neutral steroids is discarded via the ground glass end of the tube. Next 0.8 g sodium bicarbonate is added to the phenolic extract and shaken for 3 min to dissolve. The estrogens are re-extracted into 6.0 mℓ diethyl ether by shaking for 3 min. The carbonate layer is discarded. The ether extract is transferred to a clean tube and 0.1 mℓ quinol is added and evaporated under nitrogen gas, in a boiling water bath. Next 1 mℓ Kober reagent is added and the tubes are vortex mixed. They are boiled for 40 min.

Fluorimetry

After boiling, the tubes are removed and cooled in an ice bath. Following addition of 1.5 mℓ chilled distilled water to each they are vortex mixed. The contents are then added to the cooled fluorimeter tubes, to which 0.5 mℓ ice-cold Ittrich reagent has been added. Each tube is shaken manually 40 to 50 times and then centrifuged at 1500 r/min for 5 min at 0°C. Fluorescence is evaluated using the Perkin Elmer MPF3 spectrofluorimeter with xenon lamp and ellipsoid condensing system. The wavelengths measured are

1.	Excitation 530 nm	fluorescence 560	specific reading
2.	Excitation 490 nm	fluorescence 520	nonspecific reading

Calculation

The corrected fluorescence is obtainable by using the formula

$$R\ 530/560 - (K \times 490/520)$$

K is a factor used to eliminate background fluorescent impurities in the extract and is dependent on the instrument used, the lamp source, and the wavelengths selected. The factor is derived by examining the urine of a patient with a very low estrogen output. The sample is taken through the assay procedure. The fluorescence at 530 nm/560 nm is a measure of the estrogen level plus the impurities, while the fluorescence at 490 nm/520 nm provides a measure of the contribution from interfering nonestrogenic substances.

$$K = \frac{530\text{nm}/560\text{nm}}{490\text{nm}/520\text{nm}}$$

Precision — Coefficient of variation = 16%.

e. Estimation of Total Estrogens in the Urine — Method 2[18]

A semiautomated method is also available for the determination of estrogens.

Apparatus

1. Gel permeation columns
   Preparation of column for gel permeation — 25 g Sephadex® G10 are placed in 300 mℓ distilled water and left to swell overnight. The mixture is then resuspended and 25 mℓ is pipetted into each column
2. Continuous flow apparatus for color reaction
   a. Sampler Mark 11 proportioning pump and solid block heater (120°C) with 2 × 28-turn mixing coils encapsulated in silicone rubber.
   b. Pump tubing in Tygon®

Internal diameter (in.)	Color
0.025	orange/white
0.040	white/white
0.073	green/green
0.051	gray/gray
0.065	blue/blue

   c. Pump tubing in Acidflex®

Internal diameter (in.)	Color
0.073	green/green
0.100	purple/orange

   d. Glassware

Glass connections	D0 A10
Glass de-bubbler	C5
Electrolyte trap	B0
Mixing coils	105-0086-01 and 116-0103-09

   e. Fluorimeter — Perkin Elmer MPF 3 with Honeywell Electronik 15 recorder

The construction of the continuous flow system is shown in Figure 3.

Reagents

Kober reagent (2% quinol in 66% sulfuric acid)
Fluorescence reagent — 125 g trichloroacetic acid in 2 ℓ trichloromethane, analytical grade
Diluent — 10 drops Brij® 35 wetting agent is added to 2 ℓ distilled water
0.1 *M* NaOH
0.3 *M* HCl
Standards — A range of standards from 25—150 nmol/ℓ is prepared in sodium hydroxide from a stock solution containing 500 μmol/ℓ

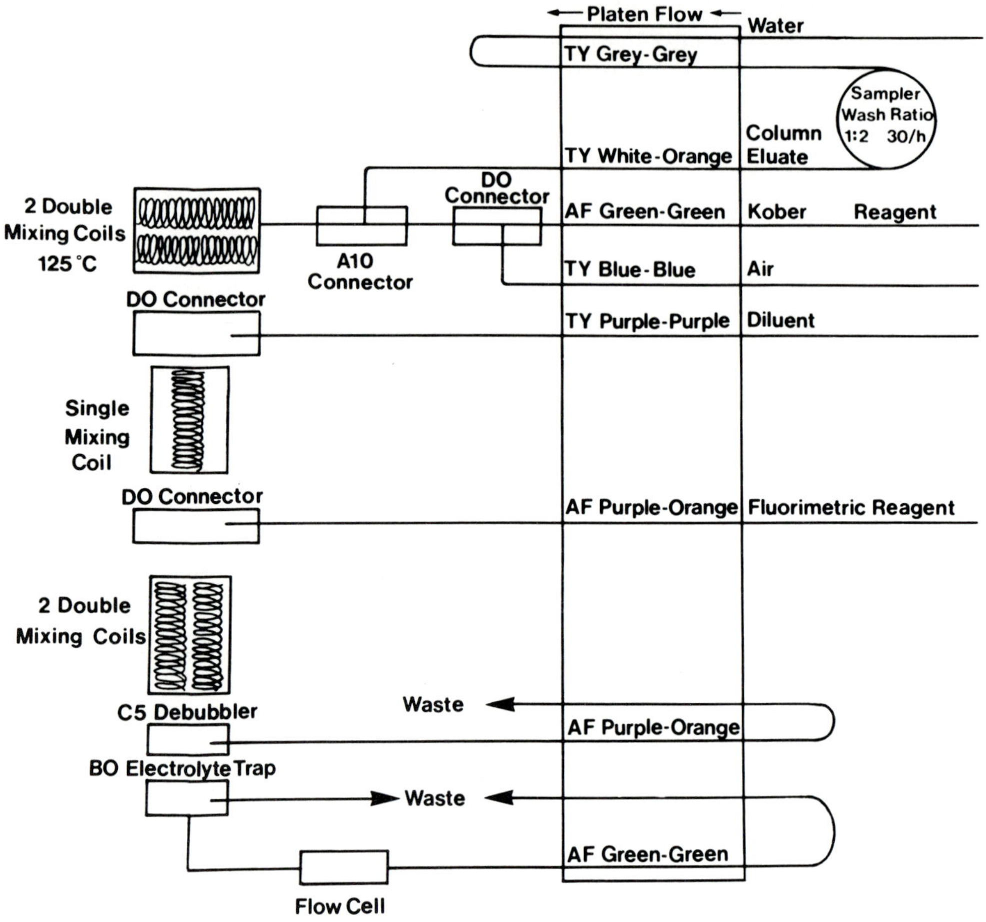

FIGURE 3. Flow diagram as used in the estimation of total nonpregnancy estrogens in the urine. TY = Tygon; AF = Acidiflex.

Method

Extraction by column: gel permeation — To 3 mℓ of urine 3 mℓ of 0.3 *M* HCl is added. They are mixed and applied to the top of the column and allowed to permeate through the column until the surface of the gel is just dry. At this point, 10 mℓ of 0.3 *M* HCl is added to the top of the column and allowed to permeate as before. This process is repeated using 10 mℓ distilled water. All the eluate is run to waste. 10 mℓ of 0.1 *M* NaOH is added to the top of the column and this eluate is collected into a glass tube. *Note:* the extraction procedure may be assisted by means of a peristaltic pump.

Fluorimetry

The heating block, fluorimeter, recorder, pump, and sampler are switched on. Diluent is pumped through the system until the heating block equilibrates at 120 to 125°C. The Kober reagent, fluorescence, and diluent are pumped into the system until equilibrium is reached. This procedure takes about 20 min.

A drift control consisting of a 50 nmol/ℓ standard is placed in the first cup. This is followed by two 25 nmol/ℓ standards, then a series of standards of 50, 75, 100, 125, and 150 nmol/ℓ. This series is followed by a urine control extract and a drift control. Eight sample extracts are placed in the next 8 cups followed by a control extract and a drift control.

Calculation

From the recorder chart, plot peak heights derived from the standard solutions as a function of concentration. Interpolate peak heights derived from the urine samples to obtain the total estrogens.

Precision — Coefficient of variation = 9%.

Note: analysis of urines estimated by this method and by that described before (method 1) gives the following relationship:

$$\text{Result by method 1} = \text{result by method } 2 \times 1.5$$

Administered compounds affecting assay of estrogens or results obtained

1. Affecting Kober procedure
   - Senna[19]
   - Cortisone[20]
   - Cascara[21]
   - Meprobamate[19]
   - Hydrochlorothiazide[20,21]
2. Affecting acid hydrolysis
   - Sugars[21]
   - Phenolphthalein[22]
   - Hydrochlorothiazide[23]
   - Mandelamine[24]
3. Affecting fluorimetric procedure
   - Cyclofenil[21]
   - Vitamin B[21]
   - Ethinyl estradiol[21]
4. In vivo effects
   - Phenothiazines[25]
   - Oral contraceptives[26]
   - Ampicillin[27]
   - Neomycin[20]

f. Biological Effect of Estrogens

Estrogens are responsible for the development and maintainence of the female sex organs, for the secondary sexual characteristics, and for maintenance of the menstrual cycle.

Genital tract — The growth and function of the uterus, cervix, ovaries, Fallopian tubes, vagina, and labia are controlled by estrogens. Changes in the genital tract during the normal cycle are discussed later.

Breasts — Estrogens are necessary for the development of the duct systems of the breasts. They also cause fat deposition in mammary tissue.

Metabolism — Estrogens increase the plasma proteins which bind steroids such as cortisol, thyroxine, and progesterone. They are mildly anabolic and lead to retention of sodium and consequently of water.

The effects of estrogens are modified by those of progestogens.

2. Progesterone and 17α-Hydroxyprogesterone

a. General

Progesterone — The main source of progesterone secretion in the ovary is the corpus luteum. Analysis of normal follicles has demonstrated the presence of progesterone in small quantities during the follicular phase of the cycle.[28] The bulk of progesterone in the circulation during this period results from conversion of adrenal pregnenolone and pregnenolone sulfate to progesterone.

Plasma progesterone levels are low in the follicular phase of the cycle but show a slight rise coincident with the LH peak. There is a major rise immediately following the LH peak reaching a maximum from 5 to 9 days after ovulation. This is due to secretion of progesterone by the cells of the corpus luteum. Levels fall to basal immediately prior to menstruation (Figure 4).

17α-Hydroxyprogesterone — During the menstrual cycle 17α-hydroxyprogesterone shows two clear-cut peaks. A significant rise in plasma level is observed on the day of the LH peak, following a fall one day after this peak. A subsequent rise is observed during the next 4 to 5 days to reach a second peak. Levels then decline progressively during the late luteal phase.

b. Radioimmunoassay of Plasma Progesterone[29]

Reagents

Phosphate buffered saline (PBS) — 0.01 *M*, pH 7.4, containing sodium azide 0.1%

0.1% gelatin in PBS freshly prepared each time

Antisera to progesterone 11 oxime BSA conjugate — For use the antisera are diluted 1/3000 in 0.1% gelatin PBS

Radioactive progesterone — (1,2,6,7-^{3}H), obtained from the Radiochemical Centre, Amersham — The specific activity of this substance is approximately 84 Ci/mmol. For use a solution is prepared in 0.1% gelatin PBS to give a count of 30,000 cpm/0.2 mℓ

Petroleum spirit — bp 60 to 80°

Dextran-coated charcoal — 250 mg charcoal (Norit A) and 25 mg Dextran T-70 are suspended in 100 mℓ 0.1% gelatin PBS. This is stirred in an ice bath for 1 hour before use.

Apparatus

Liquid scintillation counter, Packard 3380, using a PPO *bis*-MSB counting fluid.

Method

All samples tubes are set up in duplicate. Plasma (0.1 mℓ) is pipetted into polyethylene conical centrifuge tubes. To each tube is added 2 mℓ of petroleum spirit and the contents are vortex mixed for exactly 2 min. The tubes are then centrifuged at 3000 r/min for 10 min. The tubes are then stoppered and kept at −20°C for at least 1 hour. After this the petroleum spirit is decanted into glass tubes.

Standard progesterone, 50 μl in the range 0 to 95 nmol/ℓ, is pipetted into glass tubes and 2 mℓ petroleum spirit is added.

All tubes are evaporated to dryness at 37°C under nitrogen. They should be left for as short a time as possible. To all the dry tubes 100 μℓ of label is added. To all tubes, except total and blank tubes, 100 μℓ of antiserum is added and to the total and blanks 100 μℓ of 0.1% gelatin PBS is added. All the tubes are vortex mixed and incubated at 37°C for 1 hr. They are then removed and placed in an ice bath for 15 min. 500 μℓ of dextran-coated charcoal is added to each tube and they are vortex mixed and returned to the ice bath for a further 15 min. They are then centrifuged at 4°C for 10 min at 2500 r/min. Next 0.5 μℓ of the supernatant is pipetted into plastic minivials to which 4 mℓ of scinitillation fluid is added. The vials are counted.

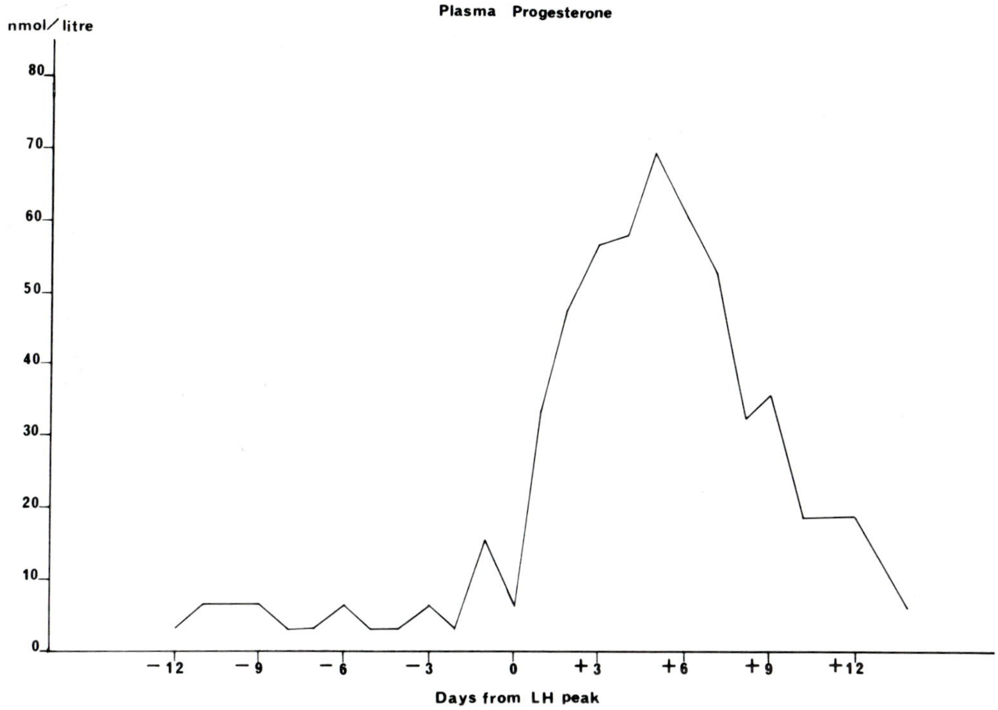

FIGURE 4. Concentration of progesterone in the peripheral plasma. Day 0 in the graph is the day of maximum LH secretion.

Total and blank tubes are prepared. Into 6 tubes are pipetted 100 $\mu\ell$ of 0.1% gelatin PBS and 100 $\mu\ell$ radioactive progesterone. Blanks are prepared by adding 500 $\mu\ell$ dextran-charcoal to three of these tubes and treating them in the same way as the samples and standards. Totals are prepared in the remaining three tubes by adding 500 $\mu\ell$ of 0.1% gelatin PBS and treating in the same way as the sample and standard tubes.

Calculation

The standard curve is calculated by using the four parameter log-logit method.[11] The concentration of progesterone in the unknown samples is calculated by reading from the graph.

Precision — Coefficient of variation = 14%.

Factors Affecting Assay

The radioimmunoassay is subject to unexpected interferences. The cleanliness of the glassware and the purity of the reagents are of the utmost importance.

c. Pregnanediol

Progesterone is transported in the blood by a specific progesterone binding protein. It is rapidly removed from the circulation and inactivated in the liver. The major metabolite is pregnanediol which is conjugated in the liver as sodium pregnanediol glucuronide and excreted in this form in the urine. Smaller amounts are excreted in the feces as the unconjugated steroid. Only 5 to 26% of progesterone is excreted as pregnanediol.[30] Levels of pregnanediol vary in the same way as progesterone during the menstrual cycle. The excretion of pregnanediol in the urine is shown in the composite diagram (Figure 5).

d. Gas-Liquid Chromatographic Method for the Estimation of Urinary Pregnanediol[31,32]

Reagents

Concentrated HCl
Acetyl chloride (analar)
Toluene (sulfur free)
Pregnanediol diacetate — 50 μg/mℓ, made up in the internal standard cholestanone 100 μg/mℓ in redistilled ethanol
Internal standard — Cholestanone 100 μg/mℓ in redistilled ethanol
The following **gases** obtained from British Oxygen: (a) high purity hydrogen, (b) oxygen-free nitrogen, and (c) compressed air.

Apparatus

1. Pye model GDC gas chromatograph equipped with a hydrogen flame ionization detector and 4 ID glass coil columns. The columns are prepared and packed with 3% SE 30 on Supelcoport® 100 to 120 mesh. The support is coated with the filtration technique.
2. S8 liquid autosampler

Method

Hydrolysis — to 5 mℓ of urine, 1 mℓ of concentrated HCl is added in a Quickfit test tube. It is placed in a boiling water bath for 12 min. It is then cooled in running water.

Extraction and acetylation — 5 mℓ of toluene is added to each tube and the tube is stoppered and vigorously shaken for 1 min. The tubes are centrifuged at 2000 r/min for 5 min and 3 mℓ of the upper toluene phase is removed and placed in a clean tube. Next, 1 mℓ of acetyl chloride is added and mixed. It is allowed to stand at room temperature for 1 hr. The solvent is evaporated in a hot water bath under a stream of compressed air. The tubes are cooled at room temperature. To each tube is added 0.2 mℓ of internal standard and the tubes are mixed on a vortex mixer. The resulting mixture is transferred into the autosampler glass tubes. A standard solution is added in every tenth tube. A control urine is processed every 11 test samples. The volume of sample injected is 5 μℓ.

Calculation

The area of each pregnanediol peak and internal standard peak is measured. The response ratio is determined by:

$$\frac{\text{area of sample peak}}{\text{area of internal standard peak}}$$

$$\text{Pregnanediol } \mu\text{mol } 1/24 \text{ hours} = \frac{\text{response ratio of sample factor volume}}{\text{response ratio of standard}}$$

The factor under these conditions = 8.2, but any variation requires a different factor volume.

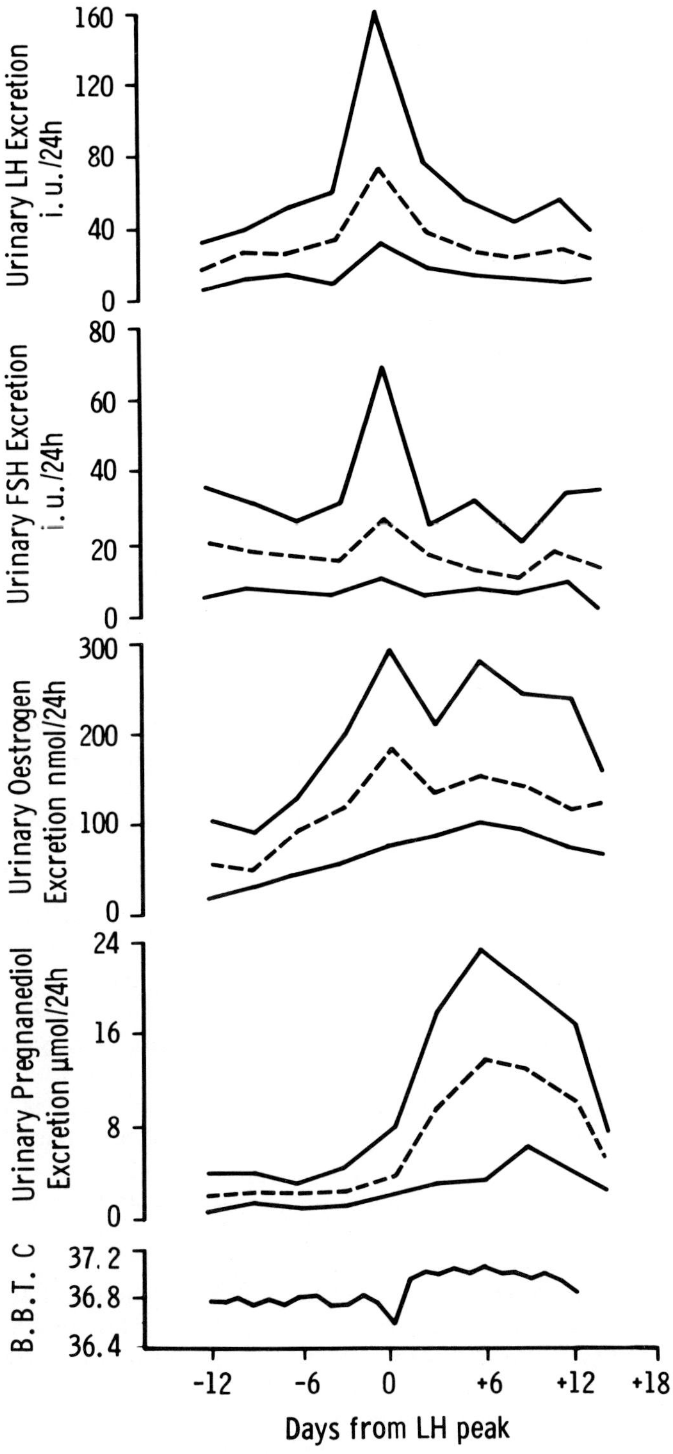

FIGURE 5. Composite diagram of urinary steroid excretion and basal body temperature during the menstrual cycle. The cycle is centered on day 0, the day of the LH peak. In normal menstruating women, 95% of all values fall within the solid lines. The broken lines represent mean excretion.

Precision — Coefficient of variation = 12%.

Factors affecting results — In vivo: ampicillin decreases levels during the luteal phase.[27]

e. The Biological Effects of Progesterone

Progesterone is the only important physiologically active progestogen. It interacts with estrogens in its effects on tissues. It exerts a strong secretory effect on the uterine endometrium which has been primed with estrogens. During the luteal phase of the menstrual cycle, progesterone, acting in conjunction with estrogen, brings about proliferation of mammary gland acini.

3. Androgens

Androstenedione is the major androgen secreted by the ovary. Androstenedione and testosterone levels are elevated in the ovulatory phase of the cycle due to augmented steroid production by the Graafian follicle, the stroma of the active ovary, and the corpus luteum.[33,34] A significant increase in levels of androstenedione has been demonstrated in the luteal phase.[35] The ovary also secretes small amounts of dehydroepiandrosterone,[36] but the quantity is masked by the large adrenal production of this steroid.

III. COMPOSITE PICTURE OF THE MENSTRUAL CYCLE

The phase of initial growth of the follicle during the follicular part of the cycle begins in the late luteal phase of the preceding cycle and ends when there is a significant increase in estrogen output, usually about 6 to 7 days before the LH surge. The chief hormonal change during this phase is the rise in level of FSH, caused by the decrease in estrogen output from the corpus luteum. An increase of smaller magnitude is noted in LH output during this phase.

During the latter half of the follicular phase, estrogen output increases, at first slowly and then more rapidly to reach a peak just before ovulation. As the levels of estrogen increase, levels of FSH fall. Output of LH increases slowly but steadily during this phase. A few days before ovulation there is an elevation of 17α-hydroxyprogesterone and androstenedione. Estrogen levels reach a peak prior to ovulation and, by positive feedback, induce release of LH within 48 hours. This rapid surge in LH output is accompanied by a smaller increase in FSH secretion. The high levels of LH persist for about 24 hours. Immediately before the follicle ruptures, estrogen levels fall and progesterone output increases slowly. Ovulation occurs approximately 24 hours after the LH peak.

Luteinization is initiated by LH, but follicular rupture and expulsion of the ovum also play a part in the process. The luteal phase of the cycle is marked by an increase in the circulating levels of progesterone, estrogens, and 17α-hydroxyprogesterone. Levels of LH and FSH are lower than during the follicular phase and are at their lowest levels at the time of maximum progesterone secretion. Unless pregnancy intervenes, the levels of estrogen and progesterone start to drop 7 to 8 days after ovulation. The drop in estrogen output results in an increase in FSH secretion and a new cycle is initiated. Coincident with the declining function of the corpus luteum and decreasing concentrations of estrogen and progesterone, necrotic changes occur in the uterine mucosa and menstrual bleeding occurs. A composite diagram of urinary steroid excretion during the cycle is shown in Figure 5.

A. Genital Tract Changes

The various changes noted in the genital tract during the menstrual cycle are related to the hormonal state. The cyclic changes in the cervical mucus either block or enhance sperm transport in the cervix. For this reason study of the cervical mucus is often undertaken during infertility studies. In addition to the changes in the cervical mucus, the cervix also undergoes anatomical changes during the cycle.[37] The secretion of mucus from the racemose glands of the endocervical canal is stimulated by estrogens and inhibited by progesterone.[38] Just after menstruation, the mucus is scanty. It progressively increases in quantity to become maximum at the time of ovulation. At ovulation the mucus is copious and clear, having its maximum elasticity (spinnbarkeit) and minimum viscosity. The extent of crystallization in mucus is reflected in the degree of ferning. Ferning is maximum at ovulation and disappears by day 22 of a regular 28-day cycle.

B. Criteria of Ovulation

The only absolute evidence of ovulation is the isolation of an ovum or an ensuing pregnancy. In view of this, the occurrence of ovulation must be inferred from associated changes.

1. Specific changes in hormonal output during the menstrual cycle. The following criteria are used to define a normal ovulatory cycle: (a) midcycle peak of LH; (b) midcycle peak of estrogen; (c) plasma progesterone levels above 16 nmol/ℓ or urine pregnanediol levels above 7.6 μmol/24 hr, 5 to 8 days after the LH peak.
2. Changes in the cervical mucus. At the time of ovulation the cervical mucus is copious, clear, and watery. Crystallization of a dried smear is at its maximum, producing a fern-leaf pattern. The maximum secretion precedes the rise in basal body temperature by 1 to 3 days.
3. Basal body temperature chart. The basal body temperature chart should show a biphasic pattern.
4. The luteal phase. A short luteal phase is defined as an interval of less than 10 days from the LH peak to the onset of menses.

IV. ABNORMALITIES IN THE MENSTRUAL CYCLE

In a cyclical system interruption of any one link in the chain of events will lead to some degree of disruption in the cycle. The menstrual cycle may be influenced by external influences such as psychological states, nutrition, stress, acute and chronic illnesses, and drug therapy.

A. Regular Cycles

1. Anovulation

An occasional anovulatory cycle is not uncommon in any normal female in the child-bearing years. Persistent anovulatory cycles may occur in regularly menstruating women and result in infertility. The condition may be diagnosed by a monophasic temperature chart, failure of midcycle peaking of LH, and failure of the rise in plasma progesterone or urinary pregnanediol in the luteal phase of the cycle. Endometrial biopsy in the luteal phase shows a persistence of proliferative phase appearances.

2. Inadequate Luteal Phase

Luteal phase deficiency is usually characterized by short cycles and may be responsible for infertility and early spontaneous abortions. It is more frequently seen immediately after the menarche and in the premenopausal years. The pathophysiology of the condition is uncertain but it may be diagnosed by measuring the luteal phase plasma progesterone.[39,40] the luteal phase urinary pregnanediol, by determination of the duration of the luteal phase,[41] and by histological dating of the endometrial biopsy.[42,43] Various reasons have been postulated for the inadequacy of the luteal phase, these include lowered secretion of FSH[41] and elevated secretion of prolactin.[44]

3. Luteinization of Unruptured Follicles

The possibility of luteinization with failure or delay of release of the ovum has been suspected for several years. In some infertile patients in whom there is normal endocrinological presumptive evidence for ovulation, for example a biphasic BBT, secretory endometrium, and elevated levels of progesterone or urinary pregnanediol, laparoscopy will indicate the absence of a corpus hemorrhagicum. In such cases of luteinization of unruptured follicles, laparoscopy is indicated for the diagnosis to be made.[45] A delay in the onset of luteinization, suggested by a delay in the rise of plasma progesterone levels and delay in the increase in BBT after the LH peak, has also been suggested as a cause of infertility in women with apparently normal function.[46]

4. Defective Follicular Phase

The defective follicular phase may be short, normal, or prolonged in duration. It is usually associated with a low estrogen production due to poor development of the follicles.[47] Long follicular phase cycles may, however, be normal in respect to hormonal production, and ovulation may occur. As women get older their menstrual cycles change and often the follicular phase becomes shorter with reduced secretion of estrogens in the follicular and luteal phases of the cycle but with normal progesterone levels.[48]

B. Oligomenorrhea

Oligomenorrhea may be defined as irregular menstruation occurring at 2 to 6 monthly intervals. In some cases ovulation may occur, the only abnormality being a prolonged follicular phase. Although it is unusual for a pathological or pharmacological cause to be identified in the hypothalamus or in the pituitary, there is often an upset in the hypothalamic-pituitary-ovarian axis.

1. Irregular Heavy Cycles

Irregular heavy bleeding may arise in disorders of the hypothalamic-pituitary-ovarian axis. In juvenile metropathia, there is a deficient production of LH relative to FSH[49] and an ovarian follicle is produced which does not rupture and which continues to produce estrogens. This leads to cystic glandular hyperplasia of the endometrium. In young girls the condition usually progresses to normal cycles without treatment. In menopausal women, a similar condition, metropathia hemorrhagica progresses slowly to secondary amenorrhea of the menopause.

2. Polycystic Ovarian Disease

Polycystic ovarian disease or Stein-Leventhal syndrome is characterized by obesity, hirsutism, chronic anovulation with oligomenorrhea or amenorrhea, and enlarged polycystic ovaries. The syndrome includes a variety of cases which manifest one or more of the preceding characteristics.

Certain abnormalities in the hypothalamic-pituitary-ovarian axis are found. Elevated levels of LH with a relatively constant and low FSH release have been demonstrated.[50] It is not known whether this pattern of gonadotropin release is due to an abnormality in the hypothalamus-pituitary system or whether it is caused by abnormal steroidogenesis in the polycystic ovary. High circulating levels of testosterone and androstenedione have been noted.[51] Dehydroepiandrosterone and dehydroepiandrosterone sulfate are present in high concentrations.[52] Estrone concentrations in peripheral plasma are elevated but estradiol levels are not elevated.[52,53] This suggests that there may be significant extraglandular production of estrogen — probably the majority of estrogen formed is derived from androstenedione.

Ovulation may be induced by clomiphene citrate, which increases the circulating levels of estradiol and FSH. Wedge resection of the ovaries may be performed and this procedure reduces ovarian secretion of androstenedione and therefore the amount of circulating estrone, enabling suppression of FSH to be lifted.

C. Amenorrhea

Physiological amenorrhea occurs in women in the reproductive age group during pregnancy and lactation when levels of FSH and LH are low. Amenorrhea is present after the menopause.

1. Primary Amenorrhea

At present the average age of the menarche in the U.K. is 13 years, with a standard deviation of about 1 year.[54] Therefore, 95% of the female population have their first menses between their 11th and 15th years. There are wide variations in the age at which the menarche occurs in different populations and in different social groups. In some parts of the world, the age at menarche has been noted to have become about 3 to 4 months earlier each decade during the past century. This trend may be stopping in certain countries.[55]

If menstruation has not occurred by the age of 18 years, this is usually taken as a manifestation of primary amenorrhea and investigations should be undertaken.

a. Patients with Normal Secondary Sexual Characteristics

Developmental abnormalities — Developmental anatomical abnormalities are found in this group of patients. These include congenital absence of the uterus and vagina, and imperforate vaginal hymen. In these patients, levels of FSH, LH estrogens, and pregnanediol are normal. Surgical measures to correct anatomical abnormalities may be indicated in this group.

Testicular feminization — Patients with this condition have normal breast development and absent secondary sexual hair The vagina is short and blind and the vulva is infantile. The uterus is absent. Karyotype testing reveals normal male 46, XY chromosomes. Testes will be found in the labial, inguinal, or abdominal position. The condition may be due to androgen insensitivity of the target organs, but as serum LH levels are elevated and plasma androgen levels are at normal or higher than normal male levels, it appears that there may be a partial insensitivity of the hypothalamic centers as well.

b. Patients with Sexual Infantilism

Turner's syndrome — Patients with this syndrome are of short stature with barrel-shaped chests, cubitus valgus, neck webbing, poor breast development, and scanty pubic hair. The external genitalia are normal but the gonads are streaks. Individuals with this condition most commonly have one X chromosome, 45, X, or chromosome type 45, X/46, XX. Levels of FSH and LH are elevated, and levels of estrogens and pregnanediol are low, reflecting the ovarian failure.

Gonadotropic hypopituitarism — Lack of or reduced secretion of gonadotropins from the pituitary gland will result in eunuchoidism. Measurements of LH, FSH, estrogen, and pregnanediol will reveal low levels. Simple delayed puberty and isolated gonadotropic deficiency are identical in the early stages. After the age of 19 years the patient should be treated as if there is a permanent defect of gonadotropic hormones. Skull X-ray and full pituitary function tests should be performed on these patients to exclude more general pituitary pathology.

Polycystic ovarian disease — Occasionally primary amenorrhea may be a feature of the polycystic ovarian syndrome. The syndrome has been discussed previously. In these patients, however, hirsutism and obesity are rare.

2. Secondary Amenorrhea

A variety of diseases have been implicated in the causation of secondary amenorrhea.[56] These include diseases of the hypothalamus and pituitary gland, diseases of the ovaries, systemic diseases, and genetic abnormalities.

a. Patients with Hypogonadism

Hypogonadism may be suspected clinically and confirmed by the measurement of estrogens and progesterone or pregnanediol, all of which will be low. In the case of ovarian lesions, gonadotropin levels are persistently abnormally increased and FSH levels are greater than the highest value seen during the normal menstrual cycle. This picture is seen in the premature menopause and following castration. In hypothalamic pituitary disorders, gonadotropin levels are low. Stimulation with clomiphene citrate produces a negative result.

Intrasellar tumors — A nonfunctioning intrasellar tumor, such as a chromophobe adenoma or a craniopharyngioma within the fossa, will be detected by X-ray examination of the sella turcica. Dynamic tests of pituitary function will yield negative responses.

Sheehan's syndrome — The diagnosis is made from the past history, the clinical features of anterior pituitary insufficiency and panhypopituitarism. In this condition, ischemic necrosis of the pituitary gland occurs, usually after parturition.

Frolich's syndrome — In this condition there is pituitary hypofunction associated with secondary hypogonadism and obesity.

Anorexia nervosa — This disease is typical of girls and young women. It is characterized by an active refusal of food which leads to a significant loss of body weight. As the whole clinical picture is reversible, a functional disorder of the hypothalamic-pituitary-ovarian axis has been postulated. The onset of amenorrhea may be preceded or followed by the weight loss. Levels of pituitary gonadotropin and estrogens are low. Clomiphene citrate gives a negative response in the stationary phase of the disease but gives a positive response after the psychological condition improves and weight gain has occurred.[57] Plasma prolactin levels are normal in these patients.[58]

b. Patients without Gonadal Deficiency

Baseline gonadotropin levels, the degree of variation of LH, and the response to clomiphene and LHRH will distinguish 2 groups of patients.[59] In the first group there are normal levels of FSH and normal or slightly elevated levels of LH without any cyclical pattern. Clomiphene and LHRH cause an increase in the levels of LH and FSH, and it is believed that the defect is a disturbance of the hypothalamic regulation of gonadotropin secretion. The second group of patients are characterized by low and stable levels of LH and a lack of response to clomiphene and an abnormal response to LHRH.

Iatrogenic causes — There are two groups of drugs which cause hypothalamic suppression and secondary amenorrhea. The phenothiazines act by depleting dopaminergic neurons[60] leading to a reduction in the production of releasing hormones and therefore pituitary gonadotropic hormones. The combined oral contraceptive pill causes inhibition of releasing hormone from the hypothalamus. In a small number of women, hypothalamic suppression continues for a long time after stopping the combined pill.[61] In this post-pill amenorrhea there appears to be a defect in the normal mechanisms involved in the feedback of ovarian steroids.

Psychological causes — Psychological stress due to bereavement, imprisonment, change of environment such as leaving home and starting college, and psychoses may result in disturbances of hypothalamic function. The stress may be acute or chronic.

Weight changes — Amenorrhea may be concomitant with either a gain in weight or a loss in weight.

c. Patients with Hyperprolactinemia

The incidence of secondary amenorrhea with hyperprolactinemia ranges from 13 to 30%.[62-64] Although amenorrhea is the most common menstrual abnormality found, irregular cycles, menorrhagia, or anovular, or defective luteal phase[65] or regular cycles may occur.

Galactorrhea is noted in 30% of hyperprolactinemic patients. The mechanism by which hyperprolactinemia may lead to hypogonadism is not known. It is postulated that prolactin acts on the gonad to partially block the action of the gonadotropins, so that there is a reduction in gonadal steroid production. Levels of steroids are at the lower end of the normal range and levels of pituitary FSH and LH are also low normal or low.

Hyperprolactinemia may occur as a result of drug therapy with dopamine receptor blocking drugs (e.g., phenothiazines), dopamine depleting drugs (e.g., reserpine), and with estrogens. Pituitary tumors are sometimes associated with hyperprolactinemia and if the basal prolactin level is considerably elevated then it is considered likely that the patient has a microadenoma of the pituitary gland.[66]

Patients with polycystic ovarian disease may demonstrate elevated output of prolactin. Raised circulating adrenal androgens have been noted in hyperprolactinemic patients.[67] Some patients with post-pill amenorrhea have elevated prolactin levels.[68]

d. Patients with Hirsutism

Hypersecretion of androgenic hormones has been demonstrated in hirsute patients suffering from a variety of conditions, which include virilizing tumors,[69] the polycystic ovary syndrome,[70] congenital adrenal hyperplasia, and ovarian stromal hyperthecosis.

Virilization ranges from a slight increase in coarse body hair, facial hair, and menstrual abnormality to the more severe manifestations including clitoromegaly, temporal balding, and deepening of the voice. Testosterone production rates increase in parallel with the severity of the virilization.[71] Plasma testosterone levels are elevated and the output of 17-oxosteroids is increased. The androgens which are present in the peripheral blood are C_{19} steroids which are either biologically active themselves or which function as prehormones or precursors of active hormones. Androstenedione is the chief prehormone which contributes 60% of the blood production rate of testosterone.[72] Androstenedione and testosterone levels in the blood of hirsuite women who have a menstrual abnormality show rapid and well-defined changes in levels which are unrelated to plasma cortisol or gonadotropin levels.[73]

Test to determine the site of excessive androgen production

It is essential to determine the site of hyperandrogenicity, which may be the adrenal gland or the ovary. For 2 days before, during, and for 2 days after the test procedure 24-hr collections of urine for estimation of 17-oxogenic steroids and free cortisol are made. After the 2 control days, the patient is given dexamethasone 8 mg/day for 6 days. On days 5 and 6, HCG 5000 IU is injected.

An ovarian origin for androgen overproduction may be recognized if HCG causes an increase in 17-oxosteroids greater than 40% as compared with the values found during dexamethasone suppression.[74] Administration of estrogens, stilbestrol 5 mg/day for 5 days, will decrease the androgenic steroids in these cases. This type of response is seen in polycystic ovarian disease and in ovarian hyperthecosis,[75,76] in which there is a morphological alteration of the ovarian stromal cells so that they resemble luteinized thecal cells.

The origin is adrenal when the 17-oxosteroid production is lowered by dexamethasone but shows no modification after injection of HCG. This response is seen in Cushing's syndrome due to bilateral adrenal hyperplasia in which hirsuitism is frequent. It is also observed in congenital adrenal hyperplasia in which urinary pregnanetriol and 17-oxosteroids are always increased. In 11-hydroxylase deficiency the 17-oxogenic steroids are also increased.

The origin may be neoplastic when the androgen levels cannot be suppressed by dexamethasone or by gonadal steroids.

The dynamic endocrine tests may not give conclusive results in all cases. Percutaneous venous catheterization studies of the adrenal and ovarian veins may be indicated in some instances in order to determine the exact site of excessive androgen production.[52] Laparoscopy and histological examination of an ovarian biopsy may also form part of the diagnostic procedures to verify that nature of the lesion.

Basal hormonal levels found in disorders of the hypothalamic-pituitary-ovarian axis are shown in Table 1.

A flow diagram which may be used in the investigation of amenorrhea or oligomenorrhea is shown in Figure 6. Note that FSH, LH, and estrogen may be estimated concurrently and that prolactin and thyroid function tests may be assayed from the same blood sample.

e. Patients with Other Endocrine Disorders

Amenorrhea may occasionally result from hyperthyroidism but it is more likely to occur in myxedematous patients, when it may be accompanied by galactorrhea. Thyroid function tests should be performed in amenorrheic patients even when overt signs of thyroid disease are not present.

Oligomenorrhea or amenorrhea may be found in diabetes mellitus. When there are obvious signs of the disease or when there is a positive family history of diabetes, a glucose tolerance test should be performed.

V. THE CLIMACTERIC

The climacteric is the transitional period between the cessation of normal reproductive capacity and old age. The physiological changes which occur during this period are a result of waning ovarian function with a resultant decrease in ovarian hormone production. The climacteric may be divided into three sections, the premenopause, the menopause, and the postmenopause. The premenopause begins with the onset of declining ovarian function and is associated with alterations in cycle length[48] and also with the quality of menstrual loss which may become more scant. During this time, as the ovaries are failing, there is an increased frequency of anovulatory cycles and so one of the first steroid hormones to be lost is progesterone. The menopause is the chief

Table 1
BASAL HORMONAL LEVELS IN DISORDERS OF THE HYPOTHALAMIC-PITUITARY-OVARIAN AXIS

	Hormone levels				
Diagnosis	**LH**	**FSH**	**Prolactin**	**Androgens**	**Estrogens**
Gonadal defects					
Ovarian failure	E	E	N	N	D
Menopause	E	E	N	N	D
Polycystic ovaries	E	N	N or E	E	N
Hypothalamic and pituitary defects					
Sheehan's syndrome	D	D	N	—	D
Anorexia nervosa	D	D	N	N	D
Pituitary tumor	D or N	D or N	D or N or E	N	D
Hyperprolactinemia	D or N	D or N	E	N	D

Note: Normal, N; decreased, D; elevated, E.

manifestation of the climacteric and is the date on which the final menstrual loss occurs. Any time after the menopause is referred to as the postmenopausal period of life.

The age of the menopause is becoming progressively later — at present it is 51 years in Caucasian women. A premature menopause may occur in women because of autoimmune reactions[77] or because of chromosomal abnormalities.[78] A premature menopause could be described as one which occurs before the age of 40 years. It has been estimated that 8% of women experience an early menopause and 7% of women do not have their last menstrual loss until after the age of 55 years.

The factors controlling the normal menopause are not fully understood but ovarian function slowly and finally ceases. In the premenopausal years, there is a gradual loss of primordial follicles and oocytes but even after the menopause, immature follicles undergoing maturation and atresia have been found.[79] A progressive thinning of the ovarian cortex occurs which is often accompanied by hyperplasia of the cortical stroma. Incubation studies have demonstrated that androgenic steroid hormones, mainly dehydroepiandrosterone, androstenedione, and testosterone, can be synthesized from the ovarian stroma.[80] Very little aromatization of androgens to estrogens occurs in this tissue.

The peripheral levels of most steroid hormones are lower in postmenopausal women than in premenopausal women. The postmenopausal ovary secretes very small amounts of estradiol. This is supported by the fact that estradiol production rates are not significantly reduced after the removal of postmenopausal ovaries.[81] In aged postmenopausal women, plasma estradiol levels are decreased by 90% and plasma estrone levels are decreased by 70%.[82] In premenopausal women, both the ovary and the adrenal contribute to the peripheral levels of estrone. In postmenopausal women, the ovarian contribution to peripheral estrone is decreased. Although some estrone is secreted directly by the adrenal in postmenopausal women, the major part is formed from the peripheral conversion of androstenedione.[83] The aromatization of androstenedione occurs in peripheral tissues, particularly in adipose tissue, and has been demonstrated in both human breast and abdominal fat.[84] The conversion of plasma androgens to estrogens is increased in obese patients and in those with liver disease.[85] The major portion of androstenedione in postmenopausal women is of adrenal gland ori-

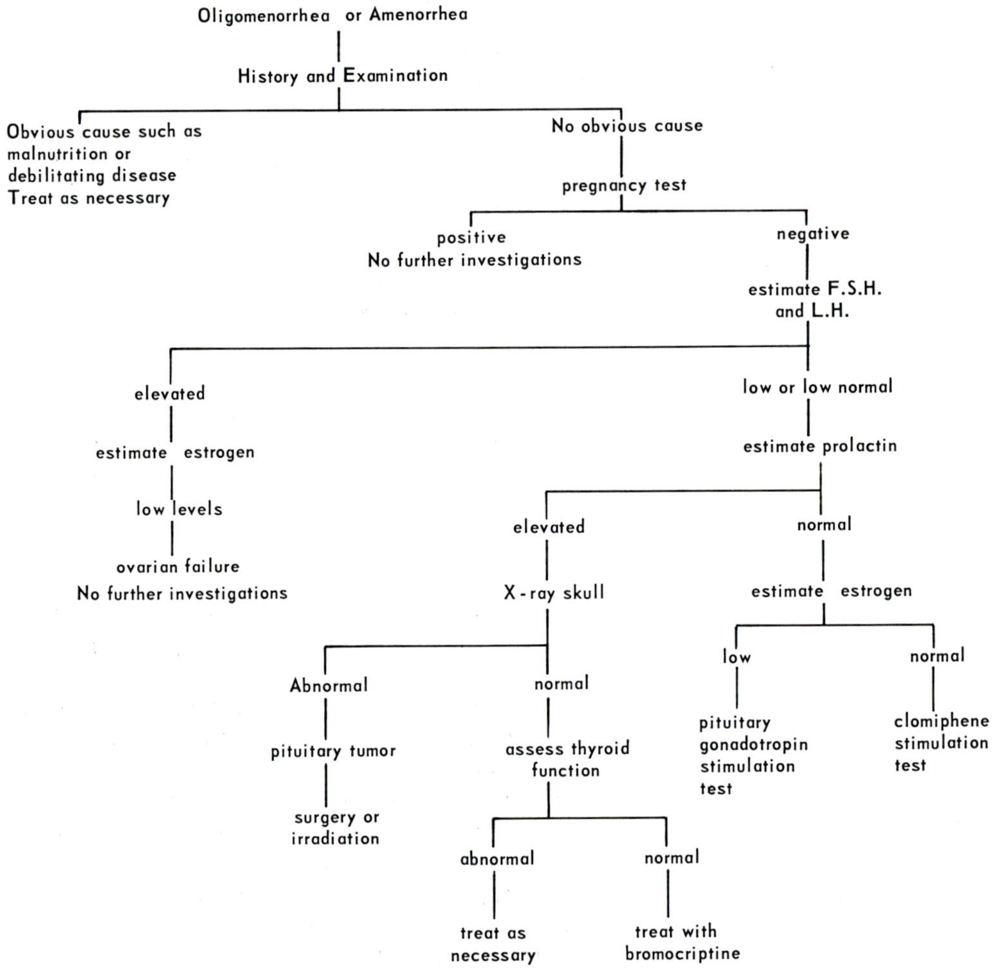

FIGURE 6. Investigation of oligomenorrhea and amenorrhea.

gin[86] and although the postmenopausal ovary secretes testosterone, androstenedione, and to a lesser extent dehydroepiandrosterone, the main source of these steroids is the adrenal cortex. In postmenopausal women 17-hydroxyprogesterone and progesterone have an almost exclusive adrenal origin.[87]

In the premenopausal years, as ovarian function is waning, there is often a shorter cycle length. During this time a significant reduction in plasma estradiol levels in the follicular and luteal phases of the cycle have been demonstrated, despite the presence of normal LH and progesterone concentrations.[48] In another study of premenopausal women who had regular ovulatory cycles, elevated FSH secretion with normal LH output and reduced plasma estradiol concentrations was demonstrated.[88] These findings may suggest that even in premenopausal women elevated gonadotropin concentrations may be secondary to reduced estrogen output. During this period sporadic ovulatory cycles may occur after a series of anovulatory cycles associated with elevated FSH and LH concentrations.[89] Eventually, the greatly diminished estrogen secretion reduces the negative feedback inhibition on the pituitary gland, and this fact combined with an increase in hypothalamic secretion of luteinizing hormone releasing factor[90] leads to the increase in production of FSH and LH.

The main changes in hormonal levels which occur after the menopause are demonstrated in Table 2. The diagnosis of the postmenopausal state should present no difficulty in that very low estrogen levels will be found combined with elevated levels of pituitary gonadotropins. The diagnosis of the premenstrual patient presents many problems. Elevated levels of LH and FSH may be found, either alone or combined, in some cycles. Low estrogen output may be demonstrated throughout the cycle although other hormone levels are normal. After many abnormal cycles a completely normal ovulatory cycle may occur. Eventually the typical elevation in FSH and LH will be noted, accompanied by reduced estrogen and pregnanediol excretion.

The metabolic changes associated with the climacteric are a consequence of failing ovarian function and diminished estrogen secretion. The feminine secondary sex characteristics are gradually lost. The effect of estrogen lack on the genital tract is marked, secretions become scant and are finally absent, and atrophic changes occur in the vagina and vulva. During the climacteric years, the "hot flush" may occur. The cause of "hot flushes" has been attributed to estrogen lack and to elevation of pituitary gonadotropins; instability of the vasomotor centers of the hypothalamus may be the root cause. Many postmenopausal women suffer from some degree of osteoporosis and a link has been demonstrated between estrogen deficiency and calcium deficiency in the etiology of this condition.

VI. OVARIAN TUMORS

Ovarian tumors are often symptomless until they reach a large size. Ovarian cancer is third in frequency in female genital cancer and carries the lowest survival rate of all gynecological malignancies. In a large proportion of cases the tumor is disseminated by the time of diagnosis. The mortality rate appears to be increasing each year at a level of 15% each decade.[91] The majority of ovarian tumors are benign (74%).[92] Ovarian tumors show a multiplicity of tumor types and the World Health Organization[93] together with the International Federation of Gynaecologists and Obstetricians[94] has produced a standardized form of classification which may allow a better comparison of data. Endocrine and metabolic changes may occur in patients with ovarian tumors but are often misleading and may not be of help in diagnosis. The tumors may be primary or secondary. Secondary deposits of malignant tumors are very common in the ovary, but those presenting primarily as ovarian tumors are much less common.

A. Epithelial Tumors

Epithelial tumors include mucinous tumors (benign and malignant), serous tumors (benign and malignant), endometroid tumors including clear cell carcinoma, mixed mesodermal tumors and carcinosarcoma, tumors of mesonephric origin, and the Brenner tumor. The most common tumors are the mucinous cystadenoma which accounts for 20% of all ovarian tumors and the serous cystadenoma which makes up for 25% of all the tumors and for 60% of all malignant ovarian tumors. Endometroid tumors may arise in the ovary in the absence of endometriosis. Estimates for the incidence of this tumor vary widely. The mesonephroma is a rather rare tumor found in women over the age of 30 years. Clinically there are no characteristic presenting symptoms or signs. The Brenner tumor accounts for less than 2% of all ovarian tumors.

Endocrine effects may occur in the presence of these epithelial tumors which are not classically considered to be functional. Of patients with mucinous cystadenomata or cystadenocarcinoma, 50% complained of irregular menstrual bleeding and postmenopausal bleeding was also noted.[95] Irregular bleeding has been noted frequently in patients with Brenner tumor[96] and endometrial hyperplasia has been recorded in just under half the cases studied.[97]

Table 2
EXCRETION OF HORMONES IN THE POSTMENOPAUSAL PERIOD COMPARED WITH EXCRETION DURING THE MENSTRUAL CYCLE

		Levels during menstrual cycle	
Hormone	Postmenopausal	Follicular phase	Maximum
FSH (IU/24 hours)	78—258	5—36	10—70
LH (IU/24 hours)	86—198	5—60	34—160
Total estrogens (nmol/24 hours)	8—56	20—195	80—300
Pregnanediol (μ mol/24 hours)	0.4—2.8	1—4.5	6—23

Hormone synthesis has been ascribed to ovarian stromal reaction resulting from the stimulus provided by the invasive epithelial tissue. The localized stromal reaction results in the formation of theca-lutein cells or of luteinized stromal cells. In cases associated with virilism the interstitial cells are normally described as luteinized thecal cells, and those presenting with hyperestrogenic symptoms and signs have cells resembling ovarian stroma. The stimulated cells may synthesize and secrete estrogen or they may secrete androstenedione which is converted peripherally to estrogen.

An elevated output of urinary estrogens has been reported in some patients with epithelial tumors.[98,99] The correlation of urinary estrogen excretion with vaginal bleeding was poor.[98]

B. Sex Cord Stromal Tumors

The sex cord stromal tumors include the granulosa cell tumor, the thecoma, and the Sertoli-Leydig cell tumors, which are generally referred to as arrhenoblastomas. It is often impossible to differentiate between the granulosa cell carcinoma and the thecoma as these tumors appear to be of mixed type.

1. Granulosa Cell Tumor

This is the commonest of the sex cord ovarian tumors, accounting for 3% of all primary ovarian tumors and 9% of all primary ovarian carcinomas.[100] The tumors may appear at any age. Many of the tumors give rise to symptoms of a pelvic neoplasm: some symptoms are related to hormonal upset. Of the tumors, 5 to 10% occur before puberty[101] and give rise to sexual precocity.[102] During the reproductive years the most common complaint is of irregular and excessive bleeding.[101] Some patients, however, give a history of amenorrhea. In the postmenopausal years uterine bleeding is the most common symptom.

Increased urinary estrogen excretion has been found in these patients with granulosa-theca cell tumors.[103,104] Greatly elevated levels of estradiol-17β have also been reported.[105] Although the tumors are commonly thought of as producing signs and symptoms of estrogen excess, virilism may also occur.[106]

2. Thecoma

The thecoma accounts for just under 2% of all ovarian tumors and for about 4% of all solid ovarian tumors.[107] It occurs most commonly in postmenopausal women and presents as postmenopausal bleeding. Increased output of estrogens in the urine has been reported.[108] and estrogen has been found in the tumor itself.[109]

3. Sertoli-Leydig Cell Tumor

This is an uncommon tumor accounting for less than 1% of all ovarian tumors. It may be seen in patients of any age but is seen most commonly in the reproductive years. The tumors are composed of the testicular elements, the Leydig and Sertoli cells in different stages of maturity. Certain of the arrhenoblastomas produce no recognizable hormonal effects although in the main they are virilizing tumors. The first symptoms may be a slow process of defeminization accompanied by progressive oligomenorrhea with scanty menstrual loss leading to amenorrhea. In 12% of cases there was no menstrual abnormality.[110] Hirsuitism is common, occurring in 79% of patients, and virilism has been seen in about 50% of cases.

High plasma testosterone and androstenedione levels have been reported which decrease postoperatively.[111,112] Excretion of 17-oxosteroid is unreliable as a reflection of the plasma androgen concentration and normal output has been reported.[110,113]

4. Hilus Cell Tumor

The hilus of the ovary contains nests of cells which are identical to the Leydig cells of the testis. Hyperplasia or neoplasia of such cells to form a tumor is associated with virilism.[114] Most of the reported cases have been in postmenopausal women although they may occur in the reproductive years. In most instances the main complaint was hirsutism. Amenorrhea may occur in younger patients. A few patients have had signs of hyperestrogenism.[115,116]

The tumor may synthesize and secrete excessive amounts of testosterone and it has been shown that the tumor has the necessary enzymic capacity for androgen biosynthesis.[117] Very high urinary testosterone sulfate concentrations have been reported in a patient with a metastatic hilus cell tumor.[118] Elevated urinary estrogen excretion has been seen in a patient with hilus cell hyperplasia.[119]

C. Lipoid Cell Tumors

"Lipoid cell tumors" is a general term used to describe tumors containing cells with a large amount of lipid in their cytoplasm and which are commonly associated with androgenic features. Numerous names have been given to this tumor such as luteoma, masculinovoblastoma, and adrenal rest tumor. The most likely origin of the lipoid cell tumor is from the ovarian stromal cells within the medulla.[120] The cells of this tumor resemble those of the zona fasciculata of the adrenal cortex. Patients with these tumors may demonstrate features of Cushing's syndrome.[121]

Elevated excretion rates of 17-oxosteroids have been reported[122] and a high output of corticosteroids has also been noted.[123] These particular biochemical features help to differentiate the lipoid cell tumors from the Sertoli-Leydig cell tumors and the hilus cell tumors. Associated biochemical findings include hypercalcemia and hyperphosphatemia, and latent or frank diabetes mellitus has been demonstrated in 45% of patients.

D. Germ Cell Tumors

These tumors, although rare, contribute significantly to the ovarian cancer mortality rate in the young.[124] Germ cells themselves may become neoplastic or they may differentiate to form tissues which are neoplastic. Many germ cell tumors are of mixed variety, containing two or more lines of neoplastic cells.

1. Dysgerminoma

This tumor may occur at any age but is seen most commonly in the second and third decades.[125] The usual mode of presentation is as a pelvic tumor but occasionally menstrual upset may be noted. The tumor itself has no particular hormonal changes ascribed to it, but is associated with other tumors, e.g., granulosa cell carcinoma,[126] choriocarinoma,[127] which may be hormone producing.

2. Cystic Teratoma

The cystic teratoma accounts for 10% of all neoplasms of the ovary.[128] There are no specific features associated with tumor. If the dermoid contains teratomatous tissue such as chorionic cells menstrual abnormalities may be noted, and HCG may be found in the blood and urine.

3. Malignant Teratoma

This is a very rare tumor which occurs in people under the age of 25 years. Deposits of chorionic tissue may be found and HCG is secreted.

4. Choriocarcinoma

This is an extremely rare ovarian tumor but it may be found as part of another germ cell tumor. Irregular menstruation may occur but more often it presents as an acute abdominal crisis. Large quantities of HCG are present in the urine.

5. Gonadoblastoma

This tumor is associated with gonadal dysgenesis and occurs in patients under 30 years of age. The commonest presentation is primary amenorrhea but occasionally oligomenorrhea or secondary amenorrhea may occur. Children may have a precocious puberty. Adult patients are phenotypic females with poorly developed breasts and often absent secondary sexual hair. The genital organs are usually immature. Of patients 89% were shown to be chromatin negative[129] and the Y chromosome was present in 96% of cases.[130]

The majority of adult patients demonstrate elevated gonadotropin output.

6. Struma Ovarii

This is a rare tumor constituting less than 1% of ovarian tumors. Pieces of thyroid tissue may be found in association with teratomata, serous cysts, and mucinous cysts. It may occur at any age. Most of these tumors are nonfunctioning but thyrotoxicosis has been reported,[131] the toxic symptoms being relieved on removal of the tumor.

7. Carcinoid Tumors

Most of the reported examples of this tumor have been associated with a teratoma. They occur in postmenopausal women. Production of serotonin has been sufficient to result in the clinical manifestations of the carcinoid syndrome.

REFERENCES

1. **Guraya, S. S.,** Interstitial gland tissue of mammalian ovary, *Acta Endocrinol. (Copenhagen),* 72 (Suppl. 171), 5, 1973.
2. **Sternberg, W. H., Segoloff, A., and Gaskill, C. J.,** Influence of chorionic gonadotrophin on human ovarian hilus cells (Leydig-like cells), *J. Clin. Endocrinol. Metab.*, 13, 139, 1953.

3. **McNatty, K. P., Hunter, W. M., McNeilly, A. S., and Sawers, R. S.,** Changes in the concentrations of pituitary and steroid hormones in the follicular fluid of human Graafian follicles throughout the menstrual cycle, *J. Endocrinol.,* 64, 555, 1975.
4. **Treloar, A. E., Boynton, R. E., Behn, B. G., and Broen, B.W.,** Variation in the human menstrual cycle throughout reproductive life, *Int. J. Fertil.,* 12, 77, 1967.
5. **McNatty, K. P. and Sawers, R. S.,** Relationship between the endocrine environment within the Graafian follicle and the subsequent rate of progesterone secretion by human granulosa cells in vitro, *J. Endocrinol.,* 66, 391, 1975.
6. **Pennington, G. W., Beazley, J. M., and Wilson, E. W.,** Ovulation — its detection and evaluation using multiple criteria in the infertile woman, *J. Obstet. Gynaecol. Brit. Commonw.,* 77, 627, 1970.
7. **Lloyd, C. W., Lobotsky, J., Baird, D. T., McCracken, J. A., Weisz, J., Pupkin, M., Zanartu, J., and Puga, J.,** Concentration of unconjugated estrogens and androgens and gestragens in ovarian and peripheral venous plasma of women: the normal menstrual cycle, *J. Clin. Endocrinol. Metab.,* 32, 155, 1971.
8. **Hawkins, R. A. and Oakey, R. E.,** Estimation of oestrone sulphate, oestradiol 17 β and oestrone in peripheral plasma: concentrations during the menstrual cycle and in man, *J. Endocrinol.,* 60, 3, 1974.
9. **Loriaux, D. L., Ruder, H. J., and Lipsett, M. B.,** The measurement of estrone sulfate in plasma, *Steroids,* 18, 463, 1971,
10. **Hammond, G., Viinikka, L., and Vihko, R.,** Automation of radioimmunoassay for some sex steroids with use of both iodinated and tritiated ligands, *Clin. Chem.,* 23, 1250, 1977.
11. **Healy, M. J. R.,** Statistical analysis of radioimmunoassay data, *Biochem. J.,* 130, 207, 1972.
12. **Anderson, D. C.,** Sex hormone binding globulin, *Clin. Endocrinol.,* 3, 69, 1974.
13. **Galvao-Teles, A., Anderson, D.C., Burke, C. W., Marshall, J. C., Corker, C. S., Bown, R. L., and Clark, M. L.,** *Lancet,* 1, 173, 1973.
14. **Anderson, D. C.,** The role of sex hormone binding globulin in health and disease, in *The Endocrine Function of the Human Ovary,* James, V. H. T., Serio, M., and Giusti, G., Eds., Academic Press, London, 1976.
15. **De Moor, P., Heyns, W., and Bouillon, R.,** Growth hormone and the steroid binding β globulin in human plasma, *J. Steroid Biochem.,* 3, 593, 1972.
16. **Gower, D. B.,** Metabolism of steroid hormones and bile acids, in *Comprehensive Biochemistry, Vol.* 20, Florkin, M. and Stotz, E. H., Eds., American Elsevier, N.Y., 1968, 63.
17. **Brown, J. B., MacCleod, S. C., MacNaughton, C., Smith, M. A., and Smyth, B.,** A rapid method for estimating oestrogens in urine using a semi-automatic extractor, *J. Endocrinol.,* 42, 5, 1968.
18. **Beastall, G. H. and McVeigh, S.,** A semi-automated method for the determination of oestrogens in early morning urine specimens from normal and infertile women, *Clin. Chim. Acta,* 70, 343, 1976.
19. **Bellon, E. M.,** Hemolytic anemia due to nalidixic acid, *Lancet,* 2, 691, 1965.
20. **Adlercreutz, H.,** Drug interference in urinary oestrogen determination, in *Proc. V Int. Symp. Quality Control Clinical Chem.,* Huber, Berne, Switzerland, 1973.
21. **Adlercreutz, H.,** Drug interference in urinary steroid hormone assay, 1st European Congress of Clin. Chem., Munich, 1974.
22. **Bolognese, R. J., Corson, S. L., and Touchstone, J. C.,** Factors affecting the yield of urinary estriol, *Obstet. Gynecol.,* 39, 683, 1972.
23. **Caraway, W. T. and Kammeyer, C.W.,** Chemical interference by drugs and other substances with clinical laboratory test procedures, *Clin. Chim. Acta,* 41, 395, 1972.
24. **Meyler, L. and Herxheimer, A.,** Eds., *Side Effects of Drugs,* Vol. 6, Excerpta Medica Foundation, Mouton, The Hague, 1968.
25. **Elking, M. P. and Kabat, H. F.,** Drug induced modifications of laboratory test values, *Am. J. Hosp. Pharm.,* 25, 485, 1968.
26. **Schwartz, M. K.,** Interferences in diagnostic biochemical procedures, *Adv. Clin. Chem.,* 16, 1, 1973.
27. **Trybuchowski, H.,** Effect of ampicillin on the urinary output of steroidal hormones in pregnant and non-pregnant women, *Clin. Chim. Acta,* 45, 9, 1973.
28. **Fowler, R. E., Chan, S. T. H., Walters, D. E., Edwards, R. G., and Steptoe, P. C.,** Steroidogenesis in human follicles approaching ovulation as judged from assays of follicular fluid, *J. Endocrinol.,* 72, 259, 1977.
29. Recommended procedure of the U.K. Supra Regional Assay Service.
30. **Collins, W. P., Koullapis, E. N., and Sommerville, I. F.,** The effect of chlormadinone acetate on progesterone secretion and metabolism, *Acta Endocrinol.,* 68, 271, 1971.
31. **Klopper, A., Mitchie, E. A., and Brown, J. B.,** A method for the determination of urinary pregnanediol, *J. Endocrinol.,* 12, 209, 1955.
32. **Podmore, D. A.,** Routine determination of urinary pregnanediol using a gas chromatograph with automatic sample application, *J. Clin. Path.,* 19, 619, 1966.

33. **Baird, D. T., Burger, P. E., Heavons-Jones, G. D., and Scaramuzzi, R. J.,** The site of secretion of androstenedione in non-pregnant women, *J. Endocrinol.*, 63, 201, 1974.
34. **de Yong, F. H., Baird, D. T., and van der Molen, H. J.,** Ovarian secretion rates of oestrogens, androgens and progesterone in normal women and in women with persistent ovarian follicles, *Acta Endocrinol. (Copenhagen)*, 77, 575, 1974.
35. **Guerrero, R., Aso, T., Brenner, P. F., Cekan, Z., Landgrew, B-M., Hagenfeldt, K., and Diczfalusy, E.,** Studies on the pattern of circulating steroids in the normal menstrual cycle, *Acta Endocrinol. (Copenhagen)*, 81, 133, 1976.
36. **Gandy, H. M.. and Peterson, R. E.,** Measurement of testosterone and 17 ketosteroids in plasma by the double isotope dilution derivative technique, *J. Clin. Endocrinol. Metab.*, 28, 949, 1968.
37. **Behrman S. J. and Kistner, R. W.,** Eds., *Progress in Infertility*, Little, Brown, Boston, 1968.
38. **Weiss, G.,** Effect of steroid hormones on cervical mucus, in *Adv. Ster. Biochem. Pharmacol.*, Briggs, M. H., Ed., 1, 137, 1970.
39. **Abraham, G. E., Maroulis, G. B., and Marshall, J. R.,** Evaluation of ovulation and corpus luteum function using measurements of plasma progesterone, *Obstet. Gynecol.*, 44, 522, 1974.
40. **Radwanska E. and Swyer, G. I. M.,** Plasma progesterone estimation in infertile women and in women under treatment with clomiphene and chorionic gonadotrophin, *J. Obstet. Gynaecol Br. Commonw.*, 81, 107, 1974.
41. **Strott, C. A., Cargille, C. M., Ross, G. T., and Lipsett, M. B.,** The short luteal phase, *J. Clin. Endocrinol. Metab.*, 30, 246, 1970.
42. **Jones, G. S.,** Luteal phase insufficiency, *Clin. Obstet. Gynecol.*, 16, 255, 1973.
43. **Reyniak, J. V.,** Luteal phase defects: recognition and management, *Bull. N.Y. Acad. Med.*, 49, 974, 1973.
44. **Seppala, M., Hirvonen, E., and Ranta, T.,** Hyperprolactinaemia and luteal insufficiency, *Lancet*, 1, 229, 1976.
45. **Marik, J. and Hulka, J.,** Luteinized unruptured follicle syndrome: a subtle cause of infertility, *Fertil. Steril.*, 29, 270, 1978.
46. **Koninckx, P. R., Heyns, W. J., Corvelyn, P. A., and Brosens, I. A.,** Delayed onset of luteinization as a cause of infertility, *Fertil. Steril.*, 29, 266, 1978.
47. **Lenton E. and Cooke, I. D.,** Other disorders of ovulation, in *Clinics in Obstetrics and Gynaecology* Vol. 1 (2), W. B. Saunders, Philadelphia, 1974, 313.
48. **Korenman, S. G. and Sherman, B. M.,** Hormonal regulation in normal and abnormal menstrual cycles, in *The Endocrine Function of the Human Ovary*, James, V.H. T., Serio, M., and Giusti, G., Eds., Academic Press, London, 1976, 359.
49. **Fraser, I. S., Michie, E. A., Baird, D. T., and Wide, L.,** Pituitary gonadotrophins and ovarian function in adolescent dysfunctional uterine bleeding, *J. Clin. Endocrinol. Metab.*, 37, 407, 1973.
50. **Yen, S. S. C., Vela, P., and Rankin, J.,** Inappropriate secretion of follicle stimulating hormone and luteinizing hormone in polycystic ovarian disease, *J. Clin. Endocrinol. Metab.*, 30, 435, 1970.
51. **Kirschner, M. A. and Jacobs, J. B.,** Combined ovarian and adrenal catheterisation. To determine the site(s) of androgen overproduction in hirsute women, *J. Clin. Endocrinol. Metab.*, 33, 199, 1971.
52. **De Vane, G. W., Czekala, N. C., Judd, H. L., and Yen, S. S. C.,** Circulating gonadotrophins, estrogens and androgens in polycystic ovarian disease, *Am. J. Obstet. Gynecol.*, 121, 496, 1975.
53. **Baird, D. T.,** The secretion of oestrogens from the ovary in normal and abnormal menstrual cycles, in *Proc. IV Int. Congr. Endocrin.*, ICS No. 182, Excerpta Medica, Amsterdam, 1972, 59.
54. **Marshall, W. A.,** Growth and sexual maturation in normal puberty, in *Clinics in Endocrinology and Metabolism*, Vol. 4, W. B. Saunders, Philadelphia, 1975, 3.
55. **Tanner, J. M.,** Trend towards earlier menarche in London, Oslo, Copenhagen, the Netherlands and Hungary, *Nature (London)*, 243, 95, 1973.
56. **Lunenfield B. and Insler V.,** Classification of amenorrhoeic states and their treatment by ovulation induction, *Clin. Endocrinol.*, 3, 223, 1974.
57. **Besser, G. M.,** Amenorrhoea — its investigation and the assessmant of the role of prolactin, in *The Endocrine Function of the Ovary*, James, V. H. T., Serio, M., and Giusti, G., Eds., Academic Press, London, 1976, 261.
58. **Borghi, A., Forti, G., Fusi, C., Vigiani, E., Calabresi, E., and Cattani, G.,** Disorders of the hypothalamic-pituitary-ovarian axis in anorexia nervosa, in *The Endocrine Function of the Ovary*, James, V. H. T., Serio, M., and Giusti, G., Eds., Academic Press, London, 1976, 291.
59. **Franchimont, P., Valcke, J. C., and Lambotte, R.,** Female gonadal disfunction, in *Clinics in Endocrinology and Metabolism*, Vol. 3, W. B. Saunders, Philadelphia, 1974, 533.
60. **Turkington, R. W.,** Inhibition of prolactin secretion and successful therapy of Forbes-Albright Syndrome with L-dopa, *J. Clin. Endocrinol. Metab.*, 34, 306, 1972.
61. **Shearman, R. P.,** Prolonged secondary amenorrhoea after oral contraceptive therapy, *Lancet*, 2, 64, 1971.

62. **Franks, S., Murray, M. A. F., Jequier, A. M., Steele, S. J., Nabarro, J. D. N., and Jacobs, H. S.,** Incidence and significance of hyperprolactinemia in women with amenorrhoea, *Clinical Endocrinol.*, 4, 597, 1975.
63. **Seppala, M., Hirvonen, E., Ranta, T., Virkkunen, P., and Leppaluoto, J.,** Raised serum prolactin levels in amenorrhoea, *Brit Med J.*, 2, 305, 1975.
64. **Bohnet, H. G., Dahlen, H. G., Wuttke, W., and Schneider, H. P. G.,** Hyperprolactinaemic anovulatory syndrome, *J. Clin. Endocrinol. Metab.*, 42, 132, 1976.
65. **Del Pozo, E., Wyss, H., Lancranjan, I., Obvlensky, W., and Varga, L.,** Prolactin-induced luteal insufficiency and its treatment with bromocriptine: preliminary results, in *Ovulation in the Human, Proc. Serono Symp.* No. 8, Grosignani, P. G. and Mishell, D. R., Eds., Academic Press, London, 1976, 297.
66. **Frantz, A. G., Habif, D. V., Hyman, G. A., Suh, H. K., Sassin, J. F., Zimmerman, E. A., Noel, G. L., and Kleinberg, D. L.,** Physiological and pharmacological factors affecting prolactin secretion, including its suppression by L-dopa in the treatment of breast cancer, in *Human Prolactin*, Pasteels, J., and Robyn, C., Eds., *Excerpta Med. Int. Congr. Ser.*, 308, 273, 1973.
67. **Thorner, M. O.,** Prolactin, in *Clinics Endocrinology and Metabolism*, Vol. 6, W. B. Saunders, Philadelphia, 1977, 201.
68. **Tyson, J. E., Andreasson, B., Huth, J., Smith, B., and Zacur, H.,** Neuroendocrine dysfunction with psychogenic implications in post pill galactorrhoea-amenorrhoea, *Obstet. Gynecol.*, 46, 1, 1975.
69. **Kirschner, M. A. and Bardin, C. W.,** Androgen production and metabolism in normal and virilized women, *Metabolism*, 21, 667, 1972.
70. **Stahl, N. L., Teeslink, C. R., and Greenblatt, R. B.,** Ovarian, adrenal and peripheral testosterone levels in the polycystic ovarian syndrome, *Am. J. Obstet. Gynecol.*, 117, 194, 1973.
71. **Kirschner, M. A., Zucker, I. R., and Jespersen, D. L.,** Ovarian and adrenal vein catheterization studies in woman with idiopathic hirsutism, in *The Endocrine Function of the Human Ovary*, James, V. H. T., Serio, M., and Giusti, G., Eds., Academic Press, London, 1976, 443.
72. **Horton, R., and Tait, J. F.,** In vivo conversion of dehydroisoandrosterone to plasma androstenedione and testosterone in man, *J. Clin. Endocrinol. Metab.*, 27, 79, 1966.
73. **James, V. H. T., Rippon, A. E., and Jacobs, H. S.,** Plasma androgens in patients with hirsutism, in *The Endocrine Function of the Human Ovary*, James, V. H. T., Serio, M., and Giusti, G., Eds., Academic Press, London, 1976, 457.
74. **Cooke, W. C., McEvoy, D., Bulaschenko, H., and Wallach, E. E.,** Andrenocortical and ovarian function in the hirsute woman, *Am. J. Obstet. Gynecol.*, 114, 65, 1972.
75. **Abraham, G. E. and Buster, J. E.,** Peripheral and ovarian steroids in ovarian hyperthecosis, *Obstet. Gynecol.*, 47, 581, 1976.
76. **Farber, M., Daoust, P. R., and Rogers, J.,** Hyperthecosis syndrome, *Obstet. Gynecol.*, 44, 35, 1974.
77. **Zarate, A., Karchmer, S., Gomez, E., and Castelazo-Ayala, L.,** Premature menopause, *Am. J. Obstet. Gynecol.*, 106, 110, 1970.
78. **Lucas, M., Dewhurst, C. J., Hurley, R., Anderson, S., and Blunt, S.,** A search for triple X females in a fertile population, *J. Obstet. Gynaec. Br. Commonw.*, 78, 1087, 1971.
79. **Ross, G. T. and Vandewiele, R. L.,** The ovaries, in *Textbook of Endocrinology*, 5th ed., Williams, R. H., Ed., W. B. Saunders, Philadelphia, 1974, 368.
80. **Mattingly, R. F. and Hwang, W. Y.,** Steroidogenesis of the menopausal and postmenopausal ovary, *Am. J. Obstet. Gynecol.*, 103, 679, 1969.
81. **Barlow, J. J., Emerson, K., and Saxena, B. B.,** Estradiol production after ovariectomy for carcinoma of the breast, *N. Engl. J. Med.*, 280, 633, 1969.
82. **Longscope, C.,** Metabolic clearance and blood production rates of oestrogens in postmenopausal women, *Am. J. Obstet. Gynecol.*, 111, 778, 1971.
83. **Grodin, J. M., Siiteri, P. K., and MacDonald, P. C.,** Source of oestrogen production in postmenopausal women, *J. Clin. Endocrinol. Metab.*, 36, 207, 1973.
84. **Nimrod, A. and Ryan, K. J.,** Aromatization of androgens by human abdominal and breast tissue, *J. Clin. Endocrinol. Metab.*, 40, 367, 1975.
85. **Hemsell, D. L., Grodin, J. M., Brenner, P. F., Siiteri, P. K., and MacDonald, P. C.,** Plasma precursors of estrogen II. Correlation of the extent of conversion of plasma androstenedione to estrone with age, *J. Clin. Endocrinol. Metab.*, 38, 476, 1974.
86. **Maroulis, G. B. and Abraham, G. E.,** Ovarian and adrenal contributions to peripheral steroid levels in postmenopausal women, *Obstet. Gynecol.*, 48, 150, 1976.
87. **Vermeulen, A.,** Postmenopausal ovarian function, in *The Endocrine Function of the Human Ovary*, James, V. H. T., Serio, M., and Giusti, G., Eds., Academic Press, London, 1976, 237.
88. **Sharman, B. M., West, J. H., and Korenman, S. G.,** The menopausal transition: analysis of LH, FSH, estradiol and progesterone concentrations during menstrual cycles of older women, *J. Clin. Endocrinol. Metab.*, 42, 629, 1976.

89. **Monroe, S. E. and Menon, K. M. J.**, Changes in reproductive hormone secretion during the climacteric and postmenopausal periods, *Clin. Obstet. Gynecol.*, 20, 113, 1977.
90. **Seyler, E. L., Jr. and Reichlin, S.**, Luteinizing hormone-releasing factor (LRF) in plasma of postmenopausal women, *J. Clin. Endocrinol. Metab.*, 37, 197, 1973.
91. **Campbell, H.**, In *Gynaecological Malignancy: Clinical and Experimental Studies*, Brush, M. G. and Taylor, R. W., Eds., Bailliere Tindall, London, 1975, 111.
92. **Taylor, C. W.**, Pathology of malignant ovarian tumours, *J. Obstet. Gynaecol. Brit. Emp.*, 57, 328, 1950.
93. International Histological Classification of Tumours, No. 9, Serov, S. E. and Scully, R. E., Eds., World Health Organization, Geneva, 1973.
94. International Federation of Gynaecologists and Obstetricians, Classification and staging of malignant tumours in the female pelvis, *Acta Obstet. Gynecol. Scand.*, 50, 1, 1971.
95. **Cariker, M. and Dockerty, M. B.**, Mucinous cystadenomas and cystadeno-carcinomas, *Cancer*, 7, 302, 1954.
96. **Jondahl, W. H., Dockerty, M. B., and Randall, L. M.**, Brenner tumours of the ovary, *Am. J. Obstet. Gynecol.*, 60, 160, 1950.
97. **Ming, S. and Goldman, H.**, Hormonal activity of Brenner tumors in post-menopausal women, *Amer. J. Obstet. Gynecol.*, 83, 666, 1962.
98. **Edwards, R. L., Nicholson, H. O., Zoidis, T., Butt, W. R., and Taylor, C. W.**, Endocrine studies in post-menopausal women with ovarian tumours, *J. Obstet. Gynaecol. Br. Commonw.*, 78, 467, 1971.
99. **Bhargava, V. L., Beischer, N. A., Brown, J. B., and Townsend, L.**, Hormonal activity of 'non-functional' ovarian tumours, *Aus. N. Z. J., Obstet. Gynecol.*, 9, 108, 1969.
100. **Morris, J. M. and Scully, R. E.**, *Endocrine Pathology of the Ovary*, C. V. Mosby, St. Louis, 1958.
101. **Haines, M. and Jackson, I.**, Granulosa cell tumour of the ovary: 40 cases, *J. Obstet. Gynaecol. Br. Emp.*, 57, 737, 1950.
102. **Pedowitz, P., Felmus, L. B., and Mackles, A.**, Precocious pseudo-puberty due to ovarian tumours, *Obstet. Gynecol. Survey*, 10, 633, 1955.
103. **Dorfman, R. I.**, in *Biological Activities of Steroids in Relation to Cancer*, Pincus, G. and Volmer, E. P., Eds., Academic Press, London, 1960, 445.
104. **Bruk, I., Dancaster, C. P., and Jackson, W. P. U.**, Granulosa cell tumours causing precocious puberty. Oestrogen fractionation in two cases, *Br. Med. J.*, 2, 26, 1960.
105. **Jenner, M. R., Kelch, R. P., Kaplan, S. L., and Grumbach, M. M.**, Hormonal changes in puberty. IV. Plasma oestradiol, LH and FSH in prepubertal children, pubertal females and in precocious puberty, premature thelarche, hypogonadism and in a child with feminising ovarian tumour, *J. Clin. Endocrinol. Metab.*, 34, 521, 1972.
106. **Norris, H. J. and Taylor, H. B.**, Virilization associated with cystic granulosa tumours, *Obstet. Gynecol.*, 34, 629, 1969.
107. **Sparling, D. W.**, Theca cell tumours, *Am. J. Obstet. Gynecol.*, 59, 1279, 1950.
108. **Sternberg, W. H. and Gaskill, C. J.**, Theca cell tumors with report of 12 new cases and observations on possible etiologic role of ovarian stromal hyperplasia, *Am. J. Obstet. Gynecol.*, 59, 575, 1950.
109. **Knight, W. R.**, Theca cell tumors of the ovary. Report of 15 cases. Review of literature, *Am. J. Obstet. Gynecol.*, 56, 311, 1948.
110. **Pedowitz, P. and O'Brien, F. B.**, Arrhenoblastoma of the ovary, *Obstet. Gynecol.*, 16, 62, 1960.
111. **Mahesh, V. B., McDonough, P. G., and Deles, C. A.**, Endocrine studies in the arrhenoblastoma, *Am. J. Obstet. Gynecol.*, 107, 183, 1970.
112. **Greenblatt, R. B., Mahesh, V. B., and Gambrell, R. D., Jr.**, Arrhenoblastoma. Three case reports, *Obstet Gynecol.*, 39, 567, 1972.
113. **Laatikainen, T., Pelkonen, R., and Vihko, R.**, Steroids in two subjects with ovarian androgen producing tumours, arrhenoblastoma and gynandroblastoma, *J. Clin. Endocrinol. Metab.*, 34, 580, 1972.
114. **Berger, L.**, Tumour of the sympathiocotropic cells of the ovary with virilization, *Rev. Can. Biol.*, 1, 539, 1942.
115. **Novak, E. R. and Mattingly, R. E.**, Hilus cell tumor of the ovary, *Obstet. Gynecol.*, 15, 425, 1960.
116. **Goodwin, J. W., Ehrmann, R. L., and Leavitt, T.**, An apparently oestrogenic hilum cell tumour of the ovary, *Obstet. Gynecol.*, 19, 467, 1962.
117. **Fahmy, D., Griffiths, K., Turnbull, A. C., and Symington, T.**, A comparision of the metabolism in vitro of ($7\alpha^3$H) dehydroepiandrosterone sulphate and ($4\ ^{14}$C) pregnenolone by tissue from a hilus cell tumour of the ovary, *J. Endocrinol.*, 41, 61, 1968.
118. **Echt, C. R. and Hada, H. E.**, Androgen excretion patterns in a patient with metastatic hilus cell tumour of the ovary, *Am. J. Obstet. Gynecol.*, 100, 1055, 1968.

119. **Hawkins, D. F. and Lawrence, C. M.,** Virilising ovarian hilus cell hyperplasia with special reference to hormone excretion, *J. Obstet. Gyanecol. Br. Commonw.*, 72, 285, 1965.
120. **Taylor, H. B. and Norris, H. J.,** Lipid cell tumors of the ovary, *Cancer,* 20, 1953, 1967.
121. **Griffin, N. B. and Peerman, C. G.,** Granulosa cell tumour of the ovary: 40 cases, *J. Obstet. Gynaecol. Br. Emp.*, 57, 737, 1950.
122. **Pedowitz, P. and Pomerance, W.,** Adrenal like tumours of the ovary. Review of the literature and report of two new cases, *Obstet. Gynecol.*, 19, 183, 1962,
123. **Koss, L. G., Rothschild, E. O., Fleisher, M., and Francis, J. E.,** Masculinizing tumour of the ovary, apparently with adreno-cortical activity, *Cancer,* 23, 1245, 1969.
124. **Lingeman, C.,** Etiology of cancer of the human ovary: a review, *J. Nat. Cancer Inst.*, 53, 1603, 1974.
125. **Fox, H. and Langley, F. A.,** *Post-graduate Obstetrical and Gynaecological Pathology,* Pergamon Press, Oxford, 1973.
126. **Mangione, P.,** Dysgerminoma and granulosa cell carcinoma-unitary histogenetic concept, *Riv. Obstet. Ginecol. Prat.*, 18, 499, 1963.
127. **Larson, N. E., Dockerty, M. B., and Pratt, J. H.,** Primary mixed choriocarcinoma and dysgerminoma of the ovary. Report of a case, *Mayo Clinic Proc.* 33, 431, 1958.
128. **Haines, M. and Taylor, C. W.,** *Gynaecological Pathology,* Churchill, London, 1962.
129. **Scully, R. E.,** Gonadoblastoma: a review of 74 cases, *Cancer,* 25, 1340, 1970.
130. **Schellas, H. F.,** Malignant potential of the dysgenetic gonad. Part 1, *Obstet. Gynecol.*, 44, 298, 1974.
131. **Smith, F. G.,** Pathology and physiology of struma ovarii, *Arch. Surg. (Chicago),* 53, 603, 1946.

Chapter 3

THE GASTROINTESTINAL HORMONES

Linda M. Morgan and Vincent Marks

TABLE OF CONTENTS

I. INTRODUCTION

The term "hormone" was first used by Bayliss and Starling in 1902[1] to describe the action of the gastrointestinal hormone, secretin, on pancreatic secretion. However, the study of gastrointestinal hormones was subsequently neglected, and it has only been over the last 10 years that the gastrointestinal tract has become firmly established as an endocrine organ. This recent upsurge of knowledge about gastrointestinal hormones has been due largely to the development of various techniques in peptide chemistry, in particular the introduction of radioimmunoassay. These have made possible the isolation and measurement of the various gastrointestinal hormones, and the study of their modes of action.

All the gut hormones so far characterized are produced by cells which possess a common set of cytochemical and ultrastructural characteristics.[2,3] These are the APUD cells, so named from the initial letters of their three most important cytochemical properties (Amine content and/or Amine Precursor Uptake or Decarboxylation). They are considered by Pearse to be derived embryologically from the neuroectoderm of the neural crest; however, the alternative view that they are of endodermal (foregut) origin is also held.[4]

Many distinct endocrine cell types have now been identified, and they are classified in Table 1 on an ultrastructural and histochemical basis. Typically, the endocrine cells are scattered singly between the gut mucosal cells and are elongated, with apical processes reaching the gut lumen, and specific endocrine granules stored in the basal portion of the cell.

Little is known about the biosynthesis and release of individual gut hormones, but it is probable that the mechanisms involved are similar to the pancreatic endocrine cells. The hormone is synthesized in the rough endoplasmic reticulum, and migrates to the Golgi apparatus where it is packaged into membrane-bound granules, which accumulate to await the hormone-releasing signal. In gastrin, the only gastrointestinal hormone so far where release has been studied in detail, both chemical and neural factors are implicated. The release of other gastrointestinal hormones is likely also to depend on both types of stimulus.

A. Classification

The gastrointestinal hormones of known structure and function and also the "candidate hormones", chemically identified peptides of, as yet unproven physiological significance[5] are listed in Table 2, together with the major activities by which they have been characterized.

The gastrointestinal hormones, with the exception of a few of the more recently discovered candidate hormones, e.g., bombesin and somatostatin, show a wide range of structural homology, and can be divided into two distinct families on the basis of similarities in their amino acid sequence. Gastrin and cholecystokinin/pancreozymin form one group, and the secretin family, consisting of secretin, gastric inhibitory poly-

Table 1
LAUSANNE (1977) CLASSIFICATION OF GASTROENTERO-PANCREATIC ENDOCRINE CELLS[a]

	Stomach		Small intestine			
Pancreas	Oxyntic	Pyloric	Upper	Lower	Large intestine	Function proposed or ascertained
[P]	P	P	P			Bombesin?
(EC)	EC	EC	EC	EC	EC	5HT (substance P, EC_1; motilin, EC_2; others? EC_n)
D_1	D_1	D_1	D_1	D_1	D_1	(Vasoactive-intestinal-polypeptide-like); disputed
PP	(PP)	(PP)	(PP)	(PP)	(PP)	Pancreatic polypeptide
D	D	D	D			Somatostatin
B						Insulin
A	[(A)]		?			Glucagon
	X	(X)				Unknown
	ECL					Unknown (or 5-hydroxy-tryptamine)
[(G)]		G	G			Gastrin
			S	S		Secretin
			I	I		Pancreozymin
			K	K		Gastric inhibitory polypeptide
				N		Neurotensin?
			L	L	L	Glucagon-like immunoreactivity

[a] Brackets indicate occurrence only in the fetus or newborn and not, or only exceptionally, in adults. (By and with the permission of the Members of the International Committee on Classification of Gut Endocrine Cells, Secretary, Dr. J. M. Polak.)

peptide, vasoactive inhibitory polypeptide, and glucagon, the second. There is also considerable overlap in the biological activity of hormones of the same group and it is generally believed that the families arose by duplication of a common ancestral gene.[6] Peptides resembling the modern gut hormones can be traced back to the earliest vertebrates and probably also their invertebrate predecessors.[7] Insulin, glucagon, pancreatic polypeptide and somatostatin, hormones isolated from the pancreas, share a common embryological origin with the gastrointestinal hormones, and their physiological activities are closely related. This chapter will, however, be confined to the discussion of those hormones secreted from the gastrointestinal tract itself.

B. Chemistry

The amino acid sequence of the known hormones are shown in Table 3. All the gastrointestinal hormones so far characterized are single chain polypeptides, and with the exception of gastrin, are basic in character. The tertiary structure of some of the hormones has been elucidated, and glucagon and secretin have found to resemble each other in having a portion of their molecule forming an α-helix.[8] Gastrin and cholecystokinin share a common C-terminal pentapeptide, but the remaining peptide sequences are dissimilar. The secretin-like family of gut hormones, however, show considerable sequence homologies throughout the whole length of the peptide chain. There are only small interspecies variations in some of the gut hormones; for example, gastrin G-34 isolated from human and porcine sources differs by only four amino acids.[9,10]

Table 2
NOMENCLATURE AND CLASSIFICATION OF INTESTINAL HORMONES

Substance	Probable distribution within gut	Characteristic activity
A. Peptides of known amino acid sequence		
Gastrin	Antrum and duodenum	Stimulation of gastric acid release
Pancreozymin	Duodenum and jejunum	Stimulation of gall bladder contraction; stimulation of pancreatic enzyme release
Secretin	Duodenum and jejunum	Stimulation of pancreatic juice secretion
Vasoactive intestinal polypeptide	Most of gastro-intestinal tract	Vasodilation
Gastric inhibitory polypeptide	Duodenum and jejunum	Inhibition of gastric acid secretion
Motilin	Duodenum	Stimulation of gastric motor activity
B. Purified peptides of unknown/partially known amino acid sequence		
Chymodenin	Duodenum	Stimulates secretion of chymotrypsin
Glucagon-like immunoreactive substance (enteroglucagon)	Duodenum	Cross-reacts with antiglucagon antisera
C. Proposed hormones without chemical evidence		
Somatostatin-like immunoreactivity	Antrum, duodenum and jejunum	Cross-reacts with antisomatostatin antisera

Recently it has become clear that most of the gut hormones exist in several molecular forms, of differing peptide chain length. The different molecular forms of gastrin have been characterized and so far five distinct peptides, mostly of greater chain length than the standard peptide, have been found.[11-14] It therefore seems probable that gut hormones are synthesized by a "prohormone" mechanism, similar to insulin, and the different molecular forms found could represent hormone precursors.

C. Assay

Early work in the gut endocrinology field was hampered by the lack of sensitive, reliable methods of estimating the individual hormones. Until recently, bioassay was the only technique available for measuring gut hormones. The limitations of bioassays were manifold; they were tedious to perform and were suitable only for small numbers of samples. They usually lacked sufficient sensitivity to permit measurement of circulating endogenous plasma levels of hormone, and in some cases, their specificity was open to doubt. The advent of radioimmunoassay, first developed for the assay of insulin by Berson and Yalow in 1960,[15] has provided a sufficiently sensitive technique for the measurement of circulating endogenous gut hormones, and its use has caused a vast increase in our knowledge of the physiology and pathology of individual hormones.

However, RIA of gut hormones has not been without its problems. To set up a suitable RIA for a peptide hormone it is necessary to have (1) an antibody of sufficient sensitivity and specificity to measure normal circulating hormone concentrations, (2) pure hormone for labeling, and (3) standards of known potency. Because the endocrine cells of the gut are scattered throughout its entire length, the isolation of pure hormone

Table 3
AMINO ACID SEQUENCES OF THE KNOWN GASTROINTESTINAL HORMONES (PORCINE)

Gastrin I	1 10 17 Glu-Gly-Pro-Tyr-Met-GLU-Glu-Glu-Glu-Glu-Ala-Tyr-Gly-Trp-Met-Asp-PheNH$_2$
Cholecystokinin	1 10 20 Lys-Ala-Pro-Ser-Gly-Arg-Val-Ser-Met-Ile-Lys-Ala-Leu-Glu-Ser-Leu-Asp-Pro-Ser-His 30 33 Arg-Ile-Ser-Asp-Arg-Asp-Tyr-Met-Gly-Trp-Met-Asp-Phe-NH$_2$ | SO$_3$
Secretin	1 10 20 His-Ser-Asp-Gly-Thr-Phe-Thr-Ser-Glu-Leu-Ser-Arg-Leu-Arg-Asp-Ser-Ala-Arg-Leu-Gln 27 Arg-Leu-Leu-Gln-Gly-Leu-Val-NH$_2$
Glucagon	1 10 20 His-Ser-Gln-Gly-Thr-Phe-Thr-Ser-Asp-Tyr-Ser-Lys-Tyr-Leu-Asp-Ser-Arg-Arg-Ala-Gln 29 Asp-Phe-Val-Gln-Trp-Leu-Met-Asn-Thr
Vasoactive intestinal polypeptide	1 10 20 His-Ser-Asp-Ala-Val-Phe-Thr-Asp-Asn-Tyr-Thr-Arg-Leu-Arg-Lys-Gln-Met-Ala-Val-Lys 27 Lys-Tyr-Leu-Asn-Ser-Ile-Asn-NH$_2$
Gastric inhibitory polypeptide	1 10 20 Tyr-Ala-Glu-Gly-Thr-Phe-Ile-Ser-Asp-Tyr-Ser-Ile-Ala-Met-Asp-Lys-Ile-Arg-Gln-Gln 40 Asp-Phe-Val-Asn-Trp-Leu-Ala-Ala-Gln-Gln-Lys-Gly-Lys-Lys-Ser-Asp-Trp-Lys-His-Asn 43 Ile-Thr-Gln
Motilin	1 10 20 22 Pro-Ile-Phe-Thr-Tyr-Gly-Glu-Leu-Gln-Arg-Met-Glu-Glu-Lys-Gln-Arg-Asn-Lys-Gly-Gln

is difficult, and therefore suitable material for raising antiserum is generally available only in small quantities. The considerable sequence homology among members of the same gut hormone family has raised problems of specificity of the antisera. The heterogeneity of the circulating forms of most gut hormones has also complicated their measurement.[16] The different molecular forms of circulating gut hormones do not necessarily have the same potency in the assay system, and it is sometimes necessary to fractionate the plasma samples in order to obtain a true estimation of hormone concentration. Several of the gut hormones do not contain any tyrosine, the amino acid residue customarily used when radiolabeling a peptide with ^{125}I. If the peptide contains histidine residues, it is possible to incorporate ^{125}I into these, but only under harsher iodination conditions which can lead to damage of the iodinated peptide and its subsequent failure to bind to the antiserum. Another way around this problem is to use synthetic hormones in which one of the amino acids has been substituted for tyrosine. In this way the peptide can be radiolabeled, but this approach is liable to differences in antiserum binding affinity between the labeled and unlabeled hormone. The stability of some of the gut hormones both in standard solution and in plasma samples has proved very variable, and care must be exercised in choosing the right conditions for storage. This has led to the widespread incorporation of various protease inhibitors[17] into the assay systems, and the use of freeze-drying for storing standards, in an attempt to increase hormone stability. In spite of these problems, RIAs have been set up in various laboratories, but even greater care than usual is needed in the validation of a new RIA for a gut hormone.

D. Clinical Significance

At the current time, the greatest clinical interest in the assay of gut hormones for diagnostic and prognostic purposes is in the detection and follow up of the various endocrine tumors of the gastrointestinal tract. The six main hormone-secreting tumors together with their clinical and biological features are listed in Table 4 and these will be discussed individually. Further information on carcinoid tumors and insulinomas, which are not discussed in detail, may be obtained from several reviews.[214,215] Some of the gut hormones themselves are used in provocative tests in the differential diagnosis of endocrine tumors, for example the secretin stimulation test in Zollinger-Ellison syndrome, and they are also used provocatively in the diagnosis of gastric and pancreatic insufficiency.

There is no doubt that the availability of these assays, discussed in greater detail later, has led to a fundamental step forward in gut endocrine tumor diagnosis and comprehension. However, a word of caution: one must be careful not to oversimplify. The measurement of circulating immunoreactive peptide does not always reflect biological activity. Sulfation of tyrosine 7 of the pancreozymin molecule, for example, is essential for full expression of biological activity but has little effect immunologically.

II. RADIOIMMUNOASSAY OF GASTRIC INHIBITORY POLYPEPTIDE; AN ILLUSTRATION OF GASTROINTESTINAL HORMONE ANALYSIS

A detailed description of the radioimmunoassay of individual gastrointestinal hormones is of limited use, as the conditions used for a given hormone are dependent on the individual antisera raised. However, the following description of a radioimmunoassay for GIP illustrates many of the particular difficulties in assaying gut hormones; problems peculiar to the assay of the other gut hormones are described in their appropriate sections. Table 5 lists the various gut hormone preparations and antisera commercially available.

A. Antiserum Production

Because of their relatively low molecular weights (approximately 2000 to 5000) the gut hormones are poor immunogens by themselves and it is usually necessary to conjugate them to a carrier protein to produce an antiserum of a high titer and avidity.

Successful GIP antiserum production in guinea pigs was achieved by Kuzio and co-workers[18] by conjugating GIP to bovine serum albumin using the carbodiimide method.[19] The conjugate was emulsified with Freund's adjuvant and injected subcutaneously, and antiserum of sufficiently high titer and avidity for RIA was obtained after a second booster immunization. We have produced GIP antisera in rabbits using porcine GIP (obtained from Dr. J. Brown, University of British Columbia, Vancouver) conjugated to ovalbumin using gluteraldehyde,[20] emulsified with Freund's complete adjuvant and injected intradermally using the low dose, multisite technique of Vaitukaitis and co-workers.[21] The animals were boosted at 5 months with 100 μg of GIP conjugate intramuscularly, at 7 months with 2.5 μg unconjugated GIP intravenously, and at 8 months with a further 100 μg i.m. of conjugated GIP. GIP is one of the larger gut hormones with a molecular weight of 5105, and the unconjugated GIP used to boost was sufficiently immunogenic to double the antiserum titer, at least for a short while. After the third boost, GIP antibodies of approximately 1/35,000 final titer and of sufficient avidity to be useful in an RIA were produced.

B. Preparation of ^{125}I-GIP

GIP contains two tyrosine residues, and can therefore be iodinated using conven-

Table 4
BIOLOGICAL AND CLINICAL FEATURES OF HORMONE-SECRETING TUMORS OF THE GI TRACT

Feature	Insulinoma	Glucagonoma	Gastrinoma	VIP-oma	Somatostatinoma	Carcinoid
Signs and symptoms	Episodes of altered consciousness, "blackouts", "faints", psychiatric and personality changes	Mild diabetes, skin rash, enlarged liver	Abdominal pain, diarrhea, GI bleeding epigastric tenderness, hepatomegaly	Profuse watery diarrhea, flushing of skin	Impaired glucose tolerance, hypochlorhydria, steatorrhea cholelithiasis	Flushing of skin, diarrhea, edema, heart lesions
Male/female ratio	45/55	10/90	60/40	25/75	4 female, 2 male	50/50
Selective radiology	Celiac axis arteriogram positive in <50% of cases	Celiac axis arteriogram positive in <50% of cases	Peptic ulcer, gastric mucosal hypertrophy	Celiac axis arteriogram positive in <50% of cases	Celiac axis arteriogram positive in <50% of cases	Negative for 1° GI tumors
Histopathology	Single benign predominantly β-adenoma in 80% of cases	Malignant predominantly α-cell carcinoma	Malignant D-cell tumor (60%), benign (20%), islet hyperplasia (20%)	"Non-β-cell" tumor (80%), islet hyperplasia (20%)	D_1-cell tumor	Malignant carcinoid
Biochemistry	Fasting hypoglycemia	Mild hyperglycemia, hyperinsulinemia, hyperglucagonemia	Resting gastrin hypersecretion and hyperacidity	Hypersecretion of VIP, hyperkalemia, hypochlorhydria, hypercalcemia (40%), impaired glucose tolerance	Hypoinsulinemia, hypoglucagonemia, hypochlorhydria, somatostatin elevated in portal or peripheral blood	Hypersecretion of 5-hydroxytryptamine (5HT), raised urinary 5-hydroxy-indoleacetic acid (5HIAA)
Diagnosis	Fasting hypoglycemia with inappropriately high plasma insulin levels	Inappropriately high plasma glucagon levels	Excessive gastric acid production and inappropriate hypergastrinemia	High plasma VIP levels	Surgical exploration	Raised plasma 5HT, raised urinary 5HIAA

Table 5
GUT HORMONE PREPARATIONS AND ANTISERA CURRENTLY AVAILABLE

Hormone	Materials for standards, iodination	Antisera, RIA kits, etc.
Gastrin	Synthetic human gastrin I (Calbiochem; Herts, U.K.) (Medical Research Council, U.K.)	Antiserum to synthetic human gastrin (Radioimmunoassay Ltd., Cardiff, U.K.) Radioimmunoassay kits (Schwarz/Mann)
	Natural porcine gastrine II (Medical Research Council, U.K.)	(Radioassay Systems Laboratories Inc., California, U.S.) (E. R. Squibb & Sons, Inc., New Jersey, U.S.)
Secretin	Synthetic porcine secretin (Squibb Institute for Medical Research, New Jersey, U.S.) Natural porcine secretin (Karolinska Institute, Stockholm, Sweden) Synthetic tryosylated secretin (Squibb Institute)	Antiserum to natural porcine secretin (Radioimmunoassay Ltd.)
Cholecystokinin/pancreozymin (CCK/PZ)	Natural porcine CCK/PZ 0.05% pure (The Boots Co. Ltd., Nottingham U.K.) Natural porcine CCK (10%, 16%, 20%, 99% pure) (Karolinska Institute) Synthetic porcine CCK/PZ octapeptide (sulfated or unsulfated) (Squibb Institute)	
Gastric inhibitory polypeptide (GIP)	Natural porcine GIP (Dr. J. Brown, University of British Columbia, Canada)	Antiserum to natural porcine GIP (Dr. J. Brown) Antiserum to natural porcine GIP (Radioimmunoassay Ltd.)
Vasoactive intestinal polypeptide (VIP)	Natural porcine VIP (Karolinska Institute)	
Motilin	Natural porcine motilin (Dr. J. Brown)	Antiserum to natural porcine motilin (Dr. J. Brown)
	Synthetic porcine motilin (Calbiochem)	Antiserum to synthetic porcine motilin (Calbiochem)

tional chloramine-T or lactoperoxidase techniques.[22,23] We have, however, found that although no difficulty is experienced in incorporating iodine into GIP, retention of immunological activity is variable. We currently employ a mild chloramine-T technique, to minimize label damage (see Table 6). The iodination is carried out at room temperature and the reaction time is 10 sec, before stopping with sodium metabisulfite. Separation of the iodinated hormone from unreacted iodide is accomplished on a 35 × 0.9 cm Sephadex® G-15 column, eluting with 0.2 *M* acetic acid containing 0.5% human serum albumin and 2% aprotinin (Trasylol®; 10,000 KI units/mℓ, Bayer Pharmaceuticals Ltd.). Albumin is added to the elution buffer to prevent absorption of the labeled protein to the column, and aprotinin to prevent breakdown of the label through protease activity. Incorporation of iodine into the protein is typically 50 to 75% and the specific activity of the iodinated GIP approximately 80 μCi/μg. A typical elution chromatograph is shown in Figure 1. The maximum immunological activity of the iodinated peptide occurs on the descending portion of the first radiolabeled peak. The labeled protein from the column is diluted 1:1 with acid ethanol (1 part concentrated hydrochloric acid in 100 parts absolute ethanol) and stored at −20° C. This method of storage is convenient for small peptides not degradable by ethanol, as some radio-

Table 6
MATERIALS USED IN THE IODINATION OF GASTRIC INHIBITORY POLYPEPTIDE, USING CHLORAMINE-T

Materials, in order of addition	Volume
1. Porcine GIP, 4 μg	Freeze-dried material
2. 0.4 *M* phosphate buffer, pH 7.5.	10 μℓ
3. 1.0 mCi ^{125}I sodium iodide	10 μℓ
4. 15.0 μg chloramine-T	5 μℓ
Mix for 10 sec with magnetic flea	
5. 40.0 μg sodium metabisulfite	20 μℓ
6. 10.0 μg potassium iodide	50 μℓ
7. Elution buffer for column chromatography (see text)	100 μℓ

active substances are less susceptible to radiation damage in the liquid state than in the solid. An alternative method of label purification is on an anion exchange column of Sephadex® QAE-25, as in the purification of iodinated glucagon.[24] However, while this method achieves excellent purification of ^{125}I-GIP, the production of a sharply defined peak of iodinated peptide from this type of column is very susceptible to small changes in column operating conditions, and we have found it difficult to obtain reproducible results.

C. Preparation of GIP Standard

Many of the purified gut hormone preparations are unstable in solution and need careful storage to retain their immunological potency. A GIP standard of 100 μg/mℓ deteriorates within 6 weeks when stored frozen at −20°C, for example, in spite of the addition of aprotinin and albumin. We currently prepare our GIP standards by dissolving a known amount of porcine GIP (J. Brown, Vancouver) in 0.05 *M* acetic acid at a concentration of 10 μg/mℓ and freeze-drying 1 μg aliquots. A fresh vial is used for each assay.

D. Preparation of Plasma Samples

The presence of proteases in normal plasma causes degradation of many gastrointestinal hormones. Iodinated hormones are particularly susceptible, and this has led to erroneous results in several gut hormone assays, notably glucagon.[17] Collection of blood into a heparinized tube containing aprotinin (1000 KI units/mℓ blood) helps prevent this, but even so the plasma should be separated immediately and stored frozen at −20°C. Plasma for GIP estimation is collected in this way, as small differences have been found in GIP level of plasma stored at −20°C for long periods of time without aprotinin.

E. Assay Protocol

A disequilibrium assay procedure[25] is necessary in order to achieve sufficient sensitivity with our anti-GIP antiserum to measure fasting GIP levels. However, extra care is needed when the addition of the labeled ligand is delayed in order to avoid a "first-come first-served" effect decreasing the specificity of the assay.[26] The GIP assay protocol used by us is shown in Table 7.

Standard curves are set up in plasma from which GIP has been removed by treating

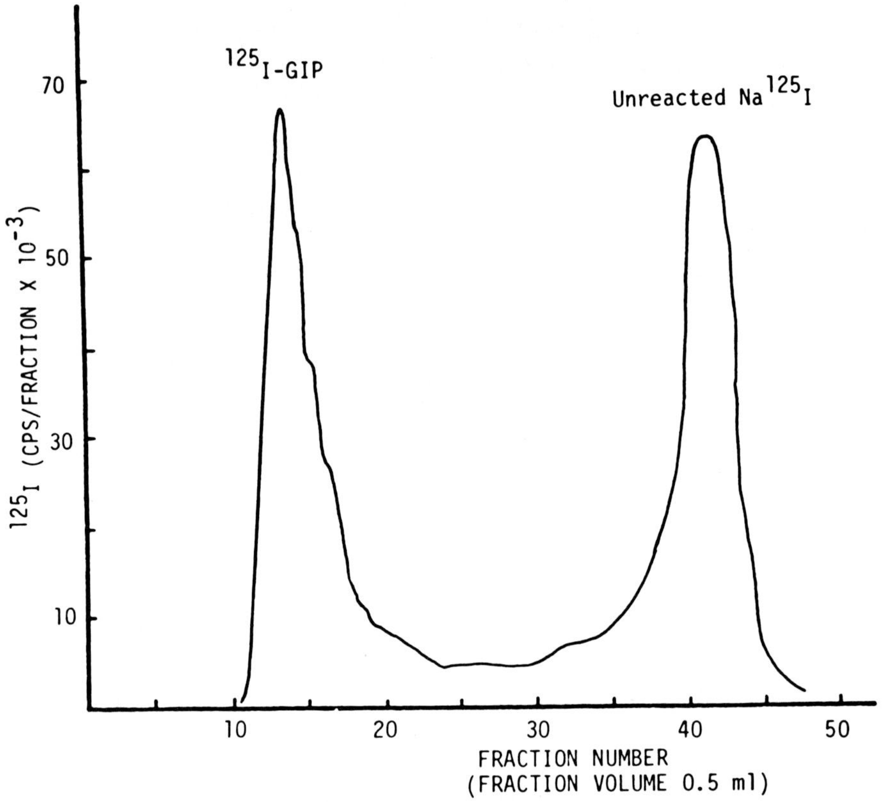

FIGURE 1. Iodination of gastric inhibitory polypeptide. Sephadex® G-15 elution chromatogram of the iodination reaction products.

with 1% charcoal at 4°C for 18 hr. This is necessary to ensure the superimposibility of a serially diluted plasma sample upon the standard curve (see Figure 2). However, charcoal treatment will extract many other low molecular weight proteins from the plasma, and difficulties in obtaining superimposibility may still be encountered. An alternative approach is to use plasma from which the hormone to be assayed has been specifically removed, as a standard diluent.[27] Aprotinin is used throughout the assay in the diluent buffer to protect against damage by proteases.

In our hands, separation of the antibody-bound from free GIP is most successful using a double antibody technique as we have encountered problems with high and variable nonspecific binding values using the charcoal method reported by Kuzio et al.[18] Separation of bound and free GIP has also been reported using ethanol.[28]

F. Assay Validation and Quality Control

The validation and quality control of a gut hormone RIA follows procedures standard to any RIA validation. They are beyond the scope of this chapter but have been the subject of several excellent reviews.[29,30] When assaying gut hormones special attention must be paid to testing out the specificity of the assay as regards the cross-reactivity with other members of the "family", e.g., secretin, glucagon, and VIP cross-reactivity in the GIP assay. Lack of superimposibility of the standard curve and a serially diluted plasma sample may be due to the presence in plasma of multiple molecular forms of the hormone possessing different binding affinities for the antiserum rather

Table 7
PROTOCOL FOR THE ASSAY OF GASTRIC INHIBITORY POLYPEPTIDE IN PLASMA

	Incubation 24 hr at 4°C				Incubation 48 hr (4°C)	Incubation 16 hr (4°C)[c]	
	Standard (μℓ)	Sample (μℓ)	Anti-GIP antiserum (μℓ 1/5000 dilution)	Buffer[a] (μℓ)	^{125}I-GIP[b] (μℓ)	Normal rabbit serum (1/135 dilution, μℓ)	Anti-rabbit antiserum (1/9 dilution, μℓ)
Totals	—	—	—	—	100	—	—
Nonspecific binding (std curve)	—	100 (hormone-free plasma)	—	300	100	50	50
Standards (0—500 pg/mℓ)	100	—	100	200	100	50	50
Sample 1	—	100	100	200	100	50	50
Nonspecific binding (sample 1)	—	100	—	300	100	50	50

[a] Buffer: 0.04 *M* phosphate pH 6.5 containing 5 g/human albumin and 500,000 KIU aprotinin per liter

[b] ^{125}I-GIP containing approx. 5000 cpm/100 μℓ (~50 pg ^{125}I-GIP/tube)

[c] After the 16-hr incubation, tubes are centrifuged at 2000 g for 20 min, the supernatants aspirated, and precipitates counted in an automatic γ counter.

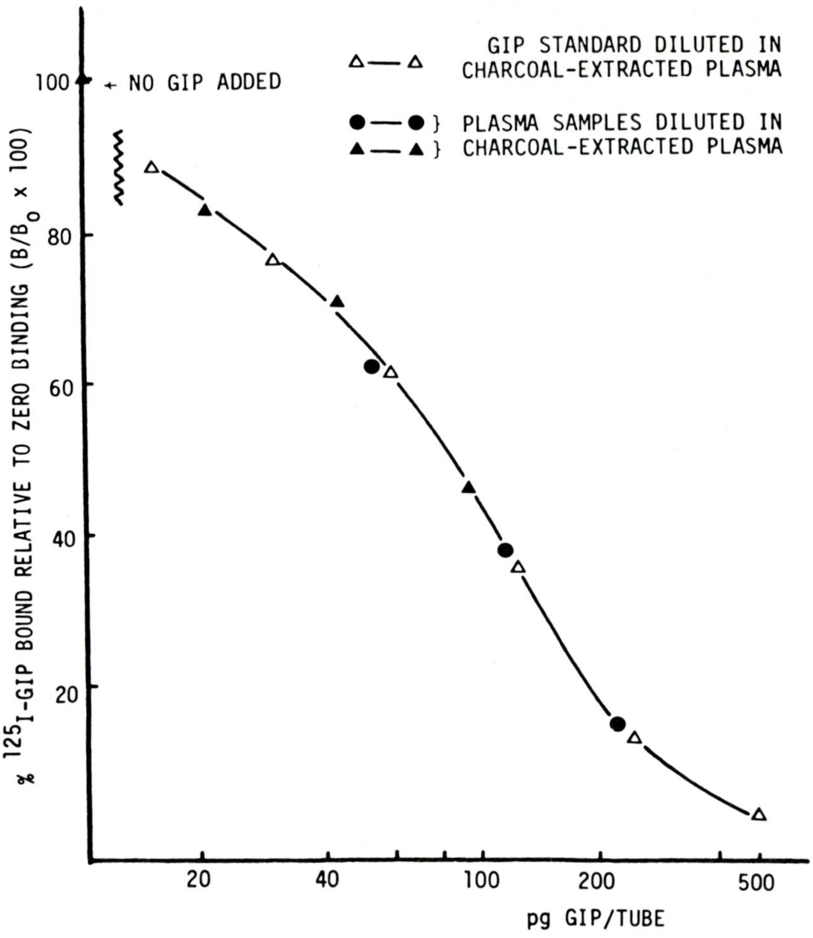

FIGURE 2. Standard curve obtained in the radioimmunoassay of gastric inhibitory polypeptide, showing the superimposibility of diluted plasma samples upon a porcine GIP standard.

than to its cross-reactivity with other hormones; fractionation of the plasma sample may occasionally be necessary to overcome this.

III. PHYSIOLOGY, ASSAY AND CLINICAL SIGNIFICANCE OF THE INDIVIDUAL GASTROINTESTINAL HORMONES

A. Gastrin

1. Physiology

The antral hormone, gastrin, was first described by Edkins in 1905[31] but it was not until 1964 that the molecular structure of porcine material was elucidated[32] and the hormone subsequently synthesized.[33] Gastrin, as then described, consisted of two acidic peptides of 17 amino acids, gastrin I and gastrin II, the difference being that the tyrosine in position 12 is sulfated in gastrin II. Gastrin is secreted mainly by the G-cells of the gastric antral mucosa, although in man the duodenum also contains a considerable amount of gastrin, and small amounts can be extracted from the more distal parts of the small intestine. Its principal physiological effects are thought to be stimulation of gastric acid secretion, pepsin secretion, and trophic effects on the gastric and duodenal mucosa.[34] Gastrin also has a number of other actions which are probably pharmacological in man, including the stimulation of pancreatic juice and enzymes[35] and the release of insulin and calcitonin.[36] Almost the complete biological activity of gastrin is obtained with the C-terminal tetrapeptide amide alone[37] and this has led to the synthesis of the pentapeptide, "pentagastrin" which has found widespread use in assessing gastric acid secretion in animals and man.

Antral gastrin release is initiated both by stimuli originating in the head (the cephalic phase) and in the stomach (the gastric phase). The cephalic phase is mediated via the vagi and is initiated by the smell and taste of food, by insulin-induced hypoglycemia and interference with glucose utilization.[38] Release of gastrin in the gastric phase is caused by distention of the stomach and the presence of partially digested protein.[39] All modes of release are inhibited by acidification of the antral mucosal area. Factors controlling the release of duodenal gastrin are less well known, but duodenal gastrin is released after meals as shown by a rise in plasma gastrin in antrectomized patients after feeding.

Since methods have become available for measuring gastrin by radioimmunoassay, it has been shown to occur in a variety of different forms.[11,12,41] Various fractions described so far range (in order of decreasing molecular weight) from "big-big" gastrin, component I, "big" gastrin (G 34, 34-amino acid chain), the heptadecapeptide G 17, to "mini" gastrins, G 14, and G 4. G 14 and G 17 are the carboxyterminal fragments of G 34; the larger components have yet to be characterized. The most abundant form of gastrin in gastrin-secreting tissues is G 17, but recently high concentrations of G 4, which is not as readily measured by radioimmunoassay, have been found in the antrum.[223] The major component of normal fasting serum is "big-big" gastrin, but after feeding it becomes G 34 or G 17. More recent studies indicate that "big-big" gastrin may be an artifact. In pernicious anemia and Zollinger-Ellison syndrome, when fasting levels are high, the most abundant form is G 34. Component I is found only in patients with Zollinger-Ellison syndrome.

2. Assay

McGuigan[42] was the first to describe the production of a gastrin antiserum of sufficiently high avidity to be suitable for RIA, and several techniques have been described subsequently. Gastrin RIAs are now available from commercial sources that are sufficiently sensitive and specific to permit measurement of both stimulated and basal gastrin levels in man.

Gastrin antiserum is generally raised against the synthetic human gastrin, G 17, coupled to a carrier protein. Earlier preparations were, however, prepared from natural material and may have been contaminated with somatostatin antibodies possibly explaining the reputed but subsequently unconfirmed reports that normal pancreatic islet D cells contain and secrete gastrin.

Most antibodies used routinely for gastrin RIA are relatively specific for the C-terminal biologically active portion of the molecule and thus also measure various other plasma gastrin components of both larger and smaller molecular size. In our own laboratory a G 17-BSA conjugate was used to immunize both rabbits and sheep. Almost all gastrin antibodies react similarly with both sulfated and nonsulfated forms of gastrin, so that the total immunoreactive gastrin concentration measured in hypergastrinemic patients is probably a reasonable reflection of the total molar concentration of gastrin components. Antibodies of unusual specificity have been used to identify circulating fragments of G 17 in patients with gastrin-secreting tumors.[43]

Iodination of synthetic human G17 can be achieved using conventional chloramine-

T methods. Earlier methods of separating iodinated protein and unreacted iodide used Sephadex® gel filtration[44] but later methods have utilized ion exchange chromatography on amino ethyl cellulose,[45] or polyacrylamide starch gel electrophoresis.[40]

Serum gastrin concentrations are usually expressed, probably correctly, in terms of pg/mℓ of G 17 standard, either synthetic human gastrin I or natural porcine gastrin II, rather than in molar terms. Actual values for serum gastrin in normal fasting subjects are generally within the range 30 to 120 pg/mℓ, and peak increments after a protein meal are variously reported as being between 50 to 500 pg/mℓ (Table 8).

Gastrin is relatively stable in plasma. Aprotinin is not required in collection of the blood and the plasma can be stored at −20°C until assayed. A detailed account of gastrin radioimmunoassay has recently been published by Hansky and Soveny.[46] Its pathophysiology has been reviewed by Walsh.[47]

Our laboratory has been involved in the organization of a National Quality Control Scheme for gastrin. At monthly intervals 36 freeze-dried plasma samples containing various levels of gastrin are sent to the participating laboratories. Over a recent 12-month period during which eight laboratories participated in the scheme, five laboratories assayed the gastrin samples with an interassay coefficient of variation of less than 10%, two laboratories with a coefficient of variation of between 10-20%, and the remaining one at 47%. An illustrative example of the range of gastrin values obtained between laboratories for a single gastrin pool is shown in Figure 3. Quality control samples "spiked" with G 17 synthetic gastrin are also sent out at intervals to assess assay accuracy.

3. Clinical Significance

Clinically, the most significant cause of a markedly raised fasting plasma gastrin level is the Zollinger-Ellison syndrome (ZE) or gastrinoma. This syndrome is caused by a gastrin-producing tumor usually situated in the pancreatic islets, but occasionally in the duodenal wall or some other ectopic site. It manifests itself clinically by severe abdominal pain associated with recurrent peptic ulceration and/or diarrhea. The most important biochemical disturbance in Zollinger-Ellison syndrome is an enormous increase in basal gastric acid secretion due to unregulated gastrin overproduction and accounts for all the clinical symptoms produced.

Fasting gastrin levels are raised in a number of other pathological conditions apart from Zollinger-Ellison. There is a general tendency for fasting gastrin levels to be inversely correlated with basal and stimulated gastric acid secretion. Thus gastric ulcer patients, who have low acid secretion, have slightly raised fasting gastrin levels. Patients with hypo- or achlorhydria, such as occurs with pernicious anemia, have greatly elevated gastrin levels. Mild hypergastrinemia is also common after vagotomy which produces hypochlorhydria.

Gastrin is destroyed in the kidney and this may be one of the reasons that patients with renal disease have elevated plasma gastrin levels. Hypergastrinemia accompanied by, and causal of, hyperacidity occurs after gastric surgery producing antral exclusion wherein the gastrin-producing mucosa of the antrum and duodenum is shielded from the gastrin suppressive effect of low pH resulting from gastric acid. Antral cell (D) hyperplasia in which hyperacidity and peptic ulceration is associated with hypergastrinemia is an uncommon condition whose very existence has been denied by some authorities.

The main clinical application of the gastrin assay is in the detection of hypergastrinemia in patients with peptic ulcer disease, and in the differential diagnosis of Zollinger-Ellison syndrome from antral cell hyperplasia or antral exclusion, the two other conditions in which hypergastrinemia and hyperacidity occur concurrently.

Table 8
VALUES OBTAINED FOR PLASMA GASTRIN IN NORMAL FASTING SUBJECTS USING VARIOUS RADIOIMMUNOASSAYS

Reported method	Antigen used for antiserum production	Standard	Iodinated hormone	Fasting plasma level	Assay sensitivity
Becker et al.[219]	Synthetic human gastrin (residues 2—17)	Synthetic human gastrin I	Synthetic human gastrin I	165 ± 4 pg/mℓ (SEM)	6.7—33 pg/mℓ
McGuigan and Trudeau[220]	Synthetic human gastrin I (residues 2—17)	Synthetic human gastrin I	Synthetic human gastrin I	425 ± 136 pg/mℓ (SD)	—
NHS Supraregional Assay Service, Guildford (1977)	Synthetic human gastrin I (ICI)	Synthetic human gastrin I (MRC)	Synthetic human gastrin I (ICI)	Undetectable — 100 pg/mℓ	25 pg/mℓ
Hansky and Soveny[46]	Synthetic human gastrin I (ICI)	Natural porcine gastrin II Synthetic human gastrin I (MRC)	Synthetic human gastrin I (ICI)	Undetectable — 160 pg/mℓ	22 pg/mℓ

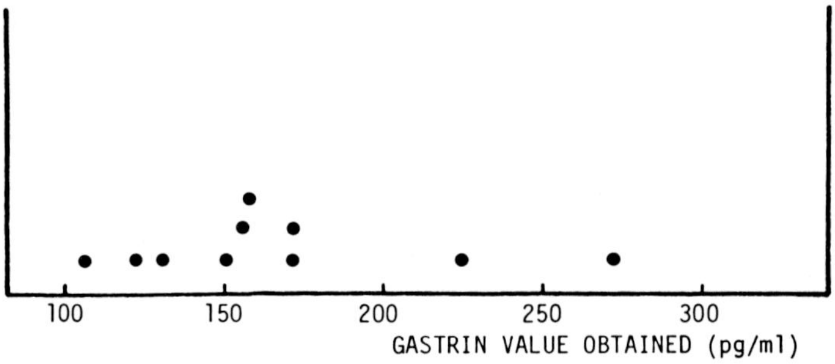

FIGURE 3. Gastrin values obtained on a single freeze-dried gastrin pool assayed in various laboratories. Each point represents results from an individual laboratory. Mean pool value = 169. Standard deviation = 47.4; coefficient of variation = 28; range 107-276.

The plasma gastrin response to intravenous calcium,[48] secretin,[49] glucagon,[164] or a protein-rich meal,[50] has been used to differentiate the various conditions. Nontumorous gastrin responds poorly to calcium and responds to secretin and glucagon with either no change or a fall in plasma levels. Zollinger-Ellison patients, on the other hand, generally show a 100% or more rise in plasma gastrin over basal levels to each of these stimuli. A high protein meal produces a marked increase in nontumorous gastrin levels but little change in Zollinger-Ellison patients.

In a comparison of the three major provocation tests in a series of hypergastrinemic patients Lamers and Van Tongeron[51] found the secretin stimulation test to be the most reliable in distinguishing Zollinger-Ellison patients from others. The protein-rich meal produced a significant increase in plasma gastrin in several of the Zollinger-Ellison patients and was the least reliable of the three tests.

B. Cholecystokinin/Pancreozymin

Ivy and Oldberg in 1928[52] obtained evidence for the existence of an intestinal hormone that could activate gall bladder contraction and to which they gave the name cholecystokinin (CCK). Later, Harper and Raper[53] isolated a substance from duodenal mucosa which stimulated pancreatic enzyme secretion. This substance they called pancreozymin (PZ). Investigation of these two hormonal activities moved independently until Jorpes and his co-workers, in 1964,[54] isolated a peptide from porcine duodenum which had the properties of both. As purification proceeded it became evident that cholecystokinin and pancreozymin were one and the same hormone.[55] Since gall bladder contraction was the first action described it is now usually called cholecystokinin or sometimes in deference to its dual origins, CCK-PZ.

CCK contains 33 amino acids, of which the five C-terminal amino acids are identical with gastrin.[56] A variant has also been identified, designated CCK-V, which consists of CCK plus an additional six amino acids at the N terminus[57] and recent work has indicated that CCK may, like gastrin, exist in multiple molecular forms.[58] CCK possesses a sulfated tyrosyl residue (C-7) similar to gastrin II, which has a sulfated tyrosine residue at C-12. Unlike gastrin, however, sulfation of CCK is essential for the full expression of its biological though not its immunological properties. Synthesis of the complete polypeptide chain has now been achieved but not its biologically active sulfated derivative.

1. Physiology

CCK-producing cells are confined to the mucosa of the upper small intestine, mainly the duodenum, where they are found in patches rather than evenly distributed.[73] High concentrations of the hormone have been isolated from the duodenum and jejunum of various mammals.[56,59] The C-terminal portion of CCK is essential for both cholecystokinin and pancreozymin-like activity.[60] Much information has been gained about the activity of the hormones from structures with cerulein, a decapeptide isolated from frog skin whose biological actions closely resemble those of porcine CCK[62,63] and which is chemically identical with the C-terminal octapeptide of CCK except for the substitution of methionine for threonine.[61]

The biological actions of CCK in addition to those by which it was discovered, include (1) insulin release,[64] (2) stimulation of intestinal motility,[65] (3) stimulation of secretion of Brunner's glands,[66] and (4) stimulation of pancreatic growth.[67] This latter effect appears to be mediated via specific receptor sites on pancreatic acinar cells.[68,69] There is also indirect evidence that the release of CCK after feeding may act as an appetite regulator by altering central nervous system electrical activity to induce satiety.[70,71]

CCK is released by various amino acids and protein hydrolysates, hydrochloric acid, and fatty acids.[72] Circulating levels of CCK are raised in man following the ingestion of a mixed meal.[59,73]

2. Assay

CCK can be measured by in vitro bioassay, using isolated rabbit gall bladder[74,75] or in vivo by measuring its effect on pancreatic enzyme secretion[76] and it is on these techniques that current views of CCK physiology are largely based.

Measurement of CCK by radioimmunoassay has proved particularly difficult, although several assays have been described.[59,73,77-80] Special problems encountered include (1) the apparent low immunogenicity of CCK, which has led to difficulties in antiserum production, (2) the nonavailability of pure human or synthetic CCK, and the subsequent lack of a reference preparation for use as standard, (3) difficulties in iodination (the only tyrosine residue in the molecule being sulfated). This has led to considerable disagreement in reported values for circulating CCK (see Table 9) and a generally unsatisfactory state of affairs.

Antisera to CCK have been produced from various crude porcine preparations used either unconjugated or conjugated to albumin or from highly purified (natural) material. The antisera produced so far have generally been of low titer, but surprisingly have shown little cross-reactivity with gastrin in the majority of cases. This suggests that the antisera recognize the nonbiologically active N-terminal portion of the CCK molecule and therefore immunological activity may not reflect biological activity. Attempts to make antisera specifically directed towards the C-terminal portion of the molecule have so far resulted in cross-reactivity with gastrin.[81]

CCK has been iodinated with conventional chloramine-T techniques, but specific activities are lower than those obtained for other gastrointestinal hormones. Higher specific activity has been obtained[73] by iodinating the naturally occurring pancreozymin variant (39 CCK) which contains a tyrosine residue with a free phenolic group. However, Rehfeld[224] has reported that chloramine-T iodination techniques cause almost complete loss of immunological activity — a possible explanation for the apparent failure to produce high-titer antisera. He recommends the nonoxidative Bolton and Hunter technique[225] for iodination. Because the clinically useful antisera to CCK have all been produced from natural preparations of the hormone, a highly purified ^{125}I-CCK is necessary for assay accuracy and specificity. Porcine CCK has become available recently in a 99% pure preparation (Karolinska Institute preparation). The radiolabeled CCK or CCK variant has been purified by gel filtration, or more recently, Amberlite® resin, which is claimed to achieve a better label purification.[82]

Table 9
VALUES OBTAINED FOR PLASMA CCK IN NORMAL FASTING SUBJECTS USING VARIOUS RADIOIMMUNOASSAYS

Reported method	Antigen used for antiserum production	Standard	Iodinated hormone	Fasting plasma level	Assay sensitivity
Go et al.[78]	10% pure porcine CCK (Karolinska)	Porcine CCK 10% pure (Karolinska)	Porcine CCK 99% pure (Karolinska)	Undetectable	—
Harvey et al.[79]	Crude porcine CCK (Boots)	Porcine CCK 99% pure (Karolinska)	Porcine CCK 99% pure (Karolinska)	25.8 ± 4.3 pg/mℓ (SEM)	5 pg/mℓ
Schlegel et al.[73]	Highly purified porcine CCK	Porcine CCK	Porcine 39-CCK (Karolinska)	222 ± 60 pg/mℓ (SD)	40 pg/mℓ
Reeder et al.[59]	Porcine CCK 85% pure (Karolinska)	CCK 17% pure (Karolinska)	Porcine CCK 10% pure (Karolinska)	731 ± 87 pg/mℓ (SD)	—
Rayford et al.[226]	Porcine CCK 16% and 99% pure (Karolinska)	Porcine CCK 99% pure (Karolinska)	Porcine 39-CCK (Karolinska)	202 ± 30 pg/mℓ (SEM)	—

Due to a lack of a standard reference preparation for CCK, different laboratories have used various porcine preparations as their working standards. This doubtless contributes to the disagreement over circulating CCK values between different RIAs.

3. Clinical Significance

There is currently little reliable information available on plasma CCK levels in different clinical conditions. Circulating CCK has been reported to rise after both milk and solid food in man.[59,79] Studies using test meals have shown that the CCK response to ingestion of food is more rapid in patients with diabetes or with duodenal ulcers than in normal subjects in whom it is said to be more prolonged.[83,84] Basal plasma CCK levels have been reported to be raised in patients with pancreatic exocrine insufficiency[79] and, if confirmed, could possibly find a place as a diagnostic tool. However, until CCK assay methods become more reliable plasma measurements are unlikely to occupy a major role in the clinical diagnosis of gut endocrine abnormalities.

C. Secretin

Bayliss and Starling[1] demonstrated that instillation of hydrochloric acid into a denervated loop of small intestine elicited the secretion of pancreatic juice. They suggested that some unidentified circulating chemical messenger to which they gave the name "secretin" might be released from the small intestine and be responsible for the effect. Half a century later the hormone was finally isolated in pure form and its amino acid sequence elucidated.[85,86]

Secretin has been localized in granular S-cells present in the mucosa between the crypts and villi throughout the length of the small intestine but at greatest concentration in the duodenum.[87] It is a strongly basic molecule containing 27 amino acids, and bears a close structural similarity to glucagon, with 14 amino acids occupying identical positions. The intact secretin molecule is needed for complete biological activity[88,89] and it has been suggested[88] that the α-helix between amino acids 5 and 13 is also necessary.

1. Physiology

Secretin exerts a wide range of biological actions, and there is considerable overlap between it and other members of the secretin family. The primary action of secretin appears to be stimulation of water and bicarbonate secretion by the pancreas.[90] However, the physiological importance of this has been questioned[91,92] largely on the basis that secretin release is stimulated by acid in the duodenum with a threshold pH of 4.5 and that after normal feeding pH levels as low as this are generally only attained in the first few centimeters of duodenum.[93] However, the extreme potency of secretin on pancreatic exocrine secretion in man together with the known ability of CCK to potentiate secretin-induced pancreatic secretion to such an extent that plasma secretin levels that are themselves too low to stimulate the pancreas become effective in the presence of physiological concentrations of CCK[94,95] may help resolve some of these objections. VIP has weak secretin-like actions on pancreatic secretion in mammals, but, unlike CCK, there is evidence to suggest that VIP is a competitive inhibitor of secretin-induced pancreatic bicarbonate secretion.[96] Other biological actions of secretin include (1) stimulation of water and bicarbonate secretion by the liver and Brunner's gland,[66] (2) stimulation of insulin release,[97,98] (3) reduction of duodenal motility,[99] and (4) inhibition of pentagastrin-induced gastric acid secretion and food stimulated gastrin release.[100-102] An exception to this inhibition of gastrin release by secretin is observed in patients with Zollinger-Ellison syndrome and hyperparathyroid patients from families with multiple endocrine adenomatosis type VI[51] in whom it is paradoxically stimulatory.

2. Assay

Early assays of secretin were based on the measurement of pancreatic juice volume or bicarbonate produced by animals injected with secretin-containing materials. This method of assay led to secretin concentrations being expressed in terms of the "Ivy Dog Unit", an arbitrary unit based on comparison with a standard reference preparation rather than on the mass of material itself. The ability of secretin to increase pancreatic volume still provides the basis of a standard test for pancreatic function in man; the secretin administered being calibrated in "Clinical Units" which were established as the smallest amount of secretin needed to elicit a satisfactory pancreatic response in man.[103] Pure, natural and synthetic porcine secretin contain between 3000 to 4000 clinical units of secretin per milligram. However, the potentiating actions of other gut hormones on pancreatic stimulation by secretin invalidate bioassays in situations where these are present, such as always occur in vivo.

The development of RIAs for secretin was hindered by difficulties encountered in radioiodinating the tyrosine-deficient molecule. These were finally overcome by Young and co-workers in 1968[104] who iodinated the histidine residue using chloramine-T at a slightly alkaline pH. This was confirmed by Teale and his colleagues[105] and several investigators have subsequently developed RIAs which are sufficiently sensitive and specific to measure circulating levels of secretin,[106-109] often with conflicting results. Both the 1 and 6 tyrosyl derivatives of synthetic secretin have also been used for radioiodination but the labeled natural compound is reported to be more immunoreactive.[110] Iodination of natural secretin by enzymic methods has also been reported using lactoperoxidase at pH 6.0.[111]

Radiolabeled secretin can be purified by a method originally introduced by Rosselin and co-workers[112] for the purification of iodinated parathyroid hormone, and depends upon binding the undamaged ^{125}I-secretin to talc which can then be washed to remove unreacted Na ^{125}I and "damaged" ^{125}I-secretin.

Secretin is an immunogenic hormone and antisera against both natural and synthetic secretin can be produced, without difficulty, with microgram quantities of the hormone either adsorbed onto charcoal or conjugated to a carrier protein. Secretin is unstable in serum because of the presence of proteases, and its breakdown is only partially prevented by the addition of Trasylol® (1,000 KIU/mℓ).[109] Blood for secretin estimation should, therefore, be collected into ice-cold plastic heparinized tubes, separated immediately, and the plasma stored at −20°C. Glass containers should be avoided as secretin binds to glass surfaces.

Synthetic secretin is generally used for radioimmunoassay standards and fasting levels in man have been reported to range from undetectable to about 500 pg/mℓ (see Table 10).

3. Clinical Significance

It is clear that bioassay methods of secretin measurement overestimated circulating levels of secretin and led to serious misconceptions about the "physiological" doses of exogenous secretin.

Acidification of the duodenum is a potent releaser of secretin, as measured by RIA, but there is disagreement over the release of secretin in response to food. Young and co-workers,[104] using an early and what would now be considered unreliable RIA, reported an increase in plasma secretin after the ingestion of 50 g glucose. Almost all others[113-115] have reported no significant change in plasma secretin levels after either oral glucose or a meal. The failure to measure a rise in secretin after food is surprising in view of the "secretin-like" pancreatic response to a meal. However, as discussed earlier, the response of the pancreas may be due to other gut hormones augmenting

Table 10
VALUES OBTAINED FOR PLASMA SECRETIN IN NORMAL FASTING SUBJECTS USING VARIOUS RADIOIMMUNOASSAYS

Reported method	Antigen used for antiserum production	Standard	Iodinated hormone	Fasting plasma level	Assay sensitivity
Boden and Chey[106]	Synthetic porcine secretin (Squibb)	Natural porcine secretin (Karolinska)	Synthetic porcine secretin	468 ± 150 pg/mℓ (SD)	100 pg/mℓ
Bloom and Ogawa[221]	Natural porcine secretin (Karolinska)	Synthetic porcine secretin	Synthetic tyrosylated secretin	Undetectable — 100 pg/mℓ	50 pg/mℓ
Byrnes[109]	Synthetic porcine secretin (Squibb)	Synthetic porcine secretin (Squibb)	Synthetic porcine secretin (Squibb)	<50 pg/mℓ	12.5—25 pg/mℓ
Chey et al.[222]	Synthetic porcine secretin	Synthetic porcine secretin	Synthetic porcine secretin	15—150 pg/mℓ	2—3 pg/mℓ

the secretory response of secretin or more likely to insensitivity of existing methods of measurement. The possibility of a portal system — either vascular or lymphatic — between the duodenum and pancreas, which are in close juxtaposition, has not been excluded, however, nor has the possibility that in man at any rate food suppresses rather than stimulates secretin secretion. Alcohol has been reported to stimulate secretin secretion in man[110] but it appears to do so by stimulation of gastric acid secretion and hence by a lowering of duodenal pH rather than by a direct stimulatory effect.

There is currently little knowledge of the involvement of secretin in pathological conditions. Bloom and Ward[116] have suggested that the secretin release after duodenal acidification is impaired in patients with duodenal ulcer, although in another study Cano and co-workers[117] reported that duodenal ulcer patients have a greater pancreatic bicarbonate response to duodenal acidification but that their secretin response was not significantly different from normal subjects. Raised plasma secretin levels have been found in conditions associated with gastric acid hypersecretion[118] and secretin assays may be clinically relevant to these situations. High plasma secretin levels have recently been reported in prolonged starvation[119] and diabetes mellitus.[120]

D. Gastric Inhibitory Polypeptide (GIP)

In 1930 Kosaka and Lim[121] postulated the existence of a hormone which they called "enterogastrone" to account for the inhibition of gastric acid secretion and delay in gastric emptying that follows the ingestion of a fat meal.

CCK was for many years the only gastrointestinal hormone known to be released in response to oral fat. But whereas certain crude preparations of porcine CCK were known to possess gastric inhibitory activity, more highly purified ones had the reverse effect and stimulated gastric secretion. This paradox led to the supposition that the "enterogastrone" activity of crude CCK preparation might be due to an impurity, and in 1969 Brown and co-workers[122] isolated a peptide with enterogastrone activity from 10% pure porcine CCK prepared at the Karolinska Institute. The peptide was subsequently purified[123] and its amino acid sequence determined.[124,125] It was named gastric inhibitory polypeptide (GIP) because of the controversy surrounding the nature of enterogastrone and the possibility that the enterogastrone effect might not be its primary action.

GIP contains 43 amino acids and is larger than other members of the secretin family. Its N-terminal end bears a close resemblance to glucagon and secretin, but the C-terminal amino acid sequence of 17 residues is not common to any other known intestinal polypeptide.

The measurement of GIP by RIA has been discussed earlier in this chapter.

GIP-immunoreactive cells have been localized in the duodenum and jejunum of man by immunohistochemical techniques,[126] and in the pancreas.[127] Brown and co-workers[128] measured the GIP content of porcine gut extracts by RIA and found that while the lower parts of the duodenum and jejunum were both rich in GIP the rest of the gastrointestinal tract contained very little.

1. Physiology

Circulating levels of immunoreactive GIP show a biphasic response to food, with an initial peak occurring about 45 min and a later peak 2 to 3 hr after eating. The early GIP response is stimulated by glucose and the later one by fat.[129] This, along with other evidence, led to the suggestion[128] that there are two forms of immunoreactive GIP which differ in their responses to the secretory stimuli of glucose or fat. The GIP produced by these two kinds of stimuli appears, however, to be identical in its immunoreactivity. Sephadex® chromatography of plasma GIP released in response to a mixed meal does reveal some heterogeneity. Three separate immunoreactive components have been separated; of these, two possess an apparent molecular weight greater than that of porcine GIP extracted from duodenal mucosa. There is controversy over the ability of amino acids or duodenal acidification to stimulate GIP release. Brown and his colleagues were unable to demonstrate any effect on GIP secretion by these agents in dogs. However, Thomas and co-workers[130] demonstrated a GIP stimulatory effect of intraduodenal amino acids in man, which we have confirmed with oral amino acid loads. Ebert et al.[226] have demonstrated GIP release by intraduodenal acidification in rat and man, but we are unable to show this in calves.

The biological actions of GIP include (1) the inhibition of pentagastrin, gastrin, insulin, and histamine-stimulated gastric acid secretion,[131] (2) inhibition of pepsin and gastrin secretion,[132,133] (3) stimulation of intestinal secretion from jejunal and ileal loops,[134] and (4) stimulation of insulin in the presence of hyperglycemia.[128]

The early rise in plasma GIP levels that follows a meal, together with the lack of GIP stimulation by duodenal acidification has led to the belief that the enterogastrone activity of GIP in man is unlikely to be physiological. It is currently thought that the insulinotropic action of GIP is the most important of its biological actions and the one most likely to be physiological.[128] It is this property of GIP which has excited the most interest and there has even been a move to rename the peptide "Glucose-mediated Insulin-releasing Polypeptide", thus conveniently retaining the abbreviated name while more accurately describing its physiological action.

As long ago as 1928 Zunz and Labarre[135] coined the term "incretin" to describe a hormone postulated to be released from the duodeno-jejunal mucosa when bathed in glucose and to stimulate the release of insulin from the pancreas. The recognition that hyperglycemia alone could not account entirely for the rise of plasma insulin observed after the ingestion of glucose[136,137] led to a search among the then-known gastrointestinal hormones for a likely "incretin" candidate. Secretin, cholecystokinin, and gastrin have all been proposed in the past as potential regulators of pancreatic endocrine function due to their ability to release insulin from the pancreas under certain conditions.[138-144] However, neither immunoassayable secretin nor gastrin appear to be released by oral glucose[145-147] and the crude preparations of CCK used to establish its insulinotropic properties in earlier work were undoubtedly contaminated with GIP. While it is by no means certain that "incretin" activity is due to a single gastrointestinal hormone, GIP currently appears to be the most likely gastrointestinal hormone to occupy this role (for further discussion of this point see Marks and Turner[148]).

2. Clinical Significance

It has been suggested that the release of GIP is regulated by and associated with the rate of absorption of nutrients from the gut. Patients with untreated celiac disease and malabsorption, for example, have a diminished plasma GIP response to a mixed meal compared with normal controls.[149] Those with chronic pancreatitis, on the other hand, show an impaired GIP response to oral fat, which is closely related to the severity of their steatorrhea but a normal or exaggerated response to a mixed meal or glucose given orally.[150,151]

The ability of GIP to potentiate insulin secretion has led to its measurement in a variety of clinical situations where insulin secretion is abnormal. Brown and co-workers[128] suggested that insulin inhibits GIP release by negative feedback control. Untreated ketotic juvenile diabetics, in whom plasma insulin levels are low, have markedly raised basal plasma GIP levels and show no further elevation after a mixed test meal.[152]

This abnormal pattern of GIP secretion becomes normal on treatment with insulin. In contrast to insulinoprivic diabetics those with maturity-onset dibetes and nondiabetic obese subjects have exaggerated GIP responses to mixed test meals[151,153] and glucose and are frequently hyperinsulinemic. However, we have found that the GIP response to oral glucose in a group of patients with insulin-secreting tumors was normal, in spite of their high circulating insulin levels.[227]

The contribution of GIP to the hyperinsulinism of obesity, the feedback control of insulin on GIP production, and speculation about its possible breakdown in obese subjects[151] is still being debated. Obese people have an exaggerated GIP response to fat and a mixed meal. The feedback control of fat-induced GIP release by insulin is defective in obesity and can be restored by food restriction or starvation.[228] The possibility must be considered[216] that GIP hyperproduction is a primary — or early secondary — event in the production of obesity. Indirect support for this suggestion also comes from the demonstration that in genetically obese mice there is GIP-cell hyperplasia throughout the gut[217] though whether this is a primary phenomenon or secondary to hyperphagia is unknown.

E. Vasoactive Intestinal Polypeptide (VIP)

Vasoactive intestinal polypeptide (VIP) was obtained in 1972 by Said and Mutt[154] from a side fraction of a crude porcine secretin preparation. It was initially isolated and characterized on the basis of its potent vasodilator and hypotensive effects, hence its name, but has since been found to have a wide range of biological actions, many of which are shared with other members of the secretin family.

The peptide contains 28 amino acids and shows considerable chemical homology with GIP, glucagon, and secretin. Like secretin, it is thought to possess a helical structure.[155] The porcine molecule has been successfully synthesized.[156] Unlike the other gastrointestinal hormones VIP is found throughout the whole length of mammalian gut from esophagus to colon.[87] Although the greatest number of VIP-containing cells are found in the small intestine[157] the hormone appears to have a widespread distribution throughout mammalian tissue and has been identified histochemically in brain and peripheral nervous tissue.[158] There is indeed some question as to whether much, if not all, of the VIP in the gut is of neural rather than of "endocrine" origin.

1. Physiology

Apart from its vasodilator and hypotensive effects[159] VIP can inhibit pentagastrin- and histamine-stimulated gastric acid secretion[96] and inhibits gastrin secretion,[160] properties it shares with GIP. VIP stimulates water and electrolyte secretion by the pancreas and increases bile flow[161] similar to secretin. Indeed in birds (but not in animals) it is a more potent stimulus to pancreatic exocrine secretion. VIP stimulates lipolysis, glycogenolysis and can, in high concentration, increase insulin release (a glucagon-like property) in the presence of moderate hyperglycemia.[162,163] The biological actions of VIP have been recently reviewed by Said.[165]

The conditions under which VIP is released into the circulation in mammals and its physiological role are still unknown. It is largely inactivated by a single passage through the liver[166] suggesting that its actions may be limited to effects upon the gastrointestinal tract and the liver. Its nonspecific tissue distribution does, however, cast doubts on its hormonal status as classically defined and currently it is being seriously considered as one of the peptide neurotransmitters.

2. Assay

A bioassay for VIP was used during isolation based on its ability to produce systemic vasodilation. RIAs have subsequently been developed that are capable of measuring circulating plasma VIP levels in pathological conditions in which they are elevated.[167,168] Recently, methods have been reported of sufficient sensitivity to measure circulating levels of VIP in normal man[169,170] (see Table 11).

There is no particular problem associated with VIP radioimmunoassay; the peptide is immunogenic and both highly purified porcine and synthetic materials are available. The presence of tyrosine residues in the molecule facilitate iodination. Conditions have been chosen similar to those described for glucagon or secretin. Antisera have been raised against porcine VIP, and both synthetic and porcine VIP have been used as RIA standards. No information is available regarding the stability of VIP in plasma but Said and Faloona[168,173] collect blood into tubes containing Trasylol®, separating and freezing quickly, as a precaution against proteolytic enzyme activity.

3. Clinical Significance

In contrast to its somewhat uncertain physiological role, the clinical significance of VIP in man has been more clearly defined than for many of the other gastrointestinal hormones. Using a RIA Bloom and co-workers[167,171] found increased plasma levels of VIP (ranging from 1030 to 1310 pg/mℓ compared with normal levels of <100 pg/mℓ) in patients with the Verner-Morrison syndrome. This syndrome (also called pancreatic cholera) exhibits symptoms of intractable watery diarrhea, hypokalemia and achlorhydria (hence WDHA), hypotension, and cutaneous flushing, and is usually associated with a pancreatic tumor. Symptoms are usually relieved by excision of the tumor where this is possible or by streptozotocin treatment when it is not. Since extracts of the excised tumors generally have a high immunoreactive VIP content Bloom[171] suggests that overproduction of VIP is responsible for the clinical syndrome and has designated the tumors vipomas.

Said and Faloona[168] measured plasma VIP levels in 28 patients with chronic watery diarrhea. In 26 of them plasma VIP levels were raised ranging from 600 to 9000 pg/mℓ. Of these exactly 50%, i.e. 13, had pancreatic islet cell tumors; four had islet-cell hyperplasia, five had bronchogenic carcinoma, and one each had a pheochromocytoma and a ganglioneuroblastoma. In four patients no etiologic diagnosis was made. Kahn and co-workers[172] obtained remission in two patients with Verner-Morrison syndrome by streptozotocin. However, plasma VIP was undetectable in one, and did not change on treatment with the other, despite remission of symptoms. Measurable amounts of VIP have recently been demonstrated in medullary thyroid carcinomas.[174] These tumors are associated with diarrhea and increased plasma levels of prostaglandins E and Fa[175] which have, hitherto, been held responsible for the abnormal bowel action. Bloom and co-workers[230] have received more than 1000 plasma samples from patients with various forms of diarrhea. Of these 34 had elevated VIP levels; in each of these cases a pancreatic tumor was found. An additional 12 patients had calcitonin-producing tumors of the thyroid, 13 had carcinoma of the lung, 4 had villous adenoma of the rectum, and 24 patients had a carcinoid tumor; none of these had elevated VIP levels. A classical Verner-Morrison syndrome occurred in 11 patients but with no tumor and normal VIP levels.

The causes of diarrhea are legion and gut endocrine adenopathies are responsible for only a small percentage of cases. However, RIA of plasma VIP levels is clearly useful in the diagnosis of VIP-secreting tumors as a cause of intractable diarrhea and might also prove useful for monitoring treatment, although elevated plasma immunoreactive VIP levels do occur unassociated with intractable diarrhea and consequently

Table 11
VALUES OBTAINED FOR PLASMA VIP IN NORMAL FASTING SUBJECTS USING VARIOUS RADIOIMMUNOASSAYS

Reported method	Antigen used for antibody production	Standard	Iodinated hormone	Fasting plasma level	Assay sensitivity
Bloom et al.[167]	Porcine VIP (Karolinska)	Porcine VIP (Karolinska)	Porcine VIP (Karolinska)	Undetectable	100 pg/mℓ
Said and Faloona[168]	Porcine VIP (Karolinska)	Porcine VIP (Karolinska)	Porcine VIP (Karolinska)	Undetectable	100—200 pg/mℓ
Ebeid et al.[169]	Porcine VIP (Karolinska)	Porcine VIP (Karolinska)	Porcine VIP (Karolinska)	96.6 ± 46.3 pg/mℓ (SD)	50 pg/mℓ
Fahrenkrug et al.[170]	Porcine VIP (Karolinska)	Porcine VIP (Karolinska)	Porcine VIP (Karolinska)	242 pg/mℓ (range undetectable — 665 pg/mℓ)	33 pg/mℓ

are not pathognomonic of Verner-Morrison syndrome. Patients with hepatic cirrhosis have markedly elevated plasma VIP levels (presumably because of failure of the liver to degrade VIP) but generally do not suffer from diarrhea or hypochlorhydria.[173]

F. Other "Candidate" Hormones of the Gut

1. Intestinal Glucagon-like Immunoreactivity

The discovery that glucagon-like peptides are secreted from the gut in response to an oral glucose load was made serendipidously as a result of an artifact in the RIA of pancreatic glucagon.[176] These gut peptides to which the names glucagon cross-reacting materials (CRM), glucagon-like immunoreactivity (GLI), or, less satisfactorily, enteroglucagon, have been given, cross-react in the RIA for pancreatic glucagon with some antipancreatic glucagon antisera but not with others. Subsequent work has tended to show that glucagon antibodies directed against the N-terminal portion of the pancreatic glucagon molecule reacted identically with gut extracts containing glucagon-like immunoreactivity (GLI), whereas those directed against the C-terminal end cross-react only very weakly.[177]

GLI has been found throughout the gastrointestinal tract in many mammalian species as well as in the pancreas itself. In most species the largest amounts are found in the jejunum and ileum, originating in mucosal cells which resemble pancreatic α-cells.[178] Various GLIs have been isolated, the only criterion for their identification being their ability to cross-react with certain glucagon antisera. Sephadex® gel filtration has separated two major immunoreactive fractions, the larger with an apparent molecular weight of 6000 to 12000 and the smaller with a molecular weight of 2500-3500.[179,180] Recently Sundby and co-workers have described the isolation and characterization of a GLI material from intestine and pancreas which has one hundred amino acid residues (hence the name glicentin) and which contains within it all the amino acids found in porcine glucagon.[218] Moody[180] postulates that the exact nature of the different GLI materials obtained from gut and pancreas depends upon the sites of cleavage of the parent compound rather than on differences in the compound itself.

Little is known about the physiology of GLI, although some of its reported biological actions are similar to those of pancreatic glucagon. GLI is released in response to a carbohydrate meal and this has led to speculation about its role as an "incretin" candidate. It has also been suggested that the exaggerated release of GLI observed in many postgastrectomy subjects is responsible for the stimulated hyperinsulinema and reactive hypoglycemia that constitutes one of the elements of the dumping syndrome.[181] However, neither possibility has been either confirmed or disproved.

Glucagon-secreting pancreatic tumors have been described[212,213] (see Table 4). The clinical diagnosis is difficult as no striking abnormalities have been associated with hyperglucagonemia although diabetes mellitus and dermopathy are often found. Basal plasma glucagon levels are raised, but this also occurs in an α-cell hyperplasia, a condition invariably associated with other endocrine abnormalities.[213] The ultimate diagnosis of glucagonoma rests with the morphological identification of tumor cells and extraction of immunoreactive glucagon from the tumor tissue.

2. Motilin

In 1967 Brown[182] observed that the intravenous injection of a crude CCK preparation caused increased motility in denervated fundal pouches of dogs. Selective purification of this impure CCK preparation led to the isolation and identification of a polypeptide containing 22 amino acids which had the ability to stimulate motor activity.[183,184] It was named motilin after the biological action by which it was first recognized. Motilin has been synthesized and it, like the natural product, has been used to produce antisera from which RIAs capable of measuring the hormone in plasma have been developed.[206]

Motilin appears to be secreted from the enterochromaffin cells of the small intestine.[185] Its biological actions include (1) increasing the motility of the fundus, antrum, and duodenum, and (2) contraction of the lower esophageal sphincter.[186] Currently very little is known about the physiological role of motilin or its involvement in pathological processes. It is probably involved in the control of normal gastrointestinal motor activity[187,188] and it might reasonably be supposed to be abnormal in certain types of "functional" bowel disorder associated with hypermotility.

3. Chymodenin

Chymodenin is a basic polypeptide recently isolated from impure preparations of porcine secretin and cholecystokinin[189] and has a molecular weight of approximately 9000. The amino acid sequence has been partly elucidated and has been found to contain sequences common to the secretin family.[231] Administration of the polypeptide to rabbits stimulates secretion of pancreatic juice selectively rich in chymotrypsinogen.[190] Much more work is needed before the hormonal status of chymodenin can be established. It is, however, of interest because it challenges the traditional view that all pancreatic enzymes are secreted in parallel. Studies with chymodenin have shown that the pancreas is capable of specific enzyme secretion, and pancreatic enzyme release may therefore be controlled by individual enzyme regulators.[191] A radioimmunoassay for chymodenin has been described, but measurement of chymodenin levels in biological materials has been hampered by the interference of nonspecific serum factors.[232]

4. Peptides of Amphibian Skin Active on the Gut, and Their Mammalian Analogues

Considerable interest has recently centered around groups of peptides found in amphibian skin which have biological actions in the mammalian gut. Some of these peptides bear close structural similarity to known gastrointestinal hormones, and the amphibian peptides are being used in mammalian systems to further elucidate the structure/activity relationships of the mammalian peptides. Moreover, amphibian peptides that are active in mammalian systems but have no mammalian counterpart have, in some cases, led to the discovery of new mammalian peptides.[192]

The amphibian skin peptides can be divided into three main groups:

(a) **The cerulein-like peptides represented by the octapeptide, cerulein, and the decapeptide, phyllocerulein.** Both bear a close structural (and pharmacological) similarity to the C-terminal of CCK, and, as mentioned previously, have been used to further elucidate the structure/activity relationships of CCK. Cerulein has also been used as a diagnostic tool in radiological examination of the gall bladder, as it causes controlled gall bladder contraction and so aids the visualization of the bile ducts and biliary calculi.[193]

(b) **The physalaemin-like peptides, or tachykinins, represented by physalaerin, uperolein, eledoisin, phyllomedusin and kassinin.** These have a spectrum of biological activity very close to a mammalian substance P, discussed in the following section. The biological action of these amphibian peptides has reinforced belief in the role of substance P in the control of gastrointestinal motility and hepatic blood flow.

(c) **The bombesin-like peptides, represented by bombesin, alytesin, ranatesin, and litorin.** Bombesin is a strong releaser of CCK and gastrin in mammals[192,194] and the biological actions of the peptide in mammalian systems are due largely to its ability to stimulate these hormones. There is some evidence, using immunohistochemical techniques, that bombesin-like peptides are present in mammalian antral or duodenal mucosa as well as in gall bladder, pancreas, and colon.[195] Bombesin-like mammalian peptides may, therefore, function as local releasing factors for gastrointestinal hormones.[196]

5. Peptides Common to Gut and Brain

When Euler and Gaddum, in 1931, attempted to study the distribution of acetylcholine in tissue extracts, they discovered an interfering substance in extracts of brain and intestine that was later identified as the peptide substance P.[197] There are now five more peptides that have been shown to be present in both gut and brain: somatostatin,[198] gastrin,[199] VIP,[200] neurotensin,[201] and enkephalin.[202] The dual distribution of these peptides is consistent with Pearse's (APUD) hypothesis that the gut, pancreatic, and most other endocrine cells are derived embryologically from neuroectoderm. The physiological significance of these peptides is still completely unknown. Most interest has centered on the physiological role of somatostatin, discussion of which is beyond the scope of this chapter, but which has been the subject of several reviews.[203-205]

A somatostatinoma syndrome attributable to overproduction of the hormone by malignant islet cell tumors has been described on several occasions[207,208,232] and is summarized in Table 4. In the first 6 reported cases all patients suffered symptoms of mild diabetes mellitus, 5 from cholelithiasis and 4 from steatorrhea. This is consistent with the known inhibitory effects of somatostatin on insulin secretion, pancreatic secretion, and gall bladder contractility. However, we have described a woman with a mixed islet-cell tumor of which the predominant cell type was somatostatin secreting, in whom the clinical presentation was markedly different from those previously reported.[234] The patient presented with hypoglycemia and the initial biochemical findings were highly suggestive of malignant insulinoma. The clinical syndrome produced in this case could not be inferred from that observed when somatostatin is administered pharmacologically. RIAs have been developed for somatostatin,[235] although there is still controversy about the feasibility of measuring somatostatin in peripheral blood. Raised pancreatic vein levels and in some cases raised peripheral somatostatic levels have, however, been reported in somatostatinoma patients.

IV. SUMMARY

In the three quarters of a century that has elapsed since discovery of the first gut hormone much as been learned about their pharmacology and a little about their physiology. Remarkably little is, however, currently known about their pathology or their usefulness as diagnostic aids. Difficulties arising as a result of their chemical complexity, their shortage of supply for investigational purposes, their exquisitely low concentration in biological fluids and inaccessibility of their secretor organ have all contributed to retard progress in this area. Events in the past few years suggest that the situation may change radically within the next decade which will see the gut takes its rightful place as the largest endocrine organ in the body.

REFERENCES

1. **Bayliss, W. M. and Starling, E. H.,** The mechanism of pancreatic secretion, *J. Physiol. (London),* 28, 325, 1902.
2. **Pearse, A.G.E.,** Common cytochemical and ultrastructural characteristics of cells producing polypeptide hormones (the APUD series) and their relevance to thyroid and ultramicrobronchial C-cells and calcitonin, *Proc. Roy. Soc. B.,* 170, 71, 1968.
3. **Carvelheira, A. F., Welsch, V., and Pearse, A. G. E.,** Cytochemical and ultrastructural observations on the argentaffin and argyrophil cells of the gastrointestinal tract in mammals and their place in the APUD series of polypeptide-secreting cells, *Histochemie,* 14, 33, 1968.
4. **Barrington, E. J. W.,** *Hormones and Evolution,* English Universities Press, London, 1964.
5. **Grossman, M. I.,** Candidate hormones of the gut, *Gastroenterology,* 67, 730, 1974.
6. **Van Noorden, S., Greenberg, J. and Pearse, A. G. E.,** Cytochemical and immunofluorescence investigations on polypeptide hormone localization in the pancreas and gut of the lamprey, *Gen. Comp. Endocrinol.,* 19, 192, 1972.
7. **Dockray, G. J.,** Molecular evolution of gut hormones. Application of comparative studies on the regulation of digestion, *Gastroenterology,* 72, 344, 1977.
8. **Bodanszky, M., Ondetti, M. A., Mutt, V. and Bodanszky, M.,** Synthesis of secretin. IV. Secondary structure in a miniature protein, *J. Am. Chem. Soc.,* 91, 944, 1969.
9. **Gregory, B. A. and Tracy, H. J.,** The constitution and properties of two gastrins extracted from hog antral mucosa, *Gut,* 5, 103, 1964.
10. **Gregory, R. A. and Tracy, H. J.,** Isolation of two "big gastrins" from Zollinger-Ellison tumour tissue, *Lancet,* 2, 797, 1972.
11. **Yalow, R. S. and Berson, S. A.,** Size and charge distinctions between endogenous human plasma gastrin in peripheral blood and heptadecapeptide gastrin, *Gastroenterology,* 58, 609, 1970.
12. **Yalow, R. S. and Berson, S. A.,** And now "big-big" gastrin, *Biochem. Biophys. Res. Commun.,* 48, 391, 1972.
13. **Rehfeld, J. F. and Stadil, F.,** Gel filtration studies on immunoreactive gastrin in serum from Zollinger-Ellison patients, *Gut,* 14, 369, 1973.
14. **Debas, H. T., Walsh, J. H., and Grossman, M. I.,** Pure human minigastrin. Secretory potency and disappearance rate, *Gut,* 15, 686, 1974.
15. **Yalow, R. S. and Berson, S. A.,** Immunoassay of endogenous plasma insulin in man, *J. Clin. Invest.,* 39, 1157, 1960.
16. **Yalow, R. S.,** Radioimmunoassay methodology: application to problems of heterogeneity of peptide hormones, *Pharmacol. Rev.,* 25, 161, 1973.
17. **Eisentraut, A. M., Whissen, N., and Unger, R. H.,** Incubation damage in the radioimmunoassay for human plasma glucagon and its prevention with "Trasylol", *Am. J. Med. Sci.,* 255, 137, 1968.
18. **Kuzio, M., Dryburgh, J. R., Malloy, K. M., and Brown, J. C.,** Radioimmunoassay for gastric inhibitory polypeptide, *Gastroenterology,* 66, 357, 1974.
19. **Parker, C. W.,** Nature of immunological responses and antigen-antibody interaction, in *Principles of Competitive Protein-Binding Assays,* Odell, W. D. and Daughaday, W. H., Eds., J. B. Lippincott, Philadephia, 1971, 25.
20. **Garaud, J. C., Moody, A. J., Eloy, R., and Grenier, J. F.,** Unusual specificities of antibodies to glucagon-gluteraldehyde-albumin conjugates, *Horm. Metab. Res.,* 8, 241, 1976.
21. **Vaitukaitis, J., Robbins, J. B., Nieschlag, E., and Ross, G. T.,** A method for producing specific antisera with small doses of immunogen, *J. Clin. Endocrinol. Metab.,* 33, 988, 1971.
22. **Hunter, W. M. and Greenwood, F. C.,** Preparation of iodine-131 labelled growth hormone of high specific activity, *Nature (London),* 194, 495, 1962.
23. **Marchalonis, J. J.,** An enzymatic method for the trace iodination of immunoglobulins and other proteins, *Biochem. J.,* 113, 299, 1969.
24. **Jørgensen, K. H. and Larsen, U. D.,** Purification of ^{125}I-glucagon by anion exchange and chromatography, *Horm. Metab. Res.,* 4, 223, 1972.
25. **Rodbard, D., Ruder, H. J., Vaitukaitis, J., and Jacobs, H. S.,** Mathematical analysis of kinetics of radioligand assays: improved sensitivity obtained by delayed addition of labelled ligand, *J. Clin. Endocrinol. Metab.,* 33, 343, 1971.
26. **Pratt, J. J. and Woldring, M. G.,** Radioimmunoassay specificity and the "first-come first-served" effect, *Clin. Chim. Acta,* 68, 87, 1976.
27. **Alford, F. P., Bloom, S. R., and Nabarro, J. D. N.,** Glucagon levels in normal and diabetic subjects: use of a specific immunoabsorbant for glucagon radioimmunoassay, *Diabetologica,* 13, 1, 1977.
28. **Moody, A. J. and Lauritzen, K.,** A sensitive radioimmunoassay for GIP, in *Proc. Int. Gastrointestinal Hormones and Pathology of the Digestive System,* Speranza, V., Basso, N., and Lezoche, E., Eds., Arti Grafiche Tris, Rome, 1977, 148.

29. **Rodbard, D.,** Statistical quality control and routine data processing for radioimmunoassay, *Clin. Chem.,* 20, 1255, 1974.
30. **Walker, W. H. C.,** An approach to immunoassay, *Clin. Chem.,* 23, 384, 1977.
31. **Edkins, J. S.,** On the chemical mechanism of gastric secretion, *Proc. Roy. Soc. London, Ser. B.,* 76, 376, 1905.
32. **Gregory, H., Hardy, P. M., Jones, D. S., Kenner, G. W., and Sheppard, R. C.,** The antral hormone, gastrin: structure of gastrin, *Nature (London),* 204, 931, 1964.
33. **Anderson, J. C., Barton, M. A., Gregory, R. A., Hardy, P. M., Kenner, J.K., Macleod, J.K., Preston, J., Sheppard, R.C., and Morley, J. S.,** Synthesis of gastrin, *Nature (London),* 204, 933, 1964.
34. **Grossman, M.,** Physiology and pathology of gastrin, in *Clinics in Endocrinology,* 3, 353, 1974.
35. **Petersen, H. and Berstad, A.,** The effect of pentagastrin on pancreatic secretion in man, *Scand. J. Gastroenterol.,* 6, 483, 1971.
36. **Rehfeld, J. F. and Stadil, F.,** The effect of gastrin on basal and glucose-stimulated insulin secretion in man, *J. Clin. Invest.,* 52, 1415, 1973.
37. **Morley, J. S., Tracey, H. J., and Gregory, R. A.,** Structure-function relationships in the active C-terminal tetrapeptide of gastrin, *Nature (London),* 207, 1356, 1965.
38. **Korman, M. G., Soveny, C. and Hansky, J.,** Radioimmunoassay of gastrin. The response of serum gastrin to insulin hypoglycaemia, *Scand. J. Gastroenterol.,* 6, 71, 1970.
39. **Debas, H. T., Walsh, J. H. and Grossman, M. I.,** Release of antral gastrin by large polypeptides, *Clin. Res.,* 22, 171A, 1974.
40. **Yalow, R. S. and Berson, S. A.,** Radioimmunoassay of gastrin, *Gastroenterology,* 58, 1, 1970.
41. **Gregory, R. A.,** Heterogeneity of the gastrins in blood and tissues, *Ciba Found. Symp.,* 41, 251, 1976.
42. **McGuigan, J. E.,** Immunochemical studies with synthetic human gastrin, *Gastroenterology,* 54, 1005, 1968.
43. **Dockray, G. J. and Walsh, J. H.,** Identification of an N-terminal fragment of heptadecapeptide gastrin in the serum of patients with Zollinger-Ellison syndrome (ZES), *Gastroenterology,* 66, 874, 1974.
44. **Young, J. D., Byrnes, D. J., Chisholm, D. J., Griffiths, F. B., and Lazarus, L.,** Radioimmunoassay of gastrin in human serum using antiserum against pentagastrin, *J. Nucl. Med.,* 10, 746, 1969.
45. **Stadil, F. and Rehfeld, J. F.,** Preparation of ^{125}I-labelled synthetic human gastrin I for radioimmunoanalysis, *Scand. J. Clin. Lab. Invest.,* 30, 361, 1972.
46. **Hansky, J. and Soveny, L.,** Radioimmunoassay of gastrin, in *Clinical and Biochemical Analysis, Vol. 5, Handbook of Radioimmunoassay,* Abraham, G., Ed., Marcel Dekker, Inc., New York, 1977, chap. 13.
47. **Walsh, J. H. and Grossman, M. I.,** Gastrin, *N. Engl. J. Med.,* 292, 1324, 1377, 1975.
48. **Passaro, E., Basso, N., and Walsh, J. H.,** Calcium challenge in the Z-E syndrome, *Surgery,* 72, 60, 1972.
49. **Thompson, J. C., Reeder, D. D., and Bunchman, H. H.,** Clinical role of serum gastrin measurements in the Zollinger-Ellison syndrome, *Am. J. Surg.,* 124, 250, 1972.
50. **Berson, S. A. and Yalow, R. S.,** Radioimmunoassay in gastroenterology, *Gastroenterology,* 62, 1061, 1972.
51. **Lamers, C. B. H. and Van Tongeron, J. H. M.,** Comparative study of the value of the calcium, secretin and meal stimulated increase in serum gastrin to the diagnosis of the Zollinger-Ellison syndrome, *Gut,* 18, 128, 1977.
52. **Ivy, A. C. and Oldberg, E.,** A hormone mechanism for gall-bladder contraction and evacuation, *Am. J. Physiol.,* 86, 599, 1928.
53. **Harper, A. A. and Raper, H. S.,** Pancreozymin, a stimulant of the secretion of pancreatic enzymes in extracts of the small intestine, *J. Physiol.,* 102, 115, 1943.
54. **Jorpes, J. E., Mutt, V., and Toczko, K.,** Further purification of cholecystokinin and pancreozymin, *Acta Chem. Scand.,* 18, 2408, 1964.
55. **Jorpes, J. E. and Mutt, V.,** Cholecystokinin and pancreozymin, one single hormone?, *Acta Physiol. Scand.,* 66, 196, 1966.
56. **Jorpes, J. E.,** Memorial lecture: the isolation and chemistry of secretin and cholecystokinin, *Gastroenterology,* 55, 157, 1968.
57. **Mutt, V. and Jorpes, J. E.,** Structure of porcine cholecystokinin-pancreozymin, *Europ. J. Biochem.,* 6, 156, 1968.
58. **Rehfeld, J. F.,** Multiple molecular forms of CCK, in *Gut Hormones: Proc. Int. Symp.,* Bloom, S. R., Ed., Churchill-Livingstone, London, 1978, 213.
59. **Reeder, D. D., Becker, H. D., and Smith, N. J.,** Measurement of endogenous release of cholecystokinin by radioimmunoassay, *Ann. Surg.,* 178, 304, 1973.

60. **Mutt, V. and Jorpes, J. E.,** Isolation and primary structure of cholecystokinin-pancreozymin, *Frontiers in Gastrointestinal Hormone Research: Proc. 15th Nobel Symp., Stockholm, 1970,* Andersson, S., Ed., Almqvist and Wiksell, Stockholm, 1973.
61. **Anastasi, A., Erspamer, V., and Endean, R.,** Isolation and structure of caerulein, an active decapeptide of the skin of *Hylacaerulea, Experimentia,* 23, 699, 1967.
62. **Bertaccini, G., Caro, G., de Endean, R., Erspamer, V., and Impicciatore, M.,** The action of caerulein on the smooth muscles of the gastrointestinal tract and the gall bladder, *Br. J. Pharmacol.,* 34, 291, 1968.
63. **Bertaccini, G., Caro, G., de Endean, R., Erspamer, V., and Impicciatore, M.,** The actions of caerulein on pancreatic secretion of the dog and biliary secretion of the dog and rat, *Br. J. Pharmacol.,* 37, 185, 1969.
64. **Unger, R. H., Ketterer, H., Dupré, J., and Eisentraut, A. M.,** The effects of secretin, pancreozymin and gastrin on insulin and glucagon secretion in anaesthetised dogs, *J. Clin. Invest.,* 46, 630, 1967.
65. **Hedner, P., Perrson, H., and Rorsman, G.,** Effect of cholecystokinin on small intestine, *Acta Physiol. Scand.,* 70, 250, 1967.
66. **Stening, G. F. and Grossman, M. I.,** Hormonal control of Brunner's glands, *Gastroenterology,* 56, 1047, 1969.
67. **Barrowman, J. A. and Mayston, P. D.,** The trophic effect of pentagastrin on the pancreas, in *Gastrointestinal Hormones: Symp.,* Thompson, J. C., Ed., University of Texas Press, Austin, 1975, 231.
68. **Galardy, R. E. and Jamieson, J. D.,** Photoaffinity labeling of secretagogue receptors in the pancreatic exocrine cell, in *Gastrointestinal Hormones: Symp.,* Thompson, J.C., Ed., University of Texas Press, Austin, 1975, 345.
69. **Klaeveman, H. L., Conlon, T. P., and Gardner, J. D.,** Effects of gastrointestinal hormones on adenylate cyclase activity in pancreatic exocrine cells, in *Gastrointestinal Hormones: Symp.,* Thompson, J. C., Ed., University of Texas Press, Austin, 1975, 321.
70. **Dafny, N. and Jacobson, E. D.,** Cholecystokinin and central nervous regulation of appetite, in *Gastrointestinal Hormones: Symp.,* Thompson, J. C., Ed., University of Texas Press, Austin, 1975, 643.
71. **Gibbs, J., Falasco, J. D., and McHugh, P. R.,** Cholecystokinin-decreased food uptake in rhesus monkeys, *Amer. J. Physiol.,* 230, 15, 1976.
72. **Meyer, J. H.,** Release of secretin and cholecystokinin, in *Gastrointestinal Hormones: Symp.,* Thompson, J. C., Ed., University of Texas Press, Austin, 1975, 475.
73. **Schlegel, W., Raptis, S., Grube, D., and Pfeiffer, F.,** Estimation of cholecystokinin-pancreozymin (CCK) in human plasma and tissue by a specific radioimmunoassay and the immunohistochemical identification of pancreozymin-producing cells in the duodenum of humans, *Clin. Chim. Acta,* 80, 305, 1977.
74. **Amer, M. S. and Becvar, W. E.,** A sensitive *in vitro* method for the assay of cholecystokinin, *J. Endocrinol.,* 43, 637, 1969.
75. **Berry, H. and Flower, R. J.,** The assay of endogenous cholecystokinin and factors influencing its release in the dog and cat, *Gastroenterology,* 60, 406, 1971.
76. **Go, V. L. W., Hofmann, A. F., and Summerskill, W. H. J.,** Pancreozymin bioassay in man based on pancreatic enzyme secretion: potency of specific amino acids and other digestive products, *J. Clin. Invest.,* 49, 1558, 1970.
77. **Young, J. D., Lazarus, L., and Chisholm, D. J.,** Radioimmunoassay of pancreozymin-cholecystokinin in human serum, *J. Nucl. Med.,* 10, 743, 1969.
78. **Go, V. L. W., Ryan, R. J., and Summerskill, W.H. J.,** Radioimmunoassay of porcine cholecystokinin-pancreozymin, *J. Lab. Clin. Med.,* 77, 684, 1971.
79. **Harvey, R. F., Donsett, L., Hartog, M., and Read, A. E.,** A radioimmunoassay for cholecystokinin-pancreozymin, *Lancet,* 2, 826, 1973.
80. **Englert, E.,** Radioimmunoassay (RIA) of cholecystokinin (CCK), *Clin. Res.,* 21, 207, 1973.
81. **Go, V. L. W. and Reilly, W. M.,** Problems encountered in the development of the cholecystokinin radioimmunoassay, in *Gastrointestinal Hormones: Symp.,* Thompson, J. C., Ed., University of Texas Press, Austin, 1975, 295.
82. **Rayford, P. L.,** Cholecystokinin assay, in *Gut Hormones: Proc. Int. Symp.,* Bloom, S. R., Ed., Churchill Livingstone, London, 1978, 208.
83. **Rayford, P. L., Fender, M. R., Ramus, N. I., Reeder, D. D., and Thompson, J. C.,** Release and half-life of CCK in man, in *Gastrointestinal Hormones: Symp.,* Thompson, J. C., Ed., University of Texas Press, Austin, 1975, 301.
84. **Thompson, J. C., Fender, H. R. and Ramus, N. I.,** Cholecystokinin metabolism in man and dogs, *Ann. Surg.,* 182, 496, 1975.
85. **Jorpes, J. E., Mutt, V., Magnusson, S. and Steele, B.,** Amino acid composition and N-terminal amino acid sequence of porcine secretin, *Biochem. Biophys. Res. Commun.,* 9, 275, 1962.

86. **Mutt, V. and Jorpes, J. E.,** Secretin: isolation and determination of structure, presented at the 4th Int. Symp. Chem. of Natural Products, Stockholm, June 26th-July 2nd, 1966.
87. **Solcia, E., Polak, J. M., Buffa, R., Capella, C., and Pearse, A. G. E.,** Endocrine cells of the intestinal mucosa, in *Gastrointestinal Hormones: Symp.,* Thompson, J. C., Ed., University of Texas Press, Austin, 1975, 155.
88. **Grossman, M. I.,** Structure of secretin, *Gastroenterology,* 57, 610, 1969.
89. **Rudman, D. and Del Rio, A. E.,** Lipolytic activity of a peptide fragment of porcine secretin, *Endocrinology,* 85, 610, 1969.
90. **Hubel, K. A.,** Secretin: a long progress role, *Gastroenterology,* 62, 318, 1972.
91. **Thomas, J. E.,** *The External Secretion of the Pancreas,* Charles C Thomas, Springfield, Illinois, 1950.
92. **Wormsley, K. G.,** Is secretin secreted?, *Gut,* 14, 743, 1973.
93. **Brooks, A. M. and Grossman, M. I.,** Postprandial pH and neutralizing capacity of the proximal duodenum in dogs, *Gastroenterology,* 59, 85, 1970.
94. **Heyer, J. H., Spingola, J., and Grossman, M. I.,** Endogenous cholecystokinin potentiates exogenous secretin in pancreas of dog, *Am. J. Physiol.,* 221, 742, 1971.
95. **Grossman, M. I. and Konturek, S. J.,** Gastric acid does drive bicarbonate secretion, *Scand. J. Gastroenterol.,* 9, 299, 1974.
96. **Konturek, S. J., Thor, P., Dembinski, A., and Krol, R.,** Vasoactive intestinal polypeptide; comparison with secretin for potency and spectrum of physiologic action, in *Gastrointestinal Hormones: Symp.,* Thompson, J. C., Ed., University of Texas Press, Austin, 1975, 611.
97. **Jorpes, J. E. and Mutt, V.,** Sekretin och glukagon som regulatorer főr insulin-insőndringen till blodet, *Nord. Med.,* 77, 301, 1967.
98. **Deckert, T.,** Stimulation of insulin secretion by glucagon and secretin, *Acta Endocrinol.,* 57, 578, 1968.
99. **Dollinger, H. C., Berz, R., and Raptis S.,** Effects of secretin and cholecystokinin on motor activity of the human jejunum: a radiotelemetering study of jejunal motility during secretin and cholecystokinin intravenous infusion, *Digestion,* 12, 9, 1975.
100. **Brooks, A. M. and Grossman, M. I.,** Effect of secretin and cholecystokinin on pentagastrin-stimulated gastric secretion in man, *Gastroenterology,* 59, 114, 1970.
101. **Bunchman, H. H., Reeder, D. D., and Thompson, J. C.,** Effect of secretin on the serum gastrin response to a meal in man and in dog, *Surg. Forum,* 22, 303, 1971.
102. **Thompson, J. C., Reeder, D. D., Bunchman, H. H., Becker, H. D., and Brandt, E. N.,** Effect of secretin on circulating gastrin, *Ann. Surg.,* 176, 384, 1972.
103. **Jorpes, J. E. and Mutt, V.,** The gastrointestinal hormones, secretin and cholecystokinin-pancreozymin, *Ann. Intern. Med.,* 55, 395, 1961.
104. **Young, J. D., Lazarus, L. and Chisholm, D. J.,** Radioimmunoassay of secretin in human serum, *J. Nucl. Med.,* 9, 641, 1968.
105. **Teale, J. D., Buchanan, K. D., and Harper, G.,** A radioimmunoassay for secretin using antibodies raised to pure natural and synthetic hormone, *Gut,* 13, 849, 1972.
106. **Boden, G. and Chey, W. Y.,** Preparation and specificity of antiserum to synthetic secretin and its use in a radioimmunoassay, *Endocrinology,* 92, 1617, 1973.
107. **Boehm, M., Lee, Y. and Chey, W. Y.,** Radioimmunoassay of secretin. I. Production of secretin antibodies and development of the radioimmunoassay, in *Endocrinology of the Gut: Int. Symp. Rec. Adv. Gastrointestinal Res.,* Chey, W. Y. and Brooks, F. P., Eds., Charles B. Slack Inc., Thorofare, New Jersey, 1974, 42.
108. **Rayford, P. L., Curtis, P. J., and Fender, H. R.,** Radioimmunoassay measurement of disappearance half-time of secretin in dogs, *Surg. Forum,* 26, 385, 1975.
109. **Byrnes, D. J.,** Radioimmunoassay of secretin, in *Handbook of Radioimmunoassay,* Abraham, G., Ed., Marcel Dekker Inc., New York, 1977, 483.
110. **Straus, E., Urbach, H. J., and Yalow, R. S.,** Comparative reactivities of ^{125}I-secretin and ^{125}I-6-tyroxyl secretin with guinea pig and rabbit anti-secretin sera, *Biochem. Biophys. Res. Comm.,* 64, 1036, 1975.
111. **Holohan, K. N., Murphy, R. F., Buchanan, K. D., and Elmore, D. T.,** Enzymic iodination of the histidyl residue of secretin: a radioimmunoassay of the hormone, *Biochim. Biophys. Acta,* 322, 178, 1973.
112. **Rosselin, G., Assan, R., Yalow, R. S., and Berson, S. A.,** Separation of antibody-bound and unbound peptide hormones labelled with iodine-131 by talcum powder and precipitated silica, *Nature (London),* 212, 355, 1966.
113. **Chey, W. Y., Tai, H. H., Rhodes, R., Lee, K. Y., and Hendricks, J.,** Radioimmunoassay of secretin; further studies, in *Gastrointestinal Hormones: Symp.,* Thompson, J. C., Ed., University of Texas Press, Austin, 1975, 269.

114. **Boden, G.,** Secretin, *Methods of Hormone Radioimmunoassay,* Jaffe, B. M. and Berman, H. R., Eds., Academic Press, New York, 1974, 275.
115. **Rayford, P. L., Miller, T. A., and Thompson, J. C.,** Secretin, cholecystokinin and newer gastrointestinal hormones, *N. Engl. J. Med.,* 294, 1093, 1976.
116. **Bloom, S. R. and Ward, A. S.,** Failure of secretin release in patients with duodenal ulcer, *Br. Med. J.,* 1, 126, 1975.
117. **Cano, R., Bloom, S. R., and Isenberg, J. I.,** Pancreatic bicarbonate secretion and serum secretin in response to graded amounts of duodenal acidification in duodenal ulcer and normal subjects, *Gastroenterology,* 68, 870, 1975.
118. **Boden, G.,** The secretin assay, in *Proc. Int. Symp. Gut Hormones,* Bloom, S. R., Ed., Churchill Livingston, London, 1978, 169.
119. **Henry, R. W., Flanagan, R. W. J., and Buchanan, K. D.,** Secretin: a new role for an old hormone, *Lancet,* 2, 202, 1975.
120. **Trimble, E. R., Buchanan, K. D., Hadden, D. R., and Montgomery, D.,** Secretin: high plasma levels in diabetes mellitus, *Acta Endocrinol.,* 85, 799, 1977.
121. **Kosaka, T. and Lim, R. K. S.,** Demonstration of the humoral agent in fat inhibition of gastric secretion, *Proc. Soc. Expl. Biol. Med.,* 27, 890, 1930.
122. **Brown, J. C., Pederson, R.A., Jorpes, J. E., and Mutt, V.,** Preparation of highly active enterogastrone, *Can. J. Physiol. Pharmacol.,* 47, 113, 1969.
123. **Brown, J. C., Mutt, V., and Pederson, R. A.,** Further purification of a polypeptide demonstrating enterogastrone activity, *J. Physiol.,* 209, 57, 1970.
124. **Brown, J. C.,** A gastric inhibitory polypeptide, I. The amino acid composition and the tryptic peptides, *Can. J. Biochem.,* 49, 255, 1970.
125. **Brown, J. C. and Dryburgh, J. R.,** A gastric inhibitory polypeptide. II. The complete amino acid sequence, *Can. J. Biochem.,* 49, 867, 1971.
126. **Polak, J. M., Bloom, S. R., Kuzio, M., Brown, J. C., and Pearse, A. G. E.,** Cellular localisation of gastric inhibitory polypeptides in the duodenum and jejunum, *Gut,* 14, 284, 1973.
127. **Smith, P. H., Merchant, F. W., Johnson, D. G., Fujimoto, W. Y., and Williams, R. H.,** Immunocytochemical localisation of a gastric inhibitory polypeptide-like material with A cells of the endocrine pancreas, *Am. J. Anat.,* 149, 585, 1977.
128. **Brown, J. C., Dryburgh, J. R., Ross, S. A., and Dupré, J.,** Identification and actions of gastric inhibitory polypeptide, *Rec. Prog. Horm. Res.,* 31, 487, 1975.
129. **Brown, J. C., Dryburgh, J. R., Moccia, P., and Pederson, R. A.,** The current status of GIP, in *Gastrointestinal Hormones: Symp.,* Thompson, J. C., Ed., University of Texas Press, Austin, 1975, 537.
130. **Thomas, F. B., Mazzaferri, E. L., Crockett, S. E., Mekhjian, M. S., Gruemer, H. D., and Cataland, S.,** Stimulation of secretion of gastric inhibitory polypeptide and insulin by intraduodenal amino acid perfusion, *Gastroenterology,* 70, 523, 1976.
131. **Pederson, R. A. and Brown, J. C.,** Inhibition of histamine-, pentagastrin-, and insulin-stimulated canine gastric secretion by pure "gastric inhibitory polypeptide", *Gastroenterology,* 62, 393, 1972.
132. **Brown, J. C., Dryburgh, J. R., and Pederson, R. A.,** Gastric inhibitory polypeptide (GIP), in *Endocrinology of the Gut: Int. Symp. Rec. Adv. Gastrointestinal Hormone Res.,* Chey, W. Y. and Brooks, F. P., Eds., Charles B. Slack, Thorofare, New Jersey, 1975, 76.
133. **Rayford, P. L., Villar, H. V., Reeder, D. D., and Thompson, J. C.,** Effect of GIP and VIP on gastrin release and gastric secretion, *Physiologist,* 17, 319, 1974.
134. **Barbezat, G. O. and Grossman, M. I.,** Intestinal secretion: stimulation by peptides, *Science,* 174, 422, 1971.
135. **Zunz, E. and Labarre, J.,** Hyerpinsulinémie consecutive a l'injection de solution de secretine non hypotensive, *C. R. Soc. Biol. (Paris),* 98, 1435, 1928.
136. **McIntyre, N., Holdsworth, D. J. and Turner, D. S.,** New interpretation of oral glucose tolerance, *Lancet,* 2, 20, 1964.
137. **Elrick, M. L., Stimmler, L. and Hlad, Y.,** Plasma insulin reponse to oral and intravenous glucose administration, *J. Clin. Endocrinol.,* 24, 1076, 1964.
138. **Dupré, J.,** An intestinal hormone affecting glucose disposal in man, *Lancet,* 2, 672, 1964.
139. **Dupré, J. and Beck, J. C.,** Stimulation of insulin release by an extract of gut mucosa, *Diabetes,* 15, 555, 1966.
140. **Dupré, J., Rojas, L., White, J. J., Unger, R. M., and Beck, J. C.,** Effects of secretin in insulin and glucagon in portal and peripheral blood in man, *Lancet,* 2, 26, 1966.
141. **Dupré, J., Curtis, D. J., Unger, R. H., Waddell, R. W., and Beck, J. C.,** Effects of secretin, pancreaozymin or gastrin on the response of the endocrine pancreas to administration of glucose or arginine in man, *J. Clin. Invest.,* 48, 745, 1969.

142. **Unger, R.H., Ketterer, H., Dupré, J., and Eisentraut, A. M.,** The effects of secretin, pancreozymin, and gastrin on insulin secretion in anaesthetised dogs, *J. Clin. Invest.*, 46, 630, 1967.
143. **Chisholm, D. J., Young, J. D., and Lazarus, L.,** The gastrointestinal stimulus to insulin release. I. Secretin, *J. Clin. Invest.*, 48, 1453, 1969.
144. **Marks, V. and Samols, E.,** Intestinal factors in the regulation of insulin secretion, *Adv. Metab. Dis.*, 4, 1, 1970.
145. **Bloom, S.,** Hormones of the gastrointestinal tract, *Br. Med. Bull.*, 30, 62, 1974.
146. **Sum, P. T. and Preshaw, R. M.,** Intraduodenal glucose infusion and pancreatic secretion in man, *Lancet*, 2, 340, 1967.
147. **Rehfeld, J. F. and Stadil, F.** The effect of gastrin on basal and glucose stimulated insulin secretion in man, *J. Clin. Invest.*, 52, 1415, 1973.
148. **Marks, V. and Turner, D. S.,** The gastrointestinal hormones with particular reference to their role in the regulation of insulin secretion, *Essays Med. Biochem.*, 3, 109, 1977.
149. **Creutzfeldt, W., Ebert, R., Arnold, R., Frerichs, H., and Brown, J. C.,** Gastric inhibtory polypeptide (GIP), gastrin and insulin: response to test meal in coeliac disease, and after duodeno-pancreatectomy, *Diabetologia*, 12, 279, 1976.
150. **Botha, J. L., Vinik, A. I., and Brown, J. C.,** Gastric inhibitory polypeptide (GIP) in chronic pancreatitis, *J. Clin. Endocrinol. Metab.*, 42, 791, 1976.
151. **Creutzfeldt, W. and Ebert, R.,** Release of gastric inhibitory polypeptide (GIP) to a test meal under normal and pathological conditions in man, Ex. Med. Int. Congr. Ser. I.D.F. Congress, New Delhi, November 1976. *Excerpta Medica* (in press).
152. **Ebert, R., Frerichs, H. and Creutzfeldt, W.,** Serum gastric inhibitory polypeptide (GIP) response in patients with maturity onset diabetes and in juvenile diabetes, *Diabetologia*, 12, 388, 1976.
153. **Crockett, S. E., Mazzaferri, E. L., and Cataland, S.,** Gastric inhibitory polypeptide (GIP) in maturity onset diabetes mellitus, *Diabetes*, 25, 931, 1976.
154. **Said, S. I. and Mutt, V.,** Isolation from porcine intestinal wall of vasoactive octosapeptide related to secretin and to glucagon, *Eur. J. Biochem.*, 28, 199, 1972.
155. **Bodanszky, M.,** The secretin family and evolution, in *Gastrointestinal Hormones: Symp.*, Thompson, J. C., Ed., University of Texas Press, Austin, 1975, 507.
156. **Bodanszky, M., Klausner, Y. S., Lin, C. Y., Mutt, V., and Said, S.,** Synthesis of the vasoactive intestinal peptide (VIP), *J. Am. Chem. Soc.*, 96, 4973, 1974.
157. **Polak, J. M., Pearse, A. G. E., Garaud, J. C., and Bloom, S. R.,** Cellular localisation of a vasoactive intestinal peptide in the mammalian and avian gastrointestinal tract, *Gut*, 15, 720, 1974.
158. **Said, S. I.,** Vasoactive intestinal polypeptide: widespread distribution in normal gastrointestinal organs, Programme of the 57th Annu. Meeting, Endocrine Society, New York, June 18—20th, 1975 (Abstr. No. 270), 1975.
159. **Said, S. I. and Mutt, V.,** Polypeptide with broad biological activity: isolation from small intestine, *Science*, 169, 1217, 1970.
160. **Villar, H. V., Fender, H. R., Rayford, P. L., Ramus, I., and Thompson, J. C.,** Inhibition of gastrin release and gastric secretion by GIP and VIP, in *Gastrointestinal Hormones: Symp.*, Thompson, J. C., Ed., University of Texas Press, Austin, 1975, 467.
161. **Makhlouf, G. M., Said, S. I., and Yau, W. M.,** Interplay of vasocative intestinal peptide (VIP) and synthetic VIP fragments with secretin and octapeptide of cholecystokinin (octa-CCK) on pancreatic and biliary secretion, *Gastroenterology*, 66, 737, 1974.
162. **Kerins, C. and Said, S. I.,** Hyperglycaemic and glycogenolytic effects of vasoactive intestinal polypeptide, *Proc. Soc. Exp. Biol. Med.*, 142, 1014, 1973.
163. **Schebalin, M., Brooks, A. M., Said, S., and Makhlouf, G. M.,** The insulinotropic effect of vasoactive intestinal peptide (VIP): direct evidence from *in vitro* studies, *Gastroenterology*, 66, 772, 1974.
164. **Korman, M. G., Soveny, C., and Hansky, J.,** The effect of glucagon on serum gastrin. II. Studies in pernicious anemia and the Zollinger-Ellison syndrome, *Gut*, 14, 459, 1973.
165. **Said, S. I.,** VIP overview, in, *Proc. Int. Symp. Gut Hormones*, Bloom, S. R., Ed., Churchill Livingstone, London, 1978, 465.
166. **Litamura, S., Yoshida, T., and Said, S. I.,** Vasoactive intestinal polypeptide: inactivation in liver and potentiation in lung of anaesthetized dogs, *Proc. Soc. Expt. Biol. Med.*, 148, 25, 1975.
167. **Bloom, S. R., Polak, J. M., and Pearse, A. G. E.,** Vasoactive intestinal peptide and watery diarrhoea syndrome, *Lancet*, 2, 14, 1973.
168. **Said, S. I. and Faloona, G. R.,** Elevated plasma and tissue levels of vasoactive intestinal polypeptide in the watery diarrhoea syndrome due to pancreatic, bronchogenic and other tumours, *N. Engl. J. Med.*, 293, 155, 1975.
169. **Ebeid, A. M., Murray, P., Hirsch, H., Wesdorp, R. I. C. and Fischer, J. E.,** Radioimmunoassay of vasoactive intestinal polypeptide, *J. Surg. Res.*, 20, 355, 1976.

170. **Fahrenkrug, J. and Muckadell, O. B.,** Radioimmunoassay of vasoactive intestinal polypeptide (VIP) in plasma, *J. Lab. Clin. Med.,* 89, 1379, 1977.
171. **Bloom, S. R. and Polak, J. M.,** The role of VIP in pancreatic cholera, in *Gastrointestinal Hormones: Symp.,* Thompson, J. C., Ed., University of Texas Press, Austin, 1975, 635.
172. **Kahn, C. R., Levy, A. G., Gardner, J. D., Miller, J. V., Gorden, P., and Schein, P. S.,** Pancreatic cholera: beneficial effects of treatment with streptozytocin, *N. Engl. J. Med.,* 292, 941, 1975.
173. **Said, S. I., Faloona, G. R., and Dean, H.,** Vasoactive intestinal polypeptide: elevated in patients with hepatic cirrhosis, *Clin. Res.,* 22, 367a, 1974.
174. **D'Orisio, T. M.,** Pathophysiology of VIP in man, in *Proc. Int. Gut Hormones,* Bloom, S. R., Ed., Churchill Livingstone, London, 1978, 484.
175. **Williams, E. D., Karim, S. S. M., and Sandler, M.,** Prostoglandin secretion by medullary carcinoma of the thyroid, *Lancet,* 1, 14, 1973.
176. **Samols, E., Tyler, J., Marri, G., and Marks, V.,** Stimulation of glucagon secretion by oral glucose, *Lancet,* 2, 1257, 1965.
177. **Flanagan, R. W. J., Buchanan, K. D., and Murphy, R. F.,** Specificity of antibodies in radioimmunoassay of glucagon, *Diabetologia,* 10, 365, 1974.
178. **Sasaki, H., Rubalcava, B., Srikant, C. B., Baetens, D., Orci, L. and Unger, R.,** Gut glucagonoid and gut glucagon, in *Gastrointestinal Hormones: Symp.,* Thompson, J. C., Ed., University of Texas Press, Austin, 1975, 519.
179. **Murphy, R. F., Buchanan, K. D., and Elmore, D. T.,** Isolation of glucagon-like immunoreactivity of gut by affinity chromatography in anti-glucagon antibodies coupled to Sepharose 4-B, *Biochim. Biophys. Acta,* 303, 118, 1973.
180. **Moody, A. J.,** Glucagons from the gut, in *Proc. Int. Symp. Gut Hormones,* Bloom, S. R., Ed., Churchill Livingstone, London, 1978, 369.
181. **Shima, K., Kuroda, K., Matsuyama, T., Tarui, S., and Nishikawa, M.,** Plasma glucagon and insulin responses to various sugars in gastrectomised and normal subjects, *Proc. Soc. Exp. Biol. Med.,* 139, 1042, 1972.
182. **Brown, J. C.,** Presence of a gastric motor-stimulating property in duodenal extracts, *Gastroenterology,* 52, 225, 1967.
183. **Brown, J. C. and Parkes, C. O.,** Effect on fundic pouch motor activity of stimulatory and inhibitory fractions separated from pancreozymin, *Gastroenterology,* 53, 731, 1967.
184. **Brown, J. C.,** Candidate hormones of the gut. IV. Motilin, *Gastroenterology,* 67, 734, 1974.
185. **Pearse, A. G. E., Polak, J. M. and Bloom, S. R.,** Enterochromaffin cells of the mammalian small intestine as the source of motilin, *Virchows Arch. B,* 16, 111, 1974.
186. **Jennewein, H. M.,** Motilin and lower esophageal sphincter, in *Proc. Int. Symp. Gut Hormones,* Bloom, S. R., Ed., Churchill Livingstone, London, 1978, 359.
187. **Strunz, U., Domschke, W., and Mitznegg, P.,** Analysis of the motor effects of 13-norleucine motilin on the rabbit, guinea-pig, rat and human alimentary tract *in vitro, Gastroenterology,* 68, 1485, 1975.
188. **Domschke, W.,** Pharmacology of motilin, in *Proc. Int. Symp. Gut Hormones,* Bloom, S. R., Ed., Churchill Livingstone, London, 1978, 335.
189. **Adelson, J. W.,** Chymodenin: an overview in *Gastrointestinal Hormones: Symp.,* Thompson, J. C., Ed., University of Texas Press, Austin, 1975, 563.
190. **Adelson, J. W. and Rothman, S. S.,** Chymodenin, a duodenal peptide: specific stimulation of chymotrypsinogen secretion, *Am. J. Physiol.,* 229, 1680, 1975.
191. **Adelson, J. W. and Rothman, S. S.,** Candidate hormones of the gut. II. Chymodenin, *Gastroenterology,* 67, 731, 1974.
192. **Erspamer, V. and Melchiorri, P.,** Polypeptides of the amphibian skin active on the gut and their mammalian analogues, in *Gastrointestinal Hormones and Pathology of the Digestive System: Proc. Int. Symp.,* Arti Grafiche Tris, Rome, 1977, 14.
193. **Sargent, E. N.,** Ceruletide in the radiologic examination of the gall bladder, in *Gastrointestinal Hormones and Pathology of the Digestive System: Proc. Int. Symp.,* Arti Grafiche Tris, Rome, 1977, 63.
194. **Fender, H. R., Curtis, P. J. and Rayford, P. L.,** Effect of bombesin on gastrin and secretin and on gastric and pancreatic secretion, *Physiologist,* 18, 212, 1975.
195. **Polak, J. M., Buchan, A. M. J., Czykowska, W., Solcia, E., Bloom, S. R., and Pearse, A.G. E.,** Bombesin in the gut, *Proc. Int. Symp. Gut Hormones,* Bloom, S. R., Ed., Churchill Livingstone, London, 1978, 541.
196. **Erspamer, V. and Melchiorri, P.,** Actions of bombesin on secretions and motility of the gastrointestinal tract in, *Gastrointestinal Hormones: Symp.,* Thompson, J. C., Ed., University of Texas Press, Austin, 1975, 575.
197. **Pearse, A. G. E. and Polak, J. M.** Immunocytochemical localisation of substance P in mammalian intestine, *Histochemistry,* 31, 373, 1975.

198. **Arimura, A., Sato, H., Dupont, A., Nishi, N., and Schally, A. V.**, Somatostatin: abundance of immunoreactive hormone in rat stomach and pancreas, *Science,* 189, 1007, 1975.
199. **Vanderhaeghen, J. J., Signeau, J. C., and Gerts, W.**, New peptide in the CNS reacting with antigastrin antibodies, *Nature (London),* 257, 604, 1975.
200. **Bryant, M. G., Bloom, S. R., Polak, J. M., Albuquerque, R. M., Modlin, I., and Pearse, A. G. E.**, Possible dual role for vasoactive intestinal peptide as gastrointestinal hormone and neurotransmitter substance, *Lancet,* 1, 991, 1976.
201. **Buchan, A. M. J., Polak, J. M., Sullivan, S., Bloom, S. R., Brown, M., and Pearce, A. G. E.**, Neurotensin in the gut, in *Proc. Int. Symp. Gut Hormones,* Bloom, S. R., Ed., Churchill Livingstone, London, 1978, 544.
202. **Polak, J. M., Sullivan, S., Buchan, A. M. J., Bloom, S. R., Facer, P., Hudson, D., and Pearse, A. G.E.**, Endorphins, in *Proc. Int. Sympt. Gut Hormones,* Bloom, S. R., Ed., Churchill Livingstone, London, 1978, 501.
203. **Vale, W., Brazeau, P., Rivier, C., Brown, M., Boss, B., Rivier, J., Burgus, R., Ling, N., and Guilleman, R.**, Somatostatin, *Rec. Progr. Horm. Res.,* 31, 365, 1975.
204. **Guilleman, R. and Gerich, J.**, Somatostatin: Physiological and clinical significance, *Ann. Rev. Med.,* 27, 379, 1976.
205. **Gerich, J.**, Somatostatin, *Arch. Intern. Med.,* 137, 659, 1977.
206. **Dryburgh, J. R. and Brown, J. C.**, Radioimmunoassay of motilin, *Gastroenterology,* 68, 1169, 1975.
207. **Larsson, K., Holst, J., Kühl, C., Lundqvist, G., Hirsch, M., Ingemansson, Z., Lindkaer Jensen, S., and Rehfeld, J.**, Pancreatic somatostatinoma, *Lancet,* 1, 666, 1977.
208. **Ganda, O., Weir, G., Stuart Soeldner, J., Legg, M., Chick, W., Patel, Y., Ebeid, A., Gabbay, K., and Reichlin, S.**, "Somatostatinoma", a somatostatin-containing tumour of the endocrine pancreas, *N. Engl. J. Med.,* 296, 963, 1977.
209. **Gerich, J. E., Lorenzi, M., Schneider, V., Karah, J. H., Riviera, J., Guilleman, R., and Forsham, P. H.**, Effects of somatostatin in plasma glucose and glucagon levels in human diabetes mellitus: pathophysiologic and therapeutic implications, *N. Engl. J. Med.,* 291, 544, 1974.
210. **Felig, P., Wahren, J., Sherwin, R., and Hendler, R.**, Insulin, glucagon and somatostatin in normal physiology and diabetes mellitus, *Diabetes,* 25, 1091, 1976.
211. **Bloom, S. R., Mortimer, C.H., Thorner, M. D., Besser, G. M., Hall, R., Gomez-Pan, A., Roy, V., Russel, R., Coy, D., Kastin, A., and Schally, A.**, Inhibition of gastrin and gastric acid secretion by growth-hormone release-inhibiting hormone, *Lancet,* 2, 1106, 1974.
212. **McGavran, M. H., Unger, R. H., Relant, L., Polk, H., Kilo, C., and Levin, M. E.**, A glucagon secreting α-cell carcinoma of the pancreas, *N. Engl. J. Med.,* 274, 1408, 1966.
213. **Croughs, R. J. M.**, Glucagonoma and A-cell hyperplasia, in *Clinics in Gastroenterology,* Vol. 3, Bonfils, S., Ed., W. B. Saunders, London, 1974, 609.
214. **Marks, V. and Samols, E.**, Insulinoma: natural history and diagnosis, in *Clinics in Gastroenterology,* Vol. 3, Bonfils, S., Ed., W. B. Saunders. 1974, 559.
215. **Malafosse, M.**, Carcinoid tumours; surgical problems, in *Clinics in Gastroenterology,* Vol. 3, Bonfils, S., Ed., W. B. Saunders, London, 1974, 711.
216. **Marks, V.**, G. P. Interview, *General Practitioner,* September 29, 1972.
217. **Polak, J. M., Pearse, A. G. E., Grimelius, L., and Marks, V.**, Gastrointestinal apudosis in obese hyperglycaemic mice, *Virchows Arch. B,* 19, 135, 1975.
218. **Jacobsen, H., Denmandt, A., Moody, A. J., and Sundby, F.**, Sequence analysis of porcine gut GLI-1, *Biochim. Biophys. Acta,* 493, 452, 1977.
219. **Becker, H. D., Reeder, D. D., and Thompson, J. C.**, Effect of glucagon on circulating gastrin, *Gastroenterology,* 65, 28, 1973.
220. **McGuigan, J. E. and Trudeau, W. L.**, Immunohistochemical measurement of elevated levels of gastrin in the serum of patients with pancreatic tumours of the Zollinger-Ellison variety, *N. Engl. J. Med.,* 278, 1308, 1968.
221. **Bloom, S. R. and Ogawa, O.**, Radioimmunoassay of human peripheral plasma secretin, *J. Endocrinol.,* 58, 24, 1973.
222. **Chey, W. Y., Tai, H., Rhodes, R., Lee, K. Y., and Hendricks, J.**, Radioimmunoassay of secretin: further studies, in *Gastrointestinal Hormones: Symp.,* Thompson, J. C., Ed., University of Texas Press, Austin, 1975, 269.
223. **Rehfeld, J. F.**, The predominating antral gastrin and intestinal cholecystokinin is their common COOH terminal tetrapeptide amide, in *Gastrins and the Vagus,* Rehfeld, J. F. and Amdrup, C., Eds., London, Academic Press, 1980.
224. **Rehfeld, J. F.**, Immunochemical studies on cholecystokinin. I. Development of sequence specific radioimmunoassays for porcine triacontatriapeptide cholecystokinin, *J. Biol. Chem.,* 253 (11), 4016, 1978.

225. **Bolton, A. E. and Hunter, W. M.,** The labelling of proteins to high specific activity by conjugation to a ^{125}I containing acylating agent, *Biochem, J.,* 133, 529, 1973.
226. **Ebert, R., Illmer, K., and Creutzfeldt, W.,** Release of gastric inhibitory polypeptide (GIP) by intraduodenal acidification in rats and humans and abolishment of the incretin effect of acid by GIP antiserum in rats, *Gastroenterology,* 76, 515, 1979.
227. **Morgan, L. M.,** Immunoassayable gastric inhibitory polypeptide: investigations into its role in carbohydrate metabolism, *Ann. Clin. Biochem.,* 16, 6, 1979.
228. **Creutzfeldt, W., Ebert, R., Willms, B., Frerichs, H., and Brown, J. C.,** Gastric inhibitory polypeptide (GIP) and insulin in obesity: increased response to stimulation and defective feedback control of serum levels, *Diabetologia,* 14, 15, 1978.
229. **Polak, J. M., Bishop, A. E., Bloom, S. R., Buchan, A. M. J., and Timson, C. M.,** The VIPergic innervation of the pancreas, *Scand. J. Gastroenterol.,* Suppl., 13, 49, 145, 1978.
230. **Bloom, S. R.,** VIP and watery diarrhoea VI, in *Gut Hormones,* Bloom, S. R., Ed., Churchill-Livingstone, Edinburgh, 1978, 583.
231. **Chang, R., Glaser, C. V., and Adelson, J. W.,** Structural studies on chymodenin, a hormone-like gastrointestinal peptide related to GIP and glucagon, *Scand. J. Gastroenterol.* Suppl. 13, 49, 36, 1978.
232. **Nelbach, M. E., Yates, G. B., and Adelson, J. W.,** Radioimmunoassay of chymodenin, with a new ^{125}I labelling method, *Scand. J. Gastroenterol.,* Suppl. 13, 49, 133, 1978.
233. **Krejs, G. J., Orci, L., Conlon, J. M., Ravazzola, M., Davis, G. R., Raskin, P., Collins, S. M., McCarthy, D. M., Baetens, D., Rubenstein, A., Aldor, T. A. M., and Unger, R. H.,** Somatostatinoma syndrome: biochemical, morphologic and clinical features, *N. Engl. J. Med.,* 301, 285, 1979.
234. **Wright, J., Abolfathi, A., Penman, E., and Marks V.,** Pancreatic somatostatinoma presenting with hypoglycaemia, *Clin. Endocrinol.,* 1980, in Press.
235. **Penman, G., Wass, J. A. H., Lund, A., Lowry, P. J., Stewart, J., Dawson, A. M., Besser, G. M., and Rees, L. M.,** Development and validation of a specific radioimmunoassay for somatostatin in human plasma, *Ann. Clin. Biochem.,* 16, 15, 1979.

Chapter 4

HORMONES OF THE ISLETS OF LANGERHANS

Norman R. Lazarus and K. J. O'Connor

TABLE OF CONTENTS

I. INTRODUCTION

Mammalian islets of Langerhans appear to be a treasure trove of peptide hormones. Insulin is found in the β cells, glucagon in α cells, and somatostatin in D cells.[1] Vasoactive intestinal peptide is also found in the islets but appears to be localized to nerve endings and probably functions as a neurotransmitter. Pancreatic polypeptide is detectable in the islets although the chief area of location, at least in humans, appears to be in the dorsal part of the duodenal lobe of the exocrine pancreas.[2] There is immunohistological evidence suggesting the presence in α cells of cholecystokinin, pancreozymin, and endorphin. However, it must be remembered that compared to radioimmunological estimations, immunocytochemical data is much less secure. Cross-reactivity of certain antibodies with related hormones cannot be excluded if the specificity of the antibody is not carefully titrated. Moreover, a false positive could be produced by hormones binding to receptor sites on the surface of the cell rather than being located intracellularly. This treatise will concern itself with the first four mentioned hormones. The presence of so many hormones in one organ poses interesting problems relating to their physiological interrelationships. Moreover, the siting of the islets of Langerhans in the midst of the exocrine pancreas suggests that exocrine and endocrine pancreatic functions may regulate each other.

II. ISLET EMBRYOLOGY

The cells of the islets of Langerhans are postulated to originate from neural-crest cells which migrate to the pancreas.[3] The hypothesis favors neural crest origin of the islets because of certain biochemical characteristics the islet cells share with other peptide secreting cells. These characteristics include: (1) fluorogenic amine content (A); (2) amine precursor uptake, i.e., 5-hydroxytryptophan and dehydroxyphenylalanine (P, U); and (3) amino acid decarboxylase (D). These three characteristics make up the acronym APUD. Other characteristics of these cells include high content of side chain carboxyl or carboxamine residues, high nonspecific esterase, high α-glycerophosphate menadione reductase, and specific immunofluorescence.

In order to test the theory, the entire ectoderm was removed from embryonic rats prior to formation of the neural-crest and the remaining mesoderm cultured for 11 days.[4] In those cases where a pancreas developed, insulin was detected or β cells were observed. These results suggest that islet cells do not originate from neural-crest cells. There is also other evidence that islet cells originate from gut endoderm during phylogeny and otogeny in different vertebrates: (1) Exo- and endocrine cells are found in the gut epithelium of *Amphioxus*;[5] (2) mixed cells containing both zymogen and endocrine granules are found in the pancreas of each class of adult Vertebrata; (3) there exists the possibility of acino-insular transformation in pancreas under experimental conditions; (4) there may be development of islet glucagon and insulin cells from the epithelium of small ducts and epithelial tubes during regeneration after partial pancreatectomy in different vertebrates.[6]

An islet-like cell has been described in the exocrine portion of the pancreas and named the "intermediate cell". These cells pose an interesting physiological problem.[7] Intermediate cells are present in both the exocrine and endocrine tissues of the normal pancreas of the rat, guinea pig, rhesus monkey, goat, chicken, and frog. Intermediate cells occur most frequently in the frog and less frequently in higher species. The widespread occurrence of these cells in the normal pancreas suggests that they represent, *ab initio,* a distinct category of cell and probably do not arise as a result of transformation of one form of specialized cell of the pancreas into another in response to metabolic demand. The feeding of dietary soya bean trypsin inhibitor to rats is accompanied by an increased prominence of acinar-intermediate cells and a reduction in the size of the islets of Langerhans.[8] Consistent with this reduction in islet cell size is a lowered insulin content of the pancreas and a lowered insulin secretion following intravenous glucose. However, release of insulin under the influence of secretin/pancreozymin is similar in both trypsin inhibitor fed rats and control rats. It is suggested that the intermediate cells secrete insulin since the granule of the intermediate cells is indistinguishable from that of the β cell granule. These cells also contain exocrine granules. That single cells are able to package and secrete different products can be demonstrated in the polymorphonuclear leucocyte[9] and in the thyroid.[10] Perhaps intermediate cells contribute to the pool of available insulin under those conditions in which there is some destruction of β cell function. Their exact role remains to be discovered.

III. EXOCRINE-ENDOCRINE PANCREATIC RELATIONSHIPS

A. Introduction

Structural studies on the vascular supply of the pancreas showed that the lobular arteries first send their blood supply into the capillary system of the islets which is then collected in efferent capillaries which form a network for the surrounding exocrine tissue.[11,12] This arrangement, together with the structural finding that exocrine acini in the vicinity of the islets differ from those at a greater distance, led to the conclusion that islet hormones influence the structure and function of the exocrine pancreas.[13] The work is hampered by an inability to measure the concentration of islet hormones that bathe the exocrine pancreas, and also by the variety of hormones that exist in the islets. Thus an integrated hypothesis of exocrine:endocrine function would have to include at a minimum insulin, glucagon, somatostatin, pancreatic polypeptide, vasoactive intestinal peptide, gut glucagon, and possibly adrenaline and acetylcholine. The following is an account of some effects of these hormones on the exocrine pancreas.

B. Insulin

Insulin is involved in the regulation of pancreatic protein synthesis and more specifically in the synthesis of amylase.[14,15] Only minimal amounts of insulin are necessary to maintain the normal function of the exocrine pancreas. Thus exocrine function is affected only in juvenile diabetics with severe deficiency but not in the adult onset type.[16,17]

There are a set of biochemical reactions which respond coordinately when the environment in which the mammalian cells are growing is altered.[18] These processes include transport into the cell of sugars, amino acids, and nucleotides, the synthesis of RNA and protein, and the degradation of protein. These reactions have been referred to as pleotropic. Pleotropic responses may be positive, i.e., an increase in substrate and macromolecular synthesis, or negative. A negative response includes decreased synthesis of RNA and protein, a decrease in polysome formation and protein degradation, and an inhibition of the uptake of nucleic acid precursors. Insulin produces a positive pleotropic response. It will stimulate the synthesis of protein and induce the enzyme tyrosine aminotransferase,[19] as well as other pleotropic reactions. The effect of insulin on the exocrine pancreas is probably part of this general pleotropic program and does not appear to explain the siting of the islets in the exocrine pancreas.

C. Glucagon

Glucagon was found to inhibit the metabolic effects of pancreaozymin, secretin, and caerulein both in animals and man.[20,21] This led to the introduction of glucagon for therapy of acute pancreatitis.[22] The treatment was not a success.[23] More recently, a 30-min infusion of glucagon (10 to 80 μg/hr) through an in vitro isolated pancreatic lobule preparation produced inhibition of protein synthesis and a discharge of stored and newly synthesized proteins with increased enzyme content. After 12 to 24 hours infusion a marked degranulation and decrease in enzyme content was observed.[24] These results are difficult to translate to the in vivo situation. The evidence that glucagon has a fundamental role in exocrine function is unconvincing.

D. Pancreatic Polypeptide

Bovine pancreatic polypeptide has both stimulatory and inhibitory actions on pancreatic secretion. Secretin induced secretion was augmented by low, (0.0125 to 0.025 $\mu g\ kg^{-1}$) and inhibited by high (1 to 50 $\mu g\ kg^{-1}$), doses of the peptide, given as a single bolus. Amylase and protein secretion were suppressed.[25]

E. Vasoactive Intestinal Peptide

This peptide causes electrolyte and water secretion by the pancreas where it also augments the response to secretin and to cholecystokinin octapeptide.[26]

F. Somatostatin

Somatostatin was administered in an intravenous bolus of 300 μg followed by a constant 60-min infusion of 5 $\mu g\ min^{-1}$, to 17 normal subjects. Somatostatin reduced the pancreatic enzyme secretion stimulated by pure cholecystokinin-pancreozymin. There was a rebound of enzyme secretion within 15 min after termination of the infusion, suggesting an outpouring of previously blocked secretory products. Bicarbonate secretion was not affected.[27]

The evidence that hormones secreted by islets of Langerhans affect exocrine pancreatic function in some special way appears to be unfounded. It should be remembered that at least three hormones are not exclusive to the islets, i.e., somatostatin, pancreatic polypeptide, and vasoactive intestinal peptide. Thus somatostatin is found in the stomach,[28] pancreatic polypeptide in the exocrine pancreas,[29] and vasoactive intestinal peptide was originally isolated from gut.[30] Reactions produced by infusion of these hormones under physiologic conditions need not necessarily be mediated via the islets. We suggest that the effects of insulin on the exocrine pancreas are part of that hormone's general pleotropic responses, while on the available evidence, glucagon does not appear to have a major exocrine function.

IV. THE BIOSYNTHESIS, CIRCULATING FORMS, AND PHYSIOLOGY OF ISLET HORMONES

A. Insulin

1. Biosynthesis

Pulse-chase experiments with insulinoma tissue and rat isolated islets showed that insulin is derived from a single chain precursor, proinsulin.[31,32] For the first 15 min only proinsulin is synthesized and then enzymic conversion causes accumulation of insulin. The proinsulin pool reaches a maximum after about 3 hr of synthesis in 17-m*M* glucose concentration. Biosynthesis is rate limiting below about 4 m*M* glucose concentration and only insulin accumulates.

The conversion of proinsulin to insulin exhibits a sharp pH optimum at pH 6.0 and a mixed exopeptidase and endopeptidase activity appears to be required to accomplish proinsulin to insulin conversion, although the enzymes responsible have not yet been purified.[33] Synthesis occurs on the ribosomes of the rough endoplasmic reticulum of the β cell and the precursor is then transferred via an energy-dependent process to the Golgi apparatus. Conversion seems to take place within the cell secretion granule and enzymic action may be terminated by co-crystallization of the products to form the dense crystalline granule core of the mature granules.

It is now well established that a precursor larger than proinsulin, preproinsulin, is the initial gene product in insulin biosynthesis.[34] The insulin messenger RNA contains coding for a further 23 amino acid residues attached to the amino end of proinsulin. The preproinsulin mRNA has been inserted into a bacterial plasmid by Ullrich et al.[35] and the total synthesis of insulin in bacteria has been accomplished.[36] The junction of the "pre"-peptide and proinsulin is an alanine-phenylalanine bond but a protease specific for this bond has not yet been identified. It has been proposed that the "pre" extension of a hormone may be necessary to confer correct charge properties to facilitate entry into the Golgi prior to granular packaging.

Proinsulin is a single chain polypeptide consisting of 81 residues in the ox and 84 in the pig. The B chain sequence of insulin comprises the amino end, and the insulin A chain, the carboxyl end of the proinsulin molecule. The two sequences are joined by the connecting peptide, which is about 30 residues long and consists of the C-peptide and two pairs of basic residues. About 5% of proinsulin is uncleaved and stored with insulin and C-peptide in the granule and thus proinsulin is subsequently released into the circulation with the insulin.

C-Peptide is stored in equimolar amounts with insulin and is secreted along with insulin and proinsulin.[37] C-Peptide primary structures in general show a higher rate of mutation acceptance than insulin. Bovine and porcine C-peptides differ by almost 35%. Although this may indicate that the only requirement for the peptide is to bridge the 8 to 10 Å gap between the C terminus of the B chain and the N terminus of the A chain, it is of interest that the C-peptide of the guinea pig is less substituted than its insulin, when compared with porcine insulin. The presence of the C-peptide sequence in proinsulin facilitates postribosomal disulfide bond formation but this is presumed to be a secondary event arising from the existence of proinsulin and not the peptide's raison d'être.

2. Circulating Forms

With the advent of immunoassay coupled with gel filtration it was demonstrated that the vast majority of circulating insulin in plasma has a molecular weight of 6000. A second insulin immunoreactive molecule in plasma, big insulin, representing about 5% of the total, is also present.[38] The ratio of big insulin to 6000-dalton insulin in the plasma of insulinoma patients is nearly always higher than the normal ratio and some insulinomas have been shown to secrete considerable quantities of newly synthesized proinsulin.[39] An insulin intermediate of slightly greater molecular weight than proinsulin has been reported in an insulinoma patient.[40] A peak of insulin-like immunoreactivity in plasma migrating on polyacrylamide gel electrophoresis between proinsulin and insulin has been reported and possibly represents partially cleaved proinsulin.[41]

3. Physiology

Insulin has a primary role in modulating fuel homeostasis in man and mammals.[42,43] Food intake stimulates insulin secretion. This leads to the uptake of nutrients by various tissues and their conversion to triglyceride, glycogen, and protein. In fasting, diminished insulin secretion causes these fuels to be mobilized.

a. Effect of Insulin on Carbohydrate Metabolism

Insulin lowers blood glucose by causing enhanced glucose entry into muscle adipose tissue and liver. Perhaps the action of insulin can best be demonstrated after the infusion into man of high (150 mg/min) and low (less than 150 mg/min) glucose.[44] Infusion of 150 mg/min glucose stimulates insulin secretion causing cessation of endogenous glucose production by the liver. Both the liver and peripheral tissues accelerate their uptake of glucose from the circulation. The nutrient is then stored either as glycogen in the liver or muscles or as fat in the fat cell. When glucose infusion rates below 150 mg/min are used, there is only a small change in blood sugar levels and a correspondingly small change in insulin secretion. Yet this small change is sufficient to decrease splanchnic glucose production promptly. There is no change in the peripheral utilization of glucose. Thus the action of insulin is both antiglycogenolytic and antigluconeogenic.

b. Effect of Insulin on Lipid Metabolism

The antilipolytic effect of insulin is not dependent upon the presence of glucose. It is mediated by levels of insulin that are below those required to effect peripheral uptake of glucose.[45,46] The molecular basis for this differential function has not been elicited. A fall in plasma insulin, mediated either by an increase in catecholamine response or by starvation, causes an increased rate of lipolysis. In starvation, the low insulin levels cause accelerated lipolysis and an increased free fatty acid load to the liver, followed by conversion of these fatty acids to ketone bodies and a decreased rate of ketone body utilization by insulin secretive tissues. Severe ketosis as seen in diabetic hyperglycemia, which occurs only when no insulin is secreted, is prevented in starvation by the small but detectable level of circulating insulin. Ketone bodies result primarily from the interplay of two organs — adipose tissue and liver, and two hormones — insulin and glucagon. Fatty acid oxidation and fatty acid biosynthesis are reciprocally controlled. A key intermediate in this balance is malonyl coA. With carbohydrate feeding, the flow of glucose to fatty acid is brisk and malonyl coA levels are high.[47] High malonyl coA suppresses carnitine acyltransferase I with the result that fatty acid oxidation is shut down. Thus malonyl coA causes a unidirectional flow of carbon from carbohydrate to fatty acid to triglyceride. In ketotic states, liver glycogen stores are depleted, malonyl coA concentrations fall, and the activity of carnitine acyltransferase I becomes derepressed. The concomitant rise in hepatic carnitine content produces maximal activity of the liver to oxidize fatty acids and to synthesize ketone bodies.

Ketone bodies are utilized as fuel sources by both the brain and heart, reducing the need for gluconeogenesis and thus sparing protein fuel. High levels of insulin will cause fatty acid synthesis from glucose and stimulate re-esterification of fatty acids to triglycerides in both the liver and adipose tissue.

c. Effect of Insulin on Protein Metabolism

Insulin accelerates the intracellular transport of amino acids, stimulates amino acid activation, facilitates the initiation of peptide chain formation, and modulates the composition of ribosomes and their aggregation into polysomes.[48] In fasting, where insulin levels are low, amino acids are mobilized from muscle tissue and enter the circulation. Thus increased mobilization of amino acids can be suppressed by small quantities of insulin. The predominant amino acids leaving the muscle are alanine and glutamine. These amino acids are the ones used for gluconeogenesis. The mechanisms of mobilization are unknown. There is some evidence that insulin can decrease proteolysis of liver proteins. A lack of insulin could generate amino acids from muscles by a similar breakdown.[48]

The biological effects of insulin are extensively described in Reference 48.

B. Glucagon

1. Biosynthesis

The biosynthesis of pancreatic glucagon proceeds via higher molecular weight intermediates. In vitro biosynthesis of 3500-dalton glucagon was demonstrated in the isolated perfused rat pancreas.[50] Subsequently, it was shown that a proglucagon of molecular weight about 20,000 daltons was initially synthesized, and that after about 2 hr the biosynthesis of 3500-dalton glucagon could be detected.[51] This proglucagon molecule was present in avian and mammalian pancreas and cross-reacted with glucagon antisera specific for the carboxyl end of glucagon.[51] It has been suggested that when proglucagon is cleaved to glucagon a 10,000-dalton fragment, produced from the remainder of the molecule, accumulates.[52] A glucagon-containing molecule of about 9000 accumulates before the appearance of 3500-dalton glucagon. The biosynthesis of this molecule does not exhibit the characteristics of a precursor when examined by pulse-chase experiments and probably represents a separate hormonal end product. The presence of 8000- and 12,000-dalton glucagons in pancreas has also been reported from immunoreactivity studies.[53] Similar sized glucagons are present in the gut and it has been suggested that all the entero- and pancreatic glucagons are present in both the gut and pancreas and that only the amounts of each differ.[54] A 12,000-dalton glucagon has been isolated and purified from porcine gut and it was shown by immunochemistry that a similar molecule was present in the pancreatic α cell.[55] The molecule consists of a 7500-dalton extension from the amino terminal end of glucagon with an eight amino acid extension from the carboxyl end. A 4500-dalton fragment containing glucagon isolated from an impure sample of pancreatic glucagon also had this same extension from the carboxyl end of glucagon. Pancreatic 20,000-dalton glucagon may be similarly extended. Another gut hormone, gastric inhibitory polypeptide, has strong primary structure similarities to glucagon. Fifteen of the first 26 amino acids of glucagon are present at the amino end of gastric inhibitory polypeptide and residues 34 to 41 of gastric inhibitory polypeptide show some analogies to the carboxyl extension of glucagon described above.

2. Circulating Forms

The 9000-dalton glucagon is present in the circulation and until further characterization the plasma form is referred to as big glucagon. Big glucagon in plasma is elevated in glucagonoma patients.[56] In normals the mean level of circulating big glucagon is about 12% of total glucagon immunoreactivity, but it is often undetectable. In glucagonoma patients the mean level is 47%. This is similar to the high circulating proinsulin level found in insulinoma patients. In chronic renal failure big glucagon represents a mean of 56% of circulating "carboxyl-end specific" glucagon immunoreactivity and it is suggested therefore that the kidneys play an important role in the metabolism of big glucagon.[57] Although 3500-dalton glucagon is the predominant immunoreactive glucagon species in diabetic ketoacidosis, big glucagon is elevated above normal values.[58] The immunoreactivity of the 20,000-dalton glucagon represents about 0.25% of total pancreatic glucagon immunoreactivity. It is stable to chaotropic agents and to elution at various pH values and cross-reacts linearly with nonspecific (that is gut glucagon cross-reacting) glucagon antibodies and also cross-reacts with "carboxyl-end specific" (that is pancreatic) glucagon antibodies. A glucagon molecule of about this molecular weight has been detected in the circulation of the dog.[51]

The majority of circulating glucagon immunoreactivity, as assessed by specific and nonspecific antisera, elutes with an approximate molecular weight of 160,000 and this material has been referred to as big plasma glucagon.[59] Big plasma glucagon levels seem to be maximal in the normal individual at approximately 29 to 65% of basal immunoreactive glucagon, although some sera have no big plasma glucagon. In glucagonoma patients big plasma glucagon is normal or reduced, with a mean of 14% of basal glucagon immunoreactivity. A family with excessive amounts of circulating big plasma glucagon has been reported. Examination of this big plasma glucagon by gel filtration showed that the major portion had a molecular weight of 160,000 eluting with the α and β globulins, but a second smaller peak was also present eluting between 10,000 to 20,000 molecular weight.[60] Big plasma glucagon levels have been reported as normal or reduced in chronic renal failure. Trypsination causes big plasma glucagon to increase slightly in immunoreactivity and this may be due to liberated immunoreactive fragments binding to larger proteins or perhaps uncovering of further immunoreactive determinants in the molecule.[61] The circulating level of big plasma glucagon does not change after administration of arginine to normal subjects whereas the 3500-dalton glucagon levels rise significantly.[60]

A glucagon species of about 2000 daltons has also been detected in plasma and may represent a degradation product of glucagon. High molecular weight components in serum which contain hormone immunoreactive determinants should be viewed as secreted hormonal forms with caution, since it has been found that radioiodinated insulin and growth hormone incubated with blood, in vivo or in vitro, resulted in the formation of high molecular weight aggregates.[62] Some of this higher molecular weight radioactivity was precipitable with antiserum to the hormone, indicating that binding of the hormone to circulating proteins was responsible.[63] Whether or not specific hormone binding proteins are involved in this phenomenon is unresolved.

3. Physiology

Glucagon was so named in 1923[64] and isolated in 1953.[65] More recently glucagon immunoreactive material was detected in the gut.[66] Gut glucagon as well as pancreatic glucagon can be secreted into the circulation under appropriate stimuli. This makes the unravelling of their physiological significance difficult. The problem has, to some extent, been resolved by the availability of antisera that can react specifically with pancreatic glucagon. However, an added complication is that gut glucagon has been detected in the islets of Langerhans.[67,68] The physiology of circulatory pancreatic glucagon is further complicated by the number of circulating species present — at least four.[69] The 9000-dalton material has been partially purified from bovine pancreas and has been show to stimulate the adenylate cyclase of mouse islets.[70] It also inhibited basal liver adenylate cyclase activity to the same extent that glucagon stimulated the enzyme. It had no effect on blood glucose concentrations in the rat. On a molar basis 9000-dalton glucagon was found to be equipotent with glucagon in stimulating lipolysis in isolated chicken fat cells. It can be predicted therefore that high levels of 9000-dalton glucagon should inhibit the glycogenolytic effect of glucagon.

The biological actions of 3500-dalton glucagon have been extensively investigated.

a. Hepatic Glycogenolysis

Glucagon is a potent hepatic glycogenolytic agent. Effects in vitro can be obtained with 1.5×10^{-11} *M*.[71] Maximal effects are found at 100 times this concentration. The onset of action is rapid and the effect brief, approximately 10 min.

b. Hepatic Gluconeogenesis

Glucagon stimulates the uptake of lactate by the liver and the conversion of lactate and pyruvate to glucose.[72] It also stimulates the uptake of amino acids from the circulation and their conversion to glucose. Although this effect of glucagon on lactate is pronounced, it cannot constitute an important mechanism for continuing support of the blood glucose level, since lactate itself is primarily derived from either glucose or glycogen. However, over the short term, there could be a substantial shift of lactate into glucose, thus providing a short-lived augmentation of circulating glucose.

Glucagon stimulates the uptake and catabolism of amino acids by the liver.[73] The effect of glucagon on gluconeogenesis from amino acid is relatively persistent (approximately 1 hr) unlike its effect on glycogenolysis. During starvation glucagon plays a role in the adaptation of the liver to increased gluconeogenesis from circulating amino acids. The mechanism of action is unclear.[74] Of these amino acids, alanine and glutamine account for approximately 50% of the amino acid release from muscle.[75] The glutamine released by muscle is taken up by the gut[76,77] which in turn releases alanine.[78] The gut may release twice as much alanine as muscle. Alanine thus accounts for half to two thirds of the glucose derived from amino acid in the liver. These experiments suggest that the gut plays a central role in adaptation to starvation. The regulators of gut adaptation are unknown.

c. Electrolyte and Renal Metabolism

In 1959 a diuretic effect of glucagon in dogs, accompanied by losses of sodium, potassium, and chloride, was described.[79,80] More recent studies have confirmed these findings and shown that magnesium, calcium, and phosphate were also excreted in increased amounts.[81] The mechanism is probably due to both an increase in glomerular filtration rate and an effect on tubular reabsorption.

d. Lipid Metabolism

Glucagon is able to stimulate glycerol and free fatty acid release from fat cells of various species at physiological concentrations. Much emphasis has been placed on the observations that in insulin-deprived diabetic subjects, the rise in plasma glucagon concentrations could be correlated with ketone body and fatty acid concentrations. Subsequent experiments showed that these latter effects could be inhibited by somatostatin. While such experiments may tend to provide a central role for glucagon it should be remembered that in pancreatectomized man (i.e., in the absence of glucagon) ketone body concentrations also rise on insulin deprivation, although at a slower rate than found in insulin deprived diabetic patients. In both cases, once insulin is present, glucagon infusion makes no difference to the ketone body concentration.

e. Glucagon and Diabetes

The circulating levels of glucagon are elevated in diabetes.[82] The secretion in response to a variety of stimuli is abnormal. Thus it was suggested that glucagon may play as important a part as insulin in the pathophysiology of diabetes.[83,84] However, hyperglycemia and hyperketonemia can develop in the absence of glucagon. Moreover there is no correlation between glucagon and circulating metabolite concentrations in this type of patient.[85] On the available evidence glucagon does not appear to play a major role in the metabolic disturbances of diabetes mellitus.[73,86]

f. Gut Glucagon

The striking aspect of gut glucagon is the lack of biological activity thus far demonstrated. The two biological effects claimed are glycogenolysis and stimulation of insulin release.[87] However, the only purified extracts thus far isolated do not cause insulin release.[88] The role of these hormones in regulation is unknown.

C. Somatostatin

1. Biosynthesis

Somatostatin is a tetradecapeptide which is synthesized and stored in the pancreatic

D cells. Work with fish islets has suggested that it is biosynthesized via an 8,000- to 15,000-dalton precursor.[89] However studies on somatostatin immunoreactive molecules in rat median eminence and neurohypophysis suggest the involvement of a somatostatin precursor of 25,000 daltons.[90]

The presence of big somatostatin-like immunoreactivity in the circulation has also been reported by a number of groups but there is, as yet, no general agreement on molecular size or stability to chaotropic agents.

2. Physiology

Somatostatin inhibits secretion of growth hormone, thyroid stimulating hormone, insulin, glucagon, gastrin, various pancreatic enzymes such as amylase, chymotrypsin, and trypsin, as well as pepsin and gastric acid.[27,91-93] Insulin release induced by arginine, glucagon, and tolbutamide is also inhibited.[94] Anatomically, in the islets of Langerhans, the somatostatin cells lie between the insulin and glucagon producing cells. This suggests that in vivo somatostatin has a role in regulating minute-by-minute output of both insulin and glucagon,[95] although experiments on cultured islets with somatostatin antisera suggest that glucagon is under greater somatostatin control than is insulin.[96] The mechanism of such an action is unknown. There is both hypertrophy and hyperplasia of somatostatin D cells in diabetes.[97] The physiological significance of this is unknown. It is possible to obtain somatostatin immunoreactivity in the perfusate of an isolated dog pancreas if the pancreas is perfused with 10 μg/mℓ of glucagon or 400 ng/mℓ of insulin for 40 to 100 min.[98] The application of these findings to normal physiological regulation is difficult to accomplish.

D. Vasoactive Intestinal Peptide

Vasoactive intestinal peptide is related in structure to glucagon, secretin, and gastric inhibitory peptide and has many biological activities. It causes vasodilation, systemic hypotension, increased cardiac output, enhancement of respiration, stimulation of glycogenolysis, and relaxation of several smooth muscle organs.[99-101] In rabbit ileal mucosa, vasoactive intestinal peptide (20 μg/mℓ) caused a prompt fivefold increase in cyclic AMP levels. An increase in cyclic AMP was observed at a concentration of 0.1 μg/mℓ with maximal levels reached at 2.0 μg/mℓ. Vasoactive intestinal peptide, when added to the serosal surface of a rabbit isolated ileum, caused net secretion of Na^+ and Cl^-. Net Cl^- secretion exceeded net Na^+ secretion. These effects are similar to those seen with cholera toxin. It is possible that the stimulatory effect of vasoactive intestinal peptide on adenylate cyclase is related to the pathogenesis of diarrhea in patients with the pancreatic cholera syndrome.[102,103] Patients with the syndrome have high circulating levels of vasoactive intestinal peptide.[104]

Vasoactive intestinal peptide probably has a role as a transmitter and/or modulator of synaptic function in the brain.[105] Its mechanism of action is unknown. It is possible that vasoactive intestinal peptide has a similar role in the islets of Langerhans. In experiments on the perfused cat pancreas it was found that vasoactive intestinal peptide at 0.5 to 5.0 μg/mℓ caused release of both insulin and glucagon.[106] The effect on glucagon release was greater than on insulin release. The glucagon response to vasoactive intestinal peptide could be blocked by increasing the glucose in the perfusate. Other workers have also found that vasoactive intestinal peptide (50 ng/kg/min for 10 min) causes increased insulin and glucagon secretion.[107] Since this result was not inhibited by propranolol it is suggested that the effect is not mediated via the β-adrenergic receptor system. Vasoactive intestinal peptide at 0.6 to 9.6 nmol/kg/hr has a secretin-like effect on pancreatic bicarbonate excretion.[108]

E. Pancreatic Polypeptide

Pancreatic polypeptide is present in exocrine and endocrine pancreatic tissue.[29] The fasting circulating level of polypeptide is 43 ± 4 pmol/ℓ.[109] In one series of experiments the polypeptide response was biphasic in normal subjects fed a protein meal. There was an eightfold increase within the first 30 min, followed by a secondary prolonged increase. The polypeptide concentration had not returned to basal within 5 hr. In another series the polypeptide response to ingestion of 500 g of cooked ground beef appears monophasic. Again the level was sustained for at least 6 hr. The intravenous infusion of a mixture of 10 essential amino acids, although raising polypeptide concentration was not nearly as effective as a protein meal. Ingestion of protein also caused release of polypeptide in elderly patients with pernicious anemia. Thus hydrochloric acid does not appear to be necessary for the protein effect. Polypeptide secretion was studied in duodenal ulcer patients who had undergone vagotomy.[109] After vagotomy the rapid response of the polypeptide to a meal was eliminated and the secondary response significantly reduced. Human polypeptide appears to be under vagal control. However another group of workers could show no difference in polypeptide secretion between duodenal ulcer patients and postvagotomy patients, where all groups were given a standard hospital lunch. Insulin hypoglycemia, while able to produce a polypeptide response in duodenal ulcer patients, could not cause secretion in those patients that had been vagotomized. Intravenous administration of glucose, amino acids, or fat did not cause polypeptide release. Thus it appears that oral but not intravenous nutrients cause release and that the vagus plays a role under specific physiological conditions.

Acute hypoglycemia, fasting, and exercise are associated with increases of polypeptide in a manner somewhat analogous to glucagon and growth hormone.

In diabetes the mean basal plasma level of polypeptide is elevated, in particular in the more severe maturity onset type requiring insulin and in the juvenile onset type.

Perhaps more intriguing than the stimuli to polypeptide secretion is its physiological role. Oral protein nutrient causes the basal level to rise to over 500 pg/mℓ. These levels are maintained for over 5 hr — i.e., until the next meal, where the ingestion of food will presumably cause the level to remain up. Thus throughout the day the circulating level of polypeptide is probably raised. Unfortunately, circadian rhythms of the peptide have not yet been published. Thus polypeptide secretion has several notable features: (1) the ingestion of protein causes high circulatory hormone levels; and (2) the hormone remains high for long periods and at least in normal patients, does not demonstrate the fluctuations in plasma levels that may be expected, for example with insulin or glucagon.

V. HORMONE RECEPTORS

A. Insulin

First studies aimed at identifying an insulin receptor were carried out in the fifties.[110] Investigations have now established the existence on cell plasma membranes of receptors to nearly all the known peptide hormones.[111-113] Rat liver insulin receptors have been purified by insulin-agarose affinity chromatography. The insulin receptor so purified has two polypeptide components with apparent molecular weight of approximately 135,000 and 45,000 daltons, respectively. It is thought that the receptor is composed of two high molecular weight subunits and two low molecular weight subunits associated by disulfide bonds.[114] While almost the whole thrust of hormone receptor studies has been directed towards the plasma membrane, there are indications that other sites of hormone action should be considered. Insulin binding sites on the Golgi were described in 1973,[115] while more recently receptors on the nuclear membrane have been found.[116] The role of these receptors is unclear. Most of the acute response of tissues to insulin can be shown to be due to interaction of the hormone at the plasma membrane. Perhaps the long term actions of insulin, e.g., enzyme induction, may be mediated by these intracellularly localized receptors.

The interaction of insulin with its receptor is complex. Analysis of insulin receptor interactions produces curvilinear Scatchard plots. It has been suggested that these plots can be explained by a single class of binding site which displays negative cooperativity in relation to the binding of insulin; i.e., the affinity of the receptor for insulin decreases with increasing levels of saturation.[117] An alternate explanation advanced is that the curvilinearity is due to the mobility of the insulin receptor in the plane of the membrane.[118] Whatever the explanation, recent data has shown that insulin is internalized after binding to its receptor; thus modifications to both theories will probably be required in order to incorporate all the experimental findings.[119] Exactly where the insulin goes and what its internal function is, is unknown. Some appears to end up in lysosomes. Perhaps the internalized insulin could be interacting with the nuclear receptors described above.

The nature of the signal by which insulin triggers its biological actions remains obscure. Searches for second messengers, e.g., cyclic AMP, have been fruitless. The effect of insulin on Ca^{2+} metabolism has also been investigated with similarly unproductive results.

A direct outcome of these studies on insulin/receptor interactions has been the definition of syndromes which produce symptomatology as a result of some factor interfering with the ability of the hormone to bind to its receptor. Such an interference is found with the syndrome associated with *Acanthosis nigricans*.[120] In this syndrome patients present with a unique form of diabetes accompanied by extreme insulin resistance. Their basal and glucose-stimulated insulin levels are 10 to 100 times normal. In order to regulate blood glucose, patients receive up to a thousand times the normal insulin dose. Investigation of the plasma of these patients reveals the presence of a protein, probably an immunoglobulin, that inhibits the binding of insulin to its receptor. It is probable that the antibody occupies the receptor site directly, or perhaps sterically hinders insulin binding. The net result is insulin resistance. Thus *Acanthosis nigricans* falls into the category of endocrine diseases whose symptomatology arises from the production of auto-antibodies, e.g., myasthenia gravis and Graves' disease.

Insulin exercises a regulating influence on the concentration of its receptor. Evidence comes from three sources: the in vitro regulation of receptors in tissue culture;[121] the in vivo control of receptors in genetically obese mice;[122,123] and from human experiments using lymphocytes and adipose tissue.[124-126] Insulin receptors are below normal in obesity and at one time it was thought that the low level of receptors may be responsible for the production of the obesity syndrome. However, most obese people have high insulin levels and it is now thought that the amount of insulin receptors is an adaptive change to the raised insulin level, i.e., the receptor alteration is a secondary and not a primary event. It should also be remembered that not all obese persons are hyperinsulinemic.[126] Thus, while receptor number plays a role in insulin insensitivity in obesity, there is also evidence of alterations of sensitivity without receptor changes. Therefore a direct correlation between receptor number and insulin sensitivity is not always apparent and the physiological relationship of receptor regulation and insulin sensitivity is not wholly clear.

B. Glucagon

Glucagon receptors on cell plasma membranes of various tissues have been well defined.[113] There seems to be general agreement that glucagon exerts its biological actions by the coupling of its receptor to adenylate cyclase, causing catalysis. Guanosine triphosphate is needed for the activation of the adenylate cyclase. The mechanism of the guanosine triphosphate activation is not completely clear and is made more difficult to assess because guanosine triphosphate seems to act in a different way to its nonmetabolizable analogues, β-α-methylene guanosine triphosphate and guanosylyl amidodiphosphate.

Various models for the interaction between receptor and enzyme have been put forward. The original model[127] postulated a permanent association between the two components, in which the catalytic unit is activated by conformational changes originating in the receptor, when the hormone is bound. The realization that membrane proteins may be able to undergo fast lateral diffusion has suggested a model in which the uncoupled receptor and the adenylate cyclase moieties can migrate independently in the plane of the membrane. Hormone binds to the plasma membrane receptor which then locks with the catalytic unit causing activation. A slightly different model has been proposed by Houslay et al.[128] In this model receptors and catalytic units are present in the membrane in approximately equal numbers. On binding glucagon, the receptor interacts with the catalytic subunit forming a large complex. After removal and readdition of glucagon, a new population of complexes are formed, which contain hybrids of active and inactive complexes of the catalytic subunit of the enzyme and of the receptors. This model is more complicated than those previously put forward. Further experimental results are awaited.

C. Vasoactive Intestinal Peptide

Receptors to vasoactive intestinal peptide have been described in rat and chicken livers.[129] These vasoactive intestinal peptide sites are distinct from glucagon. Secretin can inhibit vasoactive intestinal peptide binding to these receptors but only at concentrations a hundred times that of vasoactive intestinal peptide. Vasoactive intestinal peptide appears to activate cellular processes by also stimulating the adenylate cyclase enzyme. Probably the most interesting aspect of these findings is why receptors for vasoactive intestinal peptide exist on liver plasma membranes when the peptide is located only at nerve endings and probably functions as a neurotransmitter.

VI. CLINICAL APPLICATIONS OF IMMUNOASSAY

A. Insulin (Islet Cell Tumors)

Probably the only clinical condition in which plasma insulin needs to be measured daily is in islet cell tumor patients.

Patients with islet cell tumors generally present with symptomatology related to hypoglycemia due to inappropriate insulin release. Because the tumor is not under physiological control, insulin secretion does not diminish during fasting and hypoglycemia results. Secondly, there is an exaggerated response of the tumor to either leucine, glucagon, or tolbutamide.

When presented with a patient with suspected insulin-secreting islet cell tumor, first establish that the patient is hypoglycemic (i.e., having a blood glucose concentration below 40 mg%). Secondly, discover whether the hypoglycemia occurs on fasting or is provoked by a specific stimulus, e.g., alcohol. If hypoglycemia occurs on fasting the condition may be due to insulin secretion by an islet cell tumor or to one of a number of conditions not associated with endogenous insulin secretion.[130]

The following is a protocol to determine insulin secretion due to an islet cell tumor.

Admit the patient into hospital. Place on a diet containing 300 g carbohydrate for 3 days. On the morning of the fourth day begin a 72-hr fast. This produces a fall in blood glucose in normal adults to around 50 mg% at 72 hr. The plasma insulin from 48 hr on should be unmeasureable. If the blood glucose does not fall below 50 mg%, islet cell tumor can be excluded as a diagnosis. In order to avoid the consequences of hypoglycemia, blood glucose concentrations should be monitored often during the fast. A sensible precaution is to set up a continuous intravenous infusion of saline during the test period. This allows for frequent blood sampling and for prompt administration of glucose and/or glucagon should the occasion demand. Clinical signs of hypoglycemia, e.g., diminished mental skill or hyperactive tendon reflexes, should be watched for. If insulin is present in normal or elevated concentrations when blood glucose is below 40 mg%, the diagnosis of an islet cell tumor is most likely. A negative insulin response may not exclude islet cell tumor. It may be necessary to fast a patient on several occasions before a raised insulin level is found. When such a level is found this again confirms the diagnosis.

It is most important to carry out the hypoglycemic tests under standard conditions since many factors such as previous carbohydrate intake can influence the insulin response, especially within the first 6 hr of the test.

Another test is the response of the tumor to tolbutamide, glucagon, or leucine. Islet cell tumor patients (approximately 50%) will respond to these secretogogues with an exaggerated insulin response. The response to each test substance is independent of the response to another test substance.[131] For this reason a negative test to any one substance is not indicative of the absence of an insulin secreting tumor. Thus all three tests should be performed in suspected islet cell tumor patients. It should be borne in mind that positive leucine tests can arise in children who have an idiopathic spontaneous hypoglycemic reaction to ingested leucine. In the tolbutamide test 1 g is given i.v. Blood samples are withdrawn every 5 min for 30 min. The patient must be closely watched for hypoglycemic symptoms and appropriate treatment (see above) should be to hand.

Another test that may be used is the determination of the amount of proinsulin contributing to the circulating immunoreactive insulin. This is done by fractionation of 2 mℓ of plasma on a Sephadex® G-50 fine column (0.5 × 15 cm) in albumin-veronal buffer pH 8.6. In normals the fraction of immunoreactive material emerging in the proinsulin area should be less than 30% of that eluting in the insulin area. Many islet cell tumor patients have proinsulin-like material in excess of 30% of the total circulating immunoreactivity.[132,133]

A therapeutic trial with diazoxide may also be useful. Patients with islet cell tumors improve markedly when given diazoxide, an insulin release inhibitor. This test may be useful when other tests are inconclusive. Hypoglycemia due to the secretion of noninsulin substances will not respond to diazoxide.

The treatment for insulin secreting islet tumors is surgical removal although streptozotocin has been used successfully.

B. Glucagon

The diagnosis of glucagonoma is made with the pancreatic specific glucagon immunoassay. A random glucagon level of 1000 pg/mℓ or more after an overnight fast is suggestive of a tumor.[134,135]

C. Pancreatic Polypeptide

In 33 patients with endocrine tumors of the pancreas, 18 had very high circulating levels of pancreatic polypeptide. Thus immunoassay may be of use in the diagnosis of pancreatic endocrine tumors.[136]

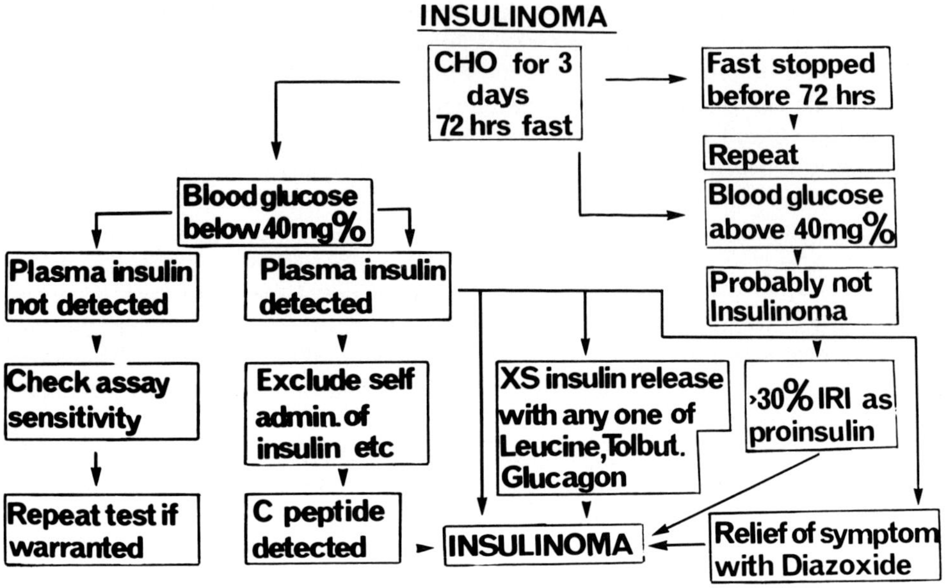

FIGURE 1. Flow diagram for the diagnosis of insulin-secreting islet cell tumors.

D. Vasoactive Intestinal Peptide

High levels of circulating vasoactive intestinal peptide produce the Vernor-Morrison syndrome.[102] These patients are characterized by having hypochlorhydria and severe and often fatal watery diarrhea. The condition is cured by the removal of the tumor.[137]

E. Circulating Serum C-Peptide

Measurement of C-peptide is useful in the diagnosis of insulinoma in those patients in which the presence of circulating antibodies to insulin interfere with the insulin assay (e.g., diabetes).[138] The assay can also be used in the diagnosis of insulinoma in patients without anti-insulin antibodies. The suppression of insulin secretion during the fasting hypoglycemia test can be monitored by observation of serum C-peptide concentrations. Insulinoma patients will show diminished or absent C-peptide suppression when compared to normals.[139] Another interesting use is in the diagnosis of self-induced hypoglycemia by exogenous insulin injection. These patients will have high insulin levels with low or unmeasureable C-peptide levels.[140]

It has been found that diabetic patients with appreciable retention of insulin secretion, as determined by C-peptide levels, are relatively "stable". Patients with complete loss of insulin secretory ability frequently have "brittle diabetes" as measured by the ability to control blood sugar and episodes of hypoglycemia and/or ketoacidosis. Thus the detection of circulating C-peptide in a patient presenting symptoms of brittle diabetes suggests that factors other than insulin deficiency may be contributory to the complications.[141] The use of the assay is limited by the nonavailability of sufficient quantities of human C-peptide.

VII. PANCREATIC HORMONE ASSAYS

A. Introduction

A prerequisite for the study of all hormones is the availability of an accurate and specific assay. Hormones may be assayed by the following methods: bioassay in vivo and in vitro; cytochemical assay; radioimmunoassay; enzyme immunoassay; and radioreceptor assay.

B. Insulin

1. Bioassay in Vivo

Insulin is bioassayed in vivo by the mouse convulsion assay.[142] Standard insulin solutions are injected intraperitoneally into mice and the time taken for the mice to convulse from hypoglycemia is recorded. Normal blood sugar is then restored by a glucose injection. A curve is obtained by plotting dose against convulsion time. Convulsion times for unknown insulin samples are obtained and by reference to the standard curve, concentrations determined. The sensitivity of the method is low, 2.5 μg/mℓ.

2. Bioassay in Vitro

The stimulation of the uptake of ^{3}H-glucose into glycerol is used as an in vitro bioassay of insulin.[143] The method is sensitive, responding to 50 pg/mℓ insulin. Fat cells are prepared from rat epididymal fat pad by collagenase digestion and incubated with ^{3}H-glucose for 1.5 hr at 37° under carbogen, in the presence of either insulin standards, ranging from 0.05 ng/mℓ to 2 ng/mℓ, or the unknown samples. A toluene scintillant is added at the end of the incubation. Because the lipid, but not the aqueous, unincorporated radioactivity dissolves in toluene, the toluene layer can be counted directly. By using polythene scintillation vials as incubation vessels, no transfer of medium need take place.

C. Glucagon

1. Bioassay in Vivo

Glucagon is measured in vivo by estimating the blood sugar rise in cats, since these animals are extremely sensitive to the hyperglycemic effect of glucagon.[144] The samples to be tested are incubated in 0.35% cysteine for 16 hr at pH 7.5 to inactivate insulin and then injected into the femoral vein. Blood is sampled immediately prior to injection and at 5 min intervals, for 25 min after injection. A standard glucagon injection is then given to the same animal and the blood sampled in the same manner. The ratio of the maximal glucose rise after the standard glucagon dose to the rise from the unknown is directly proportional to the glucagon content of the unknown sample. The assay is sensitive down to 100 ng.

2. Bioassay in Vitro

Lipolysis in the chicken fat cell is exquisitely sensitive to stimulation by glucagon.[145] Unlike the assays described for insulin or the in vivo glucagon assay, this assay appears to be highly specific for glucagon. Approximately 10 to 20 g of fat is removed from around the gizzard of 12-week-old male chickens. Fat cells are isolated by collagenase digestion. The cells are diluted to approximately 50 mg lipid per milliliter and then 500 μℓ of cells added to 1 mℓ of Kreb's Ringer phosphate buffer pH 7.4 supplemented with human serum albumin (35 g/ℓ). The glucagon standards or unknowns are now added. After 1.5 hr incubation at 37°C under carbogen, the medium is centrifuged at 100 g for 2 min and the cells aspirated from the surface. Protein is precipitated from 1 mℓ of the medium by incubation at 90°C for 2 min, followed by centrifugation. The supernatant is then assayed for glycerol content by the glycerokinase method, using a commercially available kit. Lipolysis in chick isolated fat cells is unresponsive to insulin in concentrations as high as 4 μg/mℓ and little response is shown to other hormones, used at their physiological concentrations.[146] Stimulation of lipolysis by glucagon is dose response related from less than 0.25 ng/mℓ to greater than 5 μg/mℓ.

D. Vasoactive Intestinal Peptide (VIP)

1. Bioassay in Vivo

The bioassay used in the isolation of VIP was to measure the systemic vasodilator action of the hormone in the dog.[147] Intra-arterial infusion of 40 ng/kg of the hormone increased femoral arterial flow by 50%.

VIP is a strong stimulant of water and bicarbonate secretion from the avian pancreas and this property may be worthy of examination as a potential bioassay for the hormone utilizing chicken pancreas slices.

E. Pancreatic Polypeptide

1. Bioassay in Vitro

No in vivo assay for this hormone has been reported. In our laboratories pancreatic polypeptide is bioassayed in vitro by inhibition of basal or caerulein stimulated amylase production from rabbit pancreas slices. The amylase is assayed by estimating the amount of starch hydrolyzed in a given time versus the amount of hydrolysis obtained with a known amount of purified amylase.

F. Somatostatin

1. Bioassay in Vitro

In vitro, somatostatin is bioassayed by the inhibition of growth hormone release, as measured by immunoassay, from dispersed rat pituitary cells in monolayer culture.[148] The method has been shown to be sensitive from 2 ng/mℓ up to 6 μg/mℓ.

VIII. CYTOCHEMICAL ASSAY

Cytochemical assay is a form of hormone bioassay which has not yet been developed for pancreatic hormones, but assays exist for corticotropin (ACTH)[149] and luteinizing hormone.[150] The basis of the assay is to combine the hormone effect on a biochemical parameter in the target cell with a histological assay measured by scanning microdensitometry. Luteinizing hormone can be estimated at 5 μU/mℓ which is more sensitive than the radioimmunoassay of the hormone. This type of assay has a considerable advantage over radioimmunoassay in that only biologically active forms of the hormone are measured.

IX. RADIOIMMUNOASSAY

A. Introduction

The immunoassays of the various pancreatic hormones are not described in great detail. For more information on how to set up an immunoassay as well as the theories behind the method, the reader is referred to several recently available texts.[151,152] The basic methodology of insulin and glucagon immunoassays is described and some of the major difficulties pertaining to specific hormone assays are highlighted.

B. Insulin Immunoassay

Radioimmunoassay revolutionized the measurement of hormones, both protein and nonprotein. The assay is based on competition of the hormone in the sample and hormone labeled with radioactivity for antibody raised against the hormone. An equilibrium is established, and bound and free hormone is then separated by precipitation of the antibody with an anti-gamma globulin antibody or by absorption of the unbound hormone into charcoal. Insulin was the first hormone for which the assay method was developed. The assay enables estimation of insulin at the lowest concentrations encountered in vivo.

Insulin immunoassay is carried out in a buffer of the following composition: potassium dihydrogen orthophosphate 5.4 g, bovine serum albumin 5 g, sodium chloride 9 g, thiomersal 0.243 g, made up to one liter with water adjusted to pH 7.4 with 5 *M* sodium hydroxide.

Human insulin standards are prepared by serial dilution from a stock solution stored in aliquots at −20°C. A standard range from 0.1 to 10 ng/mℓ is constructed and assayed in triplicate.

1. Preparation of Radioiodinated Insulin

The method of Hunter and Greenwood[153] is employed to iodinate 5 μg of insulin standard using chloramine-T. Sodium ^{125}I-iodide (1.5 mg) is added to 5 μg insulin, and 15 μℓ freshly prepared chloramine-T (3.5 mg/mℓ in borate buffer pH 8.0) is added. After exactly 10 sec 50 μℓ of sodium metabisulfite (9.5 mg/mℓ) and 100 μℓ of 6% bovine serum albumin are added. The reaction mixture is immediately gel filtered on a 10-cm column of Sephadex® G-25 coarse in borate buffer supplemented with 1% bovine serum albumin and 1 mℓ fractions are collected. The void volume tube obtained from the radioactivity profile is diluted to 10 mℓ and gel filtered on a 2.5 × 40 cm column of Sephadex® G-50 superfine eluted with immunoassay buffer. The peak radioactive insulin fractions are pooled and immunoassayed for insulin content using ^{131}I-insulin prepared in exactly the same manner. (The insulin content of the ^{131}I-insulin is approximated by calculation.)

2. Insulin Antisera

Insulin antisera can be raised in guinea pigs by immunization with insulin standard in Freunds' adjuvant but high affinity antisera are readily available from commercial sources. The antiserum is used at a dilution which will bind 30% of 0.25 ng of ^{125}I-insulin.

3. Assay Procedure

Standard or plasma (or serum) sample (0.1 mℓ of each) is pipetted into disposable 3-mℓ polystyrene tubes and 0.1 mℓ of antiserum is added and incubated at 4°C for 4 hr. Next 0.1 mℓ of ^{125}I-insulin (0.25 ng) is added and the assay incubated for a further 16 hr.

4. Separation of Antibody-Bound from Free Hormone

Separation of antibody-bound from free hormone is generally achieved by addition of a rabbit antiguinea pig gamma globulin antiserum to precipitate the insulin antibodies. Then 0.1mℓ of a suitable dilution of the second antibody is added and incubated for 4 hr at 4°C. The tube contents are filtered through Millipore® filters (0.45 μ) using a vacuum line and the tubes and filters washed twice with 3 mℓ of horse serum diluted 50% with assay buffer. The filters are then counted for radioactivity.

5. Treatment of Data

The standard curve data is transformed to a straight line plot by a logit transformation

$$\left(\log_e \left[\frac{\dfrac{\text{counts in the standard}}{\text{counts in the blank}}}{1 - \dfrac{\text{counts in the standard}}{\text{counts in the blank}}}\right] \text{ v. } \log_{10} \text{ dose}\right)$$

and the insulin levels in the sample read off in ng/mℓ (25 μU ≡ 1 ng).

C. Glucagon Immunoassay

Considerable difficulties were encountered in establishing a glucagon immunoassay. The difficulties are principally that glucagon is of low antigenicity due to the small molecular weight of the protein and because of the close similarity in primary structure among mammalian and avian glucagons. Conjugation of glucagon to larger molecules or polymerization of glucagon enables production of glucagon antisera, but glucagon-like immunoreactivity from the gut cross-reacts with the vast majority of these antisera. A small number of glucagon antisera have been raised against crystalline glucagon alone. Only antisera specific for the carboxyl end of 3500 molecular weight glucagon measure predominantly glucagon of pancreatic origin and such antisera are not at all common. Two further difficulties in the immunoassay of glucagon are to obtain immunologically active radiolabeled glucagon, usually ^{125}I-glucagon, and to overcome the biodegradation of glucagon in biological fluids. The radiolabeling problem has largely been solved and high quality labeled antigen can be obtaned from commercial sources. Glucagon is radioiodinated by the chloramine-T method of Hunter and Greenwood.[153] Iodination by the lactoperoxidase enzymic method has also been used.[154] A third method that is available for hormone radioiodination utilizes the Bolton-Hunter reagent, a radioiodinated phenol attached by a propyl chain to a succinimidyl residue.[155] This molecule can be conjugated to protein amino groups under very mild conditions. The biological degradation of glucagon can be reduced considerably by exercising extreme care in keeping the samples ice cold during collection and by storing them at −20°C and by addition of a proteolytic inhibitor preparation such as Trasylol® to all samples and to the assay buffer. Glucagon can be estimated at a concentration of 50 pg/mℓ which is thought to be very close to basal circulating levels of pancreatic glucagon.[152]

1. Buffer Composition

The assay buffer consists of potassium dihydrogen orthophosphate, 5.44 g; human serum albumin, 1 g; thiomersal, 0.25 g; Trasylol® aprotinin, 200 kallikrein inactivator units (KIU) per mℓ; sodium chloride, 6 g; the solution is made up to a liter and adjusted to pH 7.4 with sodium hydroxide.

2. Glucagon Standards

A standard range is constructed from 0.5 mg/mℓ aliquots of bovine or porcine glucagon dissolved in 0.001 *N* hydrochloric acid which has been stored at −80°C for no longer than 3 months. Serial dilution is used to produce standards from 31.25 pg/mℓ to 2 ng/mℓ.

3. Radioiodinated Glucagon

Glucagon is a difficult protein to iodinate. The initial procedure is the same as for insulin but only 7 sec exposure to free iodine is allowable and highly purified human serum albumin free of proteases must be substituted for bovine serum albumin. The reaction mixture is then immediately purified on QAE Sephadex® A-25 ion exchanger eluted with glucagon assay buffer. Iodinated glucagon is not bound by the column whereas free iodide is. The labeled glucagon is then gel filtered on Sephadex® G-50 in glucagon assay buffer. Radioiodinated glucagon should not be used after 1 month and repurification after 2 weeks is advisable. The labeled hormone should be stored in aliquots at −80°C.

4. Antisera Production

Two main types of glucagon antisera can be produced — glucagon carboxyl end specific which cross-reacts only with pancreatic glucagon (and a small proportion of gut glucagon) and amino end and glucagon central portion antibodies which cross-react with pancreatic and gut glucagons.

Glucagon antisera production is difficult. The hormone is usually conjugated to itself or a larger molecule such as bovine serum albumin to increase its antigenicity. The great majority of antisera produced are gut glucagon cross-reacting antisera. Pancreatic specific antisera are rarely produced. One or two are available from commercial sources at considerable expense.

5. Assay Procedure

To 0.1 mℓ of standard or plasma sample 0.1 mℓ of antiserum sufficient to bind 30% of 30 pg of radioiodinated glucagon is added. The plasma sample must be prepared from blood collected into a heparinized tube surrounded by ice and containing 0.1 mℓ of Trasylol® proteolytic inhibitor (2000 KIU) for every mℓ of blood. Immediately, 0.1 mℓ of radioiodinated glucagon (30 pg) is added and the assay incubated for 48 hr at 4°C.

6. Separation of Antibody-Bound from Free Glucagon

Separation of antibody-bound glucagon from free glucagon is achieved using dextran-coated charcoal. Sheep serum (0.1 mℓ) is added to all tubes so that sufficient protein is present to saturate any gamma globulin-binding capability of the charcoal. Next 0.5 mℓ of a mixture of activated charcoal (0.5%) and Dextran T-70 (0.25%) in 0.2 *M* glycine, which has been adjusted to pH 7.4 with sodium hydroxide, is added to each tube. After 45 min at 4°C the tubes are centrifuged at 1000 g for 20 min and 0.7 mℓ of the supernatants counted for radioactivity.

7. Treatment of Data

The data is treated the same as insulin immunoassay data; however, extra assay controls are necessary. Nonspecific binding tubes should be used for each plasma sample (antiserum substituted by buffer) and subtracted from each sample. A refinement to increase sensitivity is to use plasma freed of glucagon by incubation with charcoal in place of the assay buffer.

8. Immunoassay of Gut Glucagon

Antisera have been raised that give identical cross-reactivity with purified gut glucagon-like immunoreactivity and 3500-mol wt pancreatic glucagon. A subtraction assay is thus possible to estimate separately circulating glucagon-like immunoreactivity of gut and pancreatic origin. Glucagon immunoassay results of this type cannot be absolutely quantified, however, due to the production of a small amount of pancreatic type glucagon from the gut,[156] and gut type glucagon from the pancreas.[67,68]

D. Pancreatic Polypeptide Immunoassay

Pancreatic polypeptide immunoassay has now been established in a few laboratories[157,158] and does not appear to present any major difficulties but there is insufficient information on the heterogeneity of the hormone and on its physiology to be certain that meaningful results are being obtained.

E. Somatostatin and C-Peptide Immunoassay

Radioimmunoassay of somatostatin and C-peptide of proinsulin introduce a further complication in that an amino acid which can be readily radioiodinated, such as tyrosine, is not present in either molecule. In the case of somatostatin this difficulty was overcome by solid phase synthesis of the hormone with a tyrosine residue added to the amino end.[159] With the C-peptide immunoassay the free α-amino group of the peptide was conjugated with succinyl tyrosine.[160] Due to its small size, antisera are raised to somatostatin by conjugation of the molecule to a high molecular weight molecule such as serum α-globulin, similar to glucagon antisera production.

X. ENZYME-LINKED IMMUNOASSAY

Enzyme-linked immunoassay utilizes an enzyme covalently linked to the hormone as the tracer. The advantages lie in the long shelf-life of the labeled product and a lack of the hazards which are encountered with radioactivity labeling, coupled with the sensitivity and specificity inherent in immunoassay.

Two enzyme-linked insulin immunoassays have so far been developed. Insulin has been conjugated, using maleimide, to nonessential sulfhydryl groups of β-galactosidase.[161]

The assay is carried out as follows: The insulin-β-galactosidase complex and free insulin are made to compete for binding to anti-insulin antiserum which has itself been bound to Sepharose®. The amount of insulin-β-galactosidase complex bound to the antibody will be dependent upon the concentration of free insulin in the incubate. The insulin-β-galactosidase-Sepharose® insulin antiserum complex is recovered by centrifugation and the quantity bound estimated by assaying for β-galactosidase activity. A sensitivity of 30 pg/mℓ has been achieved. This sensitivity is comparable to that obtained with radioimmunoassay.

A further advancement of this technique is the introduction of an enzyme immunoelectrode.[162] Insulin was linked to an oxygen-utilizing enzyme, glucose oxidase, through the carbohydrate moiety of the enzyme. Insulin antibody was coupled to a nylon net and the active surface of an oxygen electrode was covered with the net. The tip of the electrode was mounted in a flow cell, and insulin, in the sample to be measured, was allowed to compete with the glucose oxidase-insulin for binding to the antibody. A pulse of glucose was then added and the change in oxygen concentration due to catalysis by the enzyme was recorded by the electrode. The amount of oxygen produced is proportional to the amount of glucose oxidase-insulin complex bound, which itself is dependent upon the free concentration of insulin in the sample to be measured. The antibody-electrode was then cleaned of antigen with a glycine wash, ready for reuse. The assay was sensitive to only about 10 μg/mℓ but the simplicity of the operation, coupled with a total assay time of less than a quarter of an hour, would indicate that this type of assay may become routine for hormone estimations.

XI. RADIORECEPTOR ASSAY

Radioreceptor hormone assay is similar to radioimmunoassay but in this case the hormone and radiolabeled hormone compete for binding to the specific hormone receptor present on the plasma membrane of a target tissue of the hormone. The bound and unbound ligands are then usually separated by Millipore® ultrafiltration. Radioreceptor assays have been described for insulin,[163] glucagon,[164] and vasoactive intestinal polypeptide.[165]

The hormone-receptor preparations for the first hormones consisted of isolated plasma membrane fraction of liver. Insulin has also been assayed with fat cell membrane and lymphocytes. Membrane preparations of a high purity are generally required and the sucrose gradient fractionation procedures of the homogenized liver are necessarily complex.[166] However, successful assays have been accomplished on less pure preparations of human adipose tissue, where the amounts of available tissue are small. For a meaningful assay it is essential that the radioiodinated hormone is bioactive. It must also be highly purified to reduce nonspecific binding. The assay is sensitive to about 5 ng/mℓ which is inferior to RIA. A considerable advantage of this technique over RIA is that only bioactive forms of the hormone are measured and the amount of displacement of a given hormone species is related to its biological activity. Thus glucagon with its N-terminal histidine removed is biologically inactive and does not displace native glucagon from its receptor in the radioreceptor assay.[167] Results obtained should be interpreted with caution since some hormones appear to be able to bind to membrane receptors other than their own. Secretin appears to bind to the vasoactive intestinal peptide liver membrane receptor, but a concentration two orders greater is required to achieve the same amount of binding as vasoactive intestinal peptide.[165]

The membrane preparations that bind insulin and glucagon also degrade the hormones and in the radioreceptor assay of glucagon this is a major problem. Incubation times should therefore be kept to a minimum. Glucagon (and vasoactive intestinal peptide) degradation can be considerably reduced by addition of bacitracin.[168]

XII. CONCLUSION

The only method of hormone assay which can compete with radioimmunoassay for convenience, sensitivity, and accuracy is that using antigen bound to enzyme. Enzyme assay is likely to be cheaper and is safer than using radioacive antigens and since the method can be just as sensitive, should become the method of choice.

REFERENCES

1. **Luft, R., Efendic, S., Hökfelt, T., Johansson, O., and Arimura, A.,** Immunohistochemical evidence for the localization of somatostatin-like immunoreactivity in a cell population of the pancreatic islets, *Med. Biol.*, 52, 211, 1976.
2. **Malaisse-Lagae, F., Stefan, Y., Cox, J., Perrelet, A., and Orci, L.,** Identification of a lobe in the adult human pancreas rich in pancreatic polypeptide, *Diabetologia*, 17, 361, 1979.
3. **Pearse, A. G. E.,** The cytochemistry and ultrastructure of polypeptide producing cells of the APUD series and the embryologic, physiologic and pathologic implications of the concept, *Histochem. Cytochem.*, 17, 303, 1969.
4. **Pictet, R. L., Rall, L. B., Phelps, P., and Rutter, R. J.,** The neural crest and the origin of the insulin-producing and other gastrointestinal hormone-producing cells, *Science*, 191, 1976.
5. **Van Noorden, S. and Pearse, A. G. E.,** The localization of immunoreactivity to insulin, glucagon and gastrin in the gut of *Amphioxus (Branchiostoma) lanceolatus*, in *The Evolution of Pancreatic Islets*, Grillo, T. A. I., Leibson, L., and Epple, A. Eds., Pergamon Press, Oxford, 1976, 163.
6. **Gerlovin, E. Sh.,** Some principles of cytodifferentiation of pancreatic islets in vertebrata during ontogeny and phylogeny from the standpoint of molecular biology and genetics, in *The Evolution of Pancreatic Islets*, Grillo, T. A. I., Leibson, L., and Epple, A., Eds., Pergamon Press, Oxford, 1976, 97.
7. **Melmed, R. N., Benitz, C. J., and Holt, S. J.,** Intermediate cells of the pancreas: ultrastructural characterization, *J. Cell Sci.*, 11, 449, 1972.
8. **Melmed, R. N., Turner, R. C., and Holt, S. J.,** Intermediate cells of the pancreas. II. Effects of dietary soya bean trypsin inhibitor on acinar-β cell structure and function in the rat, *J. Cell Sci.*, 13, 279, 1973.

9. **Bainton, D. F. and Farquhar, M. G.,** Origin of granules in polymorphonuclear leukocytes. Two types derived from opposite faces of the Golgi complex in developing granulocytes, *J. Cell Biol.*, 28, 277, 1966.
10. **Van Noorden, S., Polak, J. M., and Pearse, A. G. E.,** Single cellular origin of somatostatin and calcitonin in the rat thyroid gland, *Histochemistry*, 53, 243, 1977.
11. **Ferner, H.,** Die dissemination der Hodenzwischenzellen und der Langerhansschen Inselin als functionelles prinzip für die Samerkanälchen und das exokine Pancreas, *Z. Mikranat. Forsch.*, 63, 35, 1957.
12. **Fugita, Y., Yanatori, Y., and Murakami, T.,** Insulo-acinar axis, its vascular basis and its functional and morphological changes caused by CCK-PZ and caerulein, in *Endocrine Gut and Pancreas*, Fujita, T., Ed., Elsevier, Amsterdam, 1976, 347.
13. **Henderson, J. R.,** Why are the islets of Langerhans?, *Lancet*, 2, 469, 1969.
14. **Adler, G. and Kern, H. F.,** Regulation of exocrine pancreatic secretory process by insulin *in vivo*, *Horm. Metab. Res.*, 7, 290, 1975.
15. **Söling, H. D. and Unger, K. O.,** The role of insulin in the regulation of α-amylase synthesis in rat pancreas, *J. Clin. Invest.*, 2, 199, 1972.
16. **Chey, W. Y., Shay, H., and Schuman, C. R.,** External pancreatic secretion in diabetes mellitus, *Ann. Int. Med.*, 59, 812, 1963.
17. **Peters, N. A. P., Dick, A. P., Hales, C. N., Orrell, D. H., and Sarner, M.,** Exocrine and endocrine pancreatic function in diabetes mellitus and chronic pancreatitis, *Gut*, 7, 277, 1966.
18. **Kram, R., Mamont, P., and Tomkins, G. M.,** Pleiotypic control by adenosine 3′:5′-cyclic monophosphate: a model for growth control in animal cells, *Proc. Natl. Acad. Sci. U.S.A.*, 70, 1432, 1973.
19. **Gelehrter, T. D. and Tonkins, G. M.,** Post-transcriptional control of tyrosine aminotransferase synthesis by insulin, *Proc. Natl. Acad. Sci. U.S.A.*, 66, 390, 1970.
20. **Necheles, H., Walker, L., and Mabin, W.,** Effects of glucagon on external secretions of the pancreas, *Amer. J. Physiol.*, 191, 595, 1957.
21. **Dyck, W. P., Texter, E. C., Lasater, J. M., and Hightower, N. C.,** Influence of glucagon on pancreatic secretion in man, *Gastroenterology*, 58, 532, 1970.
22. **Knight, M. J., Condon, J. R., and Smith, R.,** Possible use of glucagon in the treatment of pancreatitis, *Br. Med. J.*, 2, 440, 1971.
23. **Kasper, H. and Fleischer, K.,** Der einflusz von glucagon auf die Lipaseakfivität im Serum bei Pankreatitis, *Dtsch. Med. Wachenschr.*, 97, 1124, 1972.
24. **Adler, G.,** Effect of glucagon on the secretory process in the rat exocrine pancreas, *Cell Tiss. Res.*, 182, 193, 1977.
25. **Lin, T.-M. and Chance, R.,** Bovine pancreatic polypeptide (BPP) and avian pancreatic polypeptide (APP), *Gastroenterology*, 67, 730, 1974.
26. **Schebalin, R., Said, S. I., and Makhlouf, G. M.,** Inhibition of gastric secretion by synthetic vasoactive intestinal peptide (VIP), *Clin. Res.*, 23, 23a, 1974.
27. **Dolliner, M. C., Raptis, S., and Pfeiffer, E. F.,** Effects of somatostatin on exocrine and endocrine pancreatic function stimulated by intestinal hormones in man, *Horm. Metab. Res.*, 8, 74, 1976.
28. **Arimura, A., Sato, H., Dupont, A., Nishi, N., and Schally, A. V.,** Abundance of immunoreactive growth hormone release inhibiting hormone in the stomach and pancreas of rat, *Fed. Proc. Am. Soc. Exp. Biol.*, 34, 273, 1975.
29. **Forssmann, W. G., Helmstaedter, V., Metz, J., Greenberg, J., and Chance, R. E.,** The identification of the F-cell in the dog pancreas as the pancreatic polypeptide producing cell, *Histochemistry*, 50, 281, 1977.
30. **Said, S. I. and Mutt, V.,** Isolation from porcine intestinal wall of a vasoactive octacosapeptide related to secretin and to glucagon, *Eur. J. Biochem.*, 28, 199, 1972.
31. **Steiner, D. F. and Oyer, P. E.,** The biosynthesis of insulin and a probable precursor of insulin by a human islet cell adenoma, *Proc. Natl. Acad. Sci. U.S.A.*, 57, 473, 1967.
32. **Lazarus, N. R., Tanese, T., Gutman, R., and Recant, L.,** Synthesis and release of proinsulin and insulin by human insulinoma tissue, *J. Clin. Endocrinol. Metab.*, 30, 273, 1970.
33. **Tager, H. S. and Steiner, D. F.,** Peptide hormones, in *Ann. Rev. Biochem.*, 43, 509, 1974.
34. **Chan, S. J., Keim, P., and Steiner, D. F.,** Cell-free synthesis of rat preproinsulins: characterization and partial amino acid sequence determination, *Proc. Natl. Acad. Sci. U.S.A.*, 73, 1964, 1976.
35. **Ullrich, A., Shine, J., Chirgwin, J., Pictet, R., Tischer, E., Rutter, W. J., and Goodman, H. M.,** Rat insulin genes: construction of plasmids containing the coding sequences, *Science*, 196, 1313, 1977.
36. **Goeddel, D. V., Kleid, D. G., Bolivar, F., Heyneker, H. L., Yansura, D. G., Crea, R., Hirose, T., Kraszewski, A., Keiichi, I., and Riggs, A. D.,** Expression in *Escherichia coli* of chemically synthesized genes for human insulin, *Proc. Natl. Acad. Sci. U.S.A.*, 76, 106, 1979.

37. **Block, M. B., Mako, M. E., Steiner, D. F., and Rubenstein, A. H.,** Circulating C-peptide immunoreactivity. Studies in normals and diabetic patients, *Diabetes,* 21, 1013, 1972.
38. **Gorden, P. and Roth, J.,** Circulating insulins. "Big" and "little", *Arch. Intern. Med.,* 123, 237, 1969.
39. **Lazarus, N. R., Gutman, R. A., Penhos, J. C., and Recant, L.,** Biologically active circulating proinsulin-like materials from an islet cell carcinoma patient, *Diabetologia,* 8, 131, 1972.
40. **Gorden, P., Freychet, P., and Nankin, H.,** A unique form of circulating insulin in human islet cell carcinoma, *J. Clin. Endocrinol. Metab.,* 33, 983, 1971.
41. **Gutman, R. A., Lazarus, N. R., and Recant, L.,** Electrophoretic characterization of circulating human proinsulin and insulin, *Diabetologia,* 8, 136, 1972.
42. **Kipnis, D. M.,** Insulin secretion in normal and diabetic individuals, in *Adv. Intern. Med.,* 16, 103, 1970.
43. **Cahill, G. F., Jr.,** Physiology of insulin in man, *Diabetes,* 20, 785, 1971.
44. **Felig, P. and Wahren, J.,** Influence of endogenous insulin secretion on splanchnic glucose and amino-acid metabolism in man, *J. Clin. Invest.,* 50, 1702, 1971.
45. **Zierler, K. and Rabinowitz, D.,** Effect of very small concentrations of insulin on forearm metabolism. Persistence of its action on potassium and free fatty acids without its effect on glucose, *J. Clin. Invest.,* 43, 950, 1964.
46. **Pozefsky, T., Felig, P., Tobin, J. D., Soeldner, J. S., and Cahill, G. F., Jr.,** Amino acid balance across tissues of the forearm in post-absorptive man of insulin at two dose levels, *J. Clin. Invest.,* 48, 2273, 1969.
47. **McGarry, J. D.,** New perspectives in the regulation of ketogenesis, *Diabetes,* 28, 517, 1979.
48. **Wool, I. G.,** Effects of insulin on cellular protein synthesis, in *Insulin,* Vol. 2, Hasselblatt, A. and Bruchhausen, F. V., Eds., Springer-Verlag, Berlin, 1975, 268.
49. **Mortimer, G. E. and Mondon, C. E.,** Inhibition by insulin of valine turnover in liver: evidence for a general control of proteolysis, *J. Biol. Chem.,* 245, 2375, 1970.
50. **O'Connor, K. J., Gay, A., and Lazarus, N. R.,** The biosynthesis of glucagon in perfused rat pancreas, *Biochem. J.,* 134, 473, 1973.
51. **O'Connor, K. J. and Lazarus, N. R.,** Studies on the biosynthesis of pancreatic glucagon in the pigeon *(Columba livia), Biochem. J.,* 156, 279, 1976.
52. **Patzelt, C., Tager, H. S., Carroll, R. J., and Steiner, D. F.,** Identification and processing of proglucagon in pancreatic islets, *Nature (London),* 282, 260, 1979.
53. **Tager, H. S. and Markese, J.,** Intestinal and pancreatic glucagon-like peptides. Evidences for identity of higher molecular weight forms, *J. Biol. Chem.,* 254, 2229, 1979.
54. **O'Connor, K. J.** Studies on the Biosynthesis and Biological Properties of the Pancreatic Glucagons, Ph.D. thesis, University of London, 1977.
55. **Jacobsen, H., Demandt, A., Moody, A. J., and Sundby, F.,** Sequence analysis of porcine gut GLI-1, *Biochim. Biophys. Acta,* 493, 452, 1977.
56. **Weir, G. C., Horton, E. S., Aoki, T. T., Slovik, D., Jaspan, J., and Rubenstein, A. H.,** Secretion by glucagonomas of a possible glucagon precursor, *J. Clin. Invest.,* 59, 325, 1977.
57. **Kuku, S. F., Jaspan, J. B., Emmanouel, D. S., Zeidler, A., Katz, A. J., and Rubenstein, A. H.,** Heterogeneity of plasma glucagon circulating components in normal subjects and patients with chronic renal failure, *J. Clin. Invest.,* 58, 742, 1976.
58. **Jaspan, J. B., Kuku, S. F., Locker, J. D., Huen, A.H.-J., Emmanouel, D. S., Katz, A. I., and Rubenstein, A. H.,** Heterogeneity of plasma glucagon in man, *Metabolism,* 25, 1397, 1976.
59. **Weir, G. C., Knowlton, S. D., and Martin, D. B.,** High molecular weight glucagon-like immunoreactivity in plasma, *J. Clin. Endocrinol. Metab.,* 40, 296, 1975.
60. **Ensink, J. W. and Palmer, J. P.,** Dominant inheritance of large molecular weight species of glucagon, *Metabolism,* 25, 1409, 1976.
61. **Valverde, I., Villanueva, M. L., Lozano, I., and Marco, J.,** Presence of glucagon immunoreactivity in the globulin fraction of human plasma ("big plasma glucagon"), *J. Clin. Endocrinol. Metab.,* 39, 1090, 1974.
62. **Antoniades, H. A.,** Metabolism of single-component and high-molecular-weight radioactive insulin in rats, *Endocrinoloy,* 99, 481, 1976.
63. **Beitins, I. Z., Rattazzi, M. C., and MacCillivray, M. H.,** Conversion of radiolabelled human growth hormone into higher molecular weight moieties in human plasma *in vivo* and *in vitro, Endocrinology,* 101, 350, 1977.
64. **Murlin, J. R., Clough, H. D., Gibbs, C. B. F., and Stokes, A. M.,** Aqueous extracts of pancreas. I. Influence on the carbohydrate metabolism of depancreatectomized animals, *J. Biol. Chem.,* 56, 253, 1923.

65. **Straub, A., Sinn, L., and Behrens, O. K.,** Purification and crystallization of hyperglycaemic glycogenolytic factor, *Science,* 117, 628, 1953.
66. **Samols, E., Tyler, J., Megyesi, C., and Marks, V.,** Immunochemical glucagon in human pancreas, gut and plasma, *Lancet,* 2, 727, 1966.
67. **Moody, A. J.,** The structural and immunological relationship between gut GLI's and glucagon, *Metabolism,* 25, 1336, 1976.
68. **Srikant, C. B. and Unger, R.H.,** Evidence for the presence of glucagon-like immunoreactivity (GLI) in the pancreas, *Endocrinology,* 99, 1655, 1976.
69. **Jaspan, J. B. and Rubenstein, A. H.,** Circulating glucagon: plasma profiles and metabolism in health and disease, *Diabetes,* 26, 887, 1977.
70. **O'Connor, K. J. and Lazarus, N. R.,** The purification and biological properties of pancreatic big glucagon, *Biochem. J.,* 156, 265, 1976.
71. **Sokal, J. E.,** Bioassay of glucagon using the isolated perfused rat liver, *Endocrinology,* 87, 1338, 1970.
72. **Exton, J. H. and Park, C. R.,** Control of gluconeogenesis in liver. II. Effects of glucagon, catecholamines and adenosine 3′5′-monophosphate on gluconeogenesis in the perfused rat liver, *J. Biol. Chem.,* 243, 4189, 1968.
73. **Felig, P., Wahrren, J., Sherwin, R., and Hendler, R.,** Insulin, glucagon and somatostatin in normal physiology and diabetes mellitus, *Diabetes,* 25, 1091, 1973.
74. **Söling, H.-D. and Kleineke, J.,** Species dependent regulation of hepatic gluconeogenesis in higher animals, in *Gluconeogenesis: Its Regulation in Mammalian Species,* Hanson, R.W. and Mehlman, M. A., Eds., John Wiley & Son, New York, 1976, 369.
75. **Mallette, L. E., Exton, J. H., and Park, C. R.,** Effects of glucagon on amino acid transport and utilization in the perfused rat liver, *J. Biol. Chem.,* 244, 5724, 1969.
76. **Felig, P.,** The glucose-alanine cycle, *Metabolism,* 22, 179, 1973.
77. **Elwyn, D. H., Parikh, H. C., and Shoemaker, W. C.,** Amino acid movements between gut, liver and periphery in anaesthetized dogs, *Am. J. Physiol.,* 215, 1260, 1968.
78. **Ruderman, N. B., Aoki, T. T., and Cahill, G. F., Jr.,** Gluconeogenesis and its disorders in man, in *Gluconeogenesis: Its Regulation in Mammalian Species,* Hanson, R. W. and Mehlman, M. A., Eds., John Wiley & Son, New York, 1976, 515.
79. **Dalle, X., Tanghe, J., and Gryspeerdt, W. I.,** Effects of glucagon on renal excretion of electrolytes, *Arch. Int. Pharmacodynamics,* 120, 505, 1959.
80. **Serratto, M. and Earle, D. P.,** Effect of glucagon on renal functions in dog, *Proc. Soc. Exp. Biol. Med.,* 102, 701, 1959.
81. **Pullman, T. N., Lavender, A. R., and Aho, I.,** Diuretic effects of glucagon on renal haemodynamics and excretion of inorganic ions, *Metabolism,* 16, 358, 1969.
82. **Unger, R. H.,** Glucagon and the insulin:glucagon ratio in diabetes and other catabolic illnesses, *Diabetes,* 20, 834, 1971.
83. **Unger, R. H. and Orci, L.,** The essential role of glucagon in the pathogenesis of the endogenous hyperglycaemia of diabetes mellitus, *Lancet,* 1, 14, 1975.
84. **Gerich, J. E., Lovenzi, M., Bier, D. M., Schneider, V., Tsalikian, E., Karam, J. H., and Forsham, P. H.,** Prevention of human diabetic ketoacidosis by somatostatin. Evidence for an essential role of glucagon, *N. Engl. J. Med.,* 292, 985, 1975.
85. **Alberti, K. G. M. M., Christensen, N. J., Iverson, J., and Øskov, H.,** Role of glucagon and other hormones in development of diabetic ketoacidosis, *Lancet,* 1, 1307, 1975.
86. **Barnes, A. J., Bloom, S. R., Machiter, K., Alford, F. P., Smythe, P., and Turnell, D.,** Glucagon and ketogenesis: studies in pancreatectomized man, *Diabetologia,* 12, 379, 1976.
87. **Gutman, R. A., Fink, G., Voyles, N., Selawry, H., Penhos, J. C., Lepp, A., and Recant, L.,** Specific biologic effects of intestinal glucagon-like substances, *J. Clin. Invest.,* 52, 1154, 1973.
88. **Murphy, R. F., Elmore, D. T., and Buchanan, K. D.,** Isolation of glucagon-like immunoreactivity of gut by affinity chromatography, *Biochem. J.,* 125, 61P, 1971.
89. **Noe, B. D., Fletcher, D. J., and Spiess, J.,** Evidence for the existence of a biosynthetic precursor for somatostatin, *Diabetes,* 28, 724, 1979.
90. **Zingg, H. H. and Patel, Y. C.,** Somatostatin precursors: evidence for presence in and release from rat median eminence and neurohypophysis, *Biochem. Biophys. Res. Comm.,* 90, 466, 1979.
91. **Hall, R., Besser, G. M., Schally, A. V., Coy, D. H., Evered, D., Goldie, D. J., Kastin, A.J., McNeilly, A. S., Mortimer, C. H., Phenekos, C., Tunbridge, W. M. C., and Weightman, D.,** Action of growth hormone release inhibiting hormone in healthy men and acromegaly, *Lancet,* 2, 581, 1973.
92. **Mortimer, C. H., Tunbridge, W. M. G., Carr, D., Yeomans, L., Lind, T., Coy, D. H., Bloom, S. R., Kastin, A., Mallison, G. N., Besser, G. M., Schally, A. V., and Hall, R.,** Effects of growth hormone release inhibiting hormone on circulating glucagon, insulin and growth hormone in normal, diabetic, acromegalic and hypopituitary patients, *Lancet,* 1, 697,1974.

93. **Gomez-Pan, A., Reed, J. D., Albinus, M., Shaw, B., Hall, R., Besser, G.M., Coy, D. H., Kastin, A. J., and Schally, A. V.**, Direct inhibition of gastric acid and pepsin secretion by growth hormone release inhibiting hormone in cats, *Lancet*, 1, 888, 1975.
94. **Efendic, S., Hökfelt, T. and Luft, R.** Somatostatin and the endocrine pancreas, *Excerpta Medica I. Congr. Ser*, 374, 151, 1976.
95. **Orci, L., Baetens, D., Rufener, C., Amherdt, M., Ravazzola, M., Struder, P., Malaisse-Lagae, F., and Unger, R. H.**, Hypertrophy and hyperplasia of somatostatin containing D-cells in diabetes, *Proc. Natl. Acad. Sci. U.S.A.*, 73, 1338, 1976.
96. **Barden, N., Lavoie, M., Dupont, A., Côté, J. and Côté, J. P.**, Stimulation of glucagon release by addition of antisomatostatin serum to islets of Langerhans *in vitro, Endocrinology*, 101, 635, 1977.
97. **Patel, Y. C. and Weir, G. C.**, Increased somatostatin content of islets from streptozotocin diabetic rats, *Clin. Endocrinol.*, 5, 191, 1976.
98. **Patton, G. S., Ipp, E., Dobbs, R. E., Orci, L., Vale, W., and Unger, R. H.**, Pancreatic immunoreactive somatostatin release, *Proc. Natl. Acad. Sci. U.S.A.*, 74, 2140, 1977.
99. **Said, S. I. and Mutt, V.**, Polypeptide with broad biological activity: isolation from small intestine, *Science*, 169, 1217, 1970.
100. **Piper, P. J., Said, S. I., and Vane, J. R.**, Effects on smooth muscle preparations of unidentified vasoactive peptides from intestine and lung, *Nature (London)*, 225, 1144, 1970.
101. **Kerins, C. and Said, S. I.**, Hyperglycaemic and glycogenolytic effects of vasoactive intestinal polypeptide, *Proc. Soc. Exp. Biol. Med.*, 142, 1014, 1973.
102. **Verner, J. V. and Morrison, A. B.**, Islet cell tumor and a syndrome of refactory watery diarrhoea and hypokalaemia, *Am. J. Med.*, 25, 374, 1958.
103. **Marks, I. N., Bank, S., and Louw, J. H.**, Islet cell tumor of the pancreas with reversible watery diarrhoea and achlorhydria, *Gastroenterology*, 52, 695, 1967.
104. **Bloom, S. R., Polak, J. M. and Pearse, A. G. E.**, Vasoactive intestinal peptide and watery diarrhoea syndrome, *Lancet*, 2, 14,1973.
105. **Said, S. I. and Rosenberg, R. N.**, Vasoactive intestinal polypeptide: abundant immunoreactivity in neural cell lines and normal nervous tissue, *Science*, 192, 907, 1976.
106. **Schebalin, M., Said, S. I., and Makhlouf, G. M.**, Stimulation of insulin and glucagon secretion by vasoactive intestinal peptide, *Am. J. Physiol.*, 232, E197, 1977.
107. **Kaneto, A., Kaneto, T., Kajinuma, H., and Kosaka, K.**, Effect of vasoactive intestinal polypeptide infused intrapancreatically on glucagon and insulin secretion, *Metab. Clin. Exp.*, 26, 781, 1977.
108. **Konturek, S. J., Domschke, S., Domschke, W., Wünsch, E., and Demling, L.**, Comparison of pancreatic responses to portal and systemic secretion and VIP in cats, *Am. J. Physiol.*, 232, E156, 1977.
109. **Schwartz, T. W., Stadil, F., Chance, R. E., Rehfeld, J. F., Larson, L.-I., and Moon, N.**, Pancreatic polypeptide response to food in duodenal ulcer patients before and after vagotomy, *Lancet*, 1, 1102, 1976.
110. **Stadie, W. C., Hangaard, N., and Vaughan, M.**, Studies of insulin binding, *J. Biol. Chem.*, 199, 729, 1952.
111. **Kono, T.**, Destruction and restoration of the insulin effector system of isolated fat cells, *J. Biol. Chem.*, 244, 5777, 1969.
112. **Cuatrecasas, P., Debuquois, B., and Krug, F.**, Insulin receptor interactions in liver cell membranes, *Biochem. Biophys. Res. Comm.*, 44, 333, 1971.
113. **Rodbell, M., Krans, H. M. J., Pohl, S. L., and Birnbaumer, L.**, The glucagon-sensitive adenyl cyclase system in plasma membranes of rat liver. III. Binding of glucagon: method of assay and specificity, *J. Biol. Chem.*, 246, 1861, 1971.
114. **Jacobs, S. and Cuatrecasas, P.**, The subunit structure of rat liver insulin receptors, abstract presented at the Endocrine Society Meeting, Washington, D.C., June 1980.
115. **Bergeron, J. J. M., Evans, W. J., and Geschwind, I. I.**, Insulin binding to rat liver golgi fractions, *J. Cell Biol.*, 59, 771, 1973.
116. **Goldfine, I. D., Smith, G. T., Wong, K. Y., and Jones, A. L.**, Cellular uptake and nuclear binding of insulin in human cultured lymphocytes. Evidence for potential intracellular sites for insulin, *Proc. Natl. Acad. Sci. U.S.A.*, 74, 1368, 1977.
117. **De Meyts, P., Bianco, A. R., and Roth, J.**, Site-site interactions among insulin receptors: characterisation of the negative co-operativity, *J. Biol. Chem.*, 251, 1877, 1976.
118. **Cuatrecasas, P.**, Membrane receptors, *Ann. Rev. Biochem.*, 43, 169, 1974.
119. **Gorden, P., Carpentier, J. L., Freychet, P., LeCam, A., and Orci, L.**, Intracellular translocation of iodine-125-labeled insulin: direct demonstration in isolated hepatocytes, *Science*, 200, 782, 1978.
120. **Flier, J. S., Kahn, C. R., Roth, J., and Bar, R. S.**, Antibodies that impair insulin receptor binding in an unusual diabetic syndrome with severe insulin resistance, *Science*, 190, 63, 1975.

121. **Gavin, J. R., III, Roth, J., Neville, D. M., Jr., De Meyts, P., and Buell, N.,** Insulin-dependent regulation of insulin receptor concentration: A direct demonstration in cell culture, *Proc. Natl. Acad. Sci. U.S.A.*, 71, 84, 1974.
122. **Baxter, D. and Lazarus, N. R.,** The control of insulin receptors in New Zealand obese mouse, *Diabetologia*, 11, 261, 1975.
123. **Kahn, C. R., Neville, D. M., Jr., and Roth, J.,** Insulin-receptor interaction in the obese hyperglycaemic mouse: a model of insulin resistance, *J. Biol. Chem.*, 248, 244, 1973.
124. **Bar, R. S., Gorden, P., Roth, J., Kahn, R., and De Meyts, P.,** Fluctuations in the affinity and concentration of insulin receptors on circulating monocytes of obese patients, *J. Clin. Invest*, 58, 1123, 1976.
125. **Olefsky, J. M.,** Decreased insulin binding to adipocytes and circulating monocytes from obese subjects, *J. Clin. Invest.*, 57, 1165, 1976.
126. **Harrison, L. C., Martin, F. I. R., and Melick, R. A.,** Correlation between insulin receptor binding in isolated fat cells and insulin sensitivity in obese human subjects, *J. Clin. Invest.*, 58, 1435, 1976.
127. **Robison, G. A., Butcher, R. W., and Sutherland, E. W.,** Adenyl cyclase as an adrenergic receptor, *Ann. N.Y. Acad. Sci.*, 139, 703, 1967.
128. **Houslay, M. D., Ellory, J. C., Smith, G. A., Hesketh, T. R., Stein, J. M., Warren, G. B., and Metcalfe, J. C.,** Exchange of partners in glucagon receptor-adenylate cyclase complexes. Physical evidence for the independent, mobile receptor model, *Biochim. Biophys. Acta*, 467, 208, 1977.
129. **Bataille, D., Besson, J., Bastard, C., Laburthe, M., and Rosselin, G.,** Specificity in hormone-receptor interaction: studies with insulin, glucagon and vasoactive intestinal peptide (VIP), in *Hormonal Receptors in Digestive Tract Physiology*, Inserm Symp. No. 3, Bonfils, S., Fromageot, P., and Rosselin, G., Eds., North-Holland Publishing Co., Amsterdam, 1977, 113.
130. **Yalow, R. and Berson, S. A.,** Dynamics of insulin secretion in hypoglycaemia, *Diabetes*, 14, 341, 1965.
131. **Floyd, J. C., Jr., Fajans, S. S., Kuopf, R. F., and Conn, J. W.,** Plasma insulin in organic hyperinsulinism; comparative effects of tolbutamide, leucine and glucose, *J. Clin. Endocrinol.*, 24, 747, 1964.
132. **Gutman, R. A., Lazarus, N. R., Penhos, J. C., Fajans, S. S., and Recant, L.,** Circulating proinsulin-like material in patients with functioning insulinomas, *N. Engl. J. Med.*, 284, 1003, 1971.
133. **Gordon, P., Sherman, B., and Roth, J.,** Proinsulin-like component of circulating insulin in the basal state and in patients and hamster with islet cell tumours, *J. Clin. Invest.*, 50, 2113, 1971.
134. **McGavran, M. H., Unger, R. H. Recant, L., Polk, H. C., Kalo, C., and Levin, M. E.,** A glucagon secreting alpha cell carcinoma of the pancreas, *N. Engl. J. Med.*, 274, 1408, 1966.
135. **Mallinson, C. N., Bloom, S. R., Warin, A. P., Salmon, P. R. and Cox, B.,** A glucagonoma syndrome, *Lancet*, 2, 1, 1974.
136. **Polak, J. M., Bloom, S. R., Adrian, T. E., Heitz, Ph., Bryant, M. G., and Pearse, A. G. E.,** Pancreatic polypeptide in insulinomas, vipomas and glucagonomas, *Lancet*, 1, 328, 1976.
137. **Bloom, S. R.,** Hormones of the gastrointestinal tract, *Br. Med. Bull.*, 30, 62, 1974.
138. **Sandler, R., Horowitz, D. L., Rubenstein, A. H., and Kuzuya, H.,** Hypoglycaemia and endogenous hyperinsulinism complicating diabetes mellitus: application of C peptide assay to diagnosis and therapy, *Amer. J. Med.*, 59, 730, 1975.
139. **Heding, L., Turner, R. C., and Harris, E.,** C peptide, proinsulin and insulin responses to fish insulin induced hypoglycaemic in the diagnosis of insulinomas, *Diabetes*, 24, Suppl. 2, 412, 1975.
140. **Service, F. J., Rubenstein, A. H., and Horwitz, D. L.,** C-peptide analysis in diagnosis of factitial hypoglycaemia in an insulin dependent diabetic, *Mayo Clin. Proc.*, 50, 697, 1975.
141. **Horwitz, D. L., Reynolds, C., and Molnar, G. D.,** Stable and unstable diabetes: differences in endogenous insulin secretion as determined by C-peptide measurement, *Clin. Res.*, 22, 471A, 1974.
142. The biological assay of insulin injection, in *British Pharmacopoeia*, Appendix XIV c, Her Majesty's Stationery Office, London, 1973, A109.
143. **Moody, A. J., Stan, M. A., and Stan, M.,** A simple free fat cell bioassay for insulin, *Horm. Metab. Res.*, 6, 12, 1974.
144. **Sokal, J. E.,** Bioassay for glucagon, in *Glucagon: Molecular Physiology, Clinical and Therapeutic Implications*, Lefebvre, P. J. and Unger, R. H., Eds., Pergamon Press, Oxford, 1972, 277.
145. **Langslow, D. R.,** The action of gut glucagon-like immunoreactivity and other intestinal hormones on lipolysis in chicken adipocytes, *Horm. Metab. Res.*, 5, 428, 1973.
146. **Langslow, D. R. and Hales, C. N.,** Lipolysis in chicken adipose tissue in vitro, *J. Endocr.*, 43, 285, 1969.
147. **Said, S. I. and Mutt, V.,** Potent peripheral and splanchnic visodilator peptide from normal gut, *Nature (London)*, 225, 863, 1970.

148. **Brazeau, P., Wylie, V., Burgus, R., Ling, N., Butcher, M., Rivier, J., and Guillemin, R.**, Hypothalamic polypeptide that inhibits the secretion of immunoreactive pituitary growth hormone, *Science,* 179, 77, 1973.
149. **Daly, J. R., Loveridge, N., Bitensky, L., and Chayen, J.**, The cytochemical bioassay of corticotropin, *Clin. Endocrinol.,* 3, 311, 1974.
150. **Rees, L. H., Holdaway, I. M., Kramer, R., McNeilly, A. S., and Chard, T.**, New bioassay for luteinizing hormone, *Nature (London),* 244, 232, 1973.
151. **Yalow, R. S. and Berson, S. A.**, Radioimmunoassay, in *Methods in Investigative and Diagnostic Endocrinology,* 2B, Part III, Non-Pituitary Hormones, Berson, S. A. and Yalow, R. S., Eds., North-Holland, Amsterdam, 1973, 864.
152. **Jaffe, B. M., and Behrman, H. R., Eds.**, *Methods of Hormone Radioimmunoassay,* Academic Press, New York, 1974, Chap. 17 and 18.
153. **Hunter, W. M. and Greenwood, F. C.**, Preparation of iodine- ^{131}-labelled growth hormone of high specific activity, *Nature (London),* 194, 495, 1962.
154. **Miyachi, Y., Vaitukaitis, J. L., Neischlag, E., and Lipsett, M. B.**, Enzymatic radioiodination of gonadotropins, *J. Clin. Endocrinol.,* 34, 23, 1972.
155. **Bolton, A. E. and Hunter, W. M.**, The labelling of proteins to high specific radioactivities by conjugation to a ^{125}I-containing acylating agent. Application to the radioimmunoassay, *Biochem. J.,* 133, 529, 1973.
156. **Vranic, M., Engerman, R., Doi, K., Morita, S., and Yip, C. C.**, Extrapancreatic glucagon in the dog, *Metab. Clin. Exp.,* 25, 1469, 1976.
157. **Adrian, T. E., Bloom, S. R., Bryant, M. G., Polak, J. M., Heitz, P. H., and Barnes, A. J.**, Distribution and release of human pancreatic polypeptide, *Gut,* 17, 940, 1976.
158. **Villanueva, M. L., Hedo, J. A., and Marco, J.**, Heterogeneity of pancreatic polypeptide immunoreactivity in human plasma, *FEBS Lett.,* 80, 99, 1977.
159. **Arimura, A., Sato, H., Coy, D. H., and Schally, A. V.**, Radioimmunoassay for GH-release inhibiting hormone, *Proc. Soc. Exp. Biol. Med.,* 148, 784, 1975.
160. **Melani, F., Rubenstein, A. H., Oyer, P. E., and Steiner, D. F.**, Identification of proinsulin and C-peptide in human serum by a specific immunoassay, *Proc. Natl. Acad. Sci. U.S.A.,* 67, 148, 1970.
161. **Kato, K., Hamaguchi, Y., Fukui, H., and Ishikawa, E.**, Enzyme-linked immunoassay. I. Novel method for the synthesis of the insulin-β-D-galactosidase conjugate and its applicability for insulin assay, *J. Biochem.,* 78, 235, 1975.
162. **Mattiasson, B. and Nilsson, H.**, An enzyme immunoelectrode assay of human serum albumin and insulin, *FEBS Lett.,* 78, 251, 1977.
163. **Gavin, J. R., III, Kahn, C. R., Gorden, P., Roth, J., and Neville, D. M., Jr.**, Radioreceptor assay of insulsin: comparison of plasma and pancreatic insulins and proinsulins, *J. Clin. Endocrinol. Metab.,* 41, 438, 1975.
164. **Holst, J. J.**, A radioreceptor assay for glucagon: binding of enteroglucagon to liver plasma membranes, *Diabetologia,* 11, 211, 1975.
165. **Desbuquois, B.**, The interaction of vasoactive intestinal polypeptide and secretin with liver-cell membranes, *Eur. J. Biochem.,* 46, 439, 1974.
166. **Neville, D. M., Jr.**, The isolation of a cell membrane fraction from rat liver, *J. Biophys. Biochem. Cytol.,* 8, 413, 1960.
167. **Rodbell, M., Birnbaumer, L., Pohl, S. L., and Sundby, F.**, The reaction of glucagon with its receptor: evidence for discreet regions of activity and binding in the glucagon molecule, *Proc. Natl. Acad. Sci. U.S.A.,* 68, 909, 1971.
168. **Desbuquois, B., Krug, F., and Cuatrecasas, P.**, Inhibitors of glucagon inactivation. Effect of glucagon-receptor interactions and glucagon-stimulated adenylate cyclase activity in liver cell membranes, *Biochim. Biophys. Acta,* 343, 101, 1974.

Chapter 5

THE HORMONES OF PREGNANCY

George W. Pennington and Sandra Naik

TABLE OF CONTENTS

I. INTRODUCTION

The fetus may be in jeopardy long before the onset of labor, and adverse antenatal factors may affect postnatal growth and development. Continued improvements in population health and in antenatal care have led to a reduction in fetal and neonatal mortality. During the last decade biochemical tests have become an integral part of antenatal care. They have contributed to the improved perinatal mortality figures, by indicating those patients in whom early induction of labor was desirable. Biochemical tests also warn of incipient fetoplacental distress and so may prevent neonatal morbidity including mental retardation.[1] Tests may also be of value in early pregnancy when early warning of fetal abnormality may enable an abortion to be performed.

Although the formation of some hormones produced during pregnancy is the result of interplay between the placenta and the fetus, the majority of hormones are produced by the placenta alone.

The placenta is probably the most versatile endocrine organ in the body and any single test of placental function can at best only examine a small fraction of placental activity. The placenta may mirror a fault elsewhere, for example a deficiency in the blood supply to the uterus and not a deficiency within the placenta itself.

Hormones may be measured in either the blood or the urine. The significance of a particular level of hormone in a body fluid is rarely understood. The amounts found in blood and urine represent minor and variable fractions of the end products of complex reactions in the organs and therefore can give only a rough guide to the activity of the hormone at its site of action.

II. PLACENTAL PROTEIN HORMONES

A. Human Chorionic Gonadotropin

Human chorionic gonadotropin (HCG) is produced by Langhans cells of the cytotrophoblast[2] and large amounts are stored in the syncytiotrophoblast.[3] HCG is a glycoprotein with a molecular weight of 38,000. It can be dissociated into α and β subunits. Assay of the β subunit of HCG differentiates the hormone from luteinizing hormone (LH) with which it cross-reacts. The rate of production of HCG at its peak output is 26 mg/day. The half-life of HCG is between 5 to 11 hr.

HCG has been detected in the maternal blood within 48 hr of implantation.[4] The early detection of HCG in the urine is the basis for methods of pregnancy testing.

1. Immunological Tests of Pregnancy

Indirect Slide Tests — Urine is added to an HCG antiserum. The HCG antibody is neutralized if HCG is present in the urine. Therefore when polystyrene latex particles coated with HCG are added no flocculation occurs. A positive test is indicated by a failure of flocculation. These tests are performed on slides and results are obtained within 2 min.

Direct slide tests — These are tests in which polystyrene latex particles are coated with HCG antibody. When urine containing HCG is added, flocculation occurs. A positive test is indicated by flocculation. These tests are performed on slides and results are obtained within 3 min.

Hemagglutination inhibition tests — HCG is coated onto red blood cells. Urine is added to an HCG antiserum. If HCG is present in the sample the HCG antibody is neutralized, so that when the red blood cells coated with HCG are added no agglutination occurs. A positive test is indicated by the absence of agglutination. The test is performed in test tubes and the result obtained within 2 to 10 hr.

2. Levels of HCG in Blood and Urine

The levels of HCG in the blood and urine mirror the levels in the placental tissue. The level increases rapidly after conception, the maximum excretion in the urine being observed 50 to 80 days after the last menstrual period. Subsequently HCG output falls rapidly, a sharp drop occurring at 17 to 19 weeks. After this there is a fairly constant level until term (Figure 1). There are large individual variations in HCG output and a wide normal range of hormone levels at all stages of pregnancy.

3. Spontaneous Abortion

Most first trimester abortions are due to abnormalities of the fetus. It has been found in patients with habitual abortion that urinary levels of HCG have no definite relationship to the eventual outcome of pregnancy.[5] Patients with threatened abortion who have low or falling levels of HCG usually abort, whereas those with normal excretion patterns generally proceed to full term delivery.

4. Ectopic Pregnancy

The HCG excretion may provide some help in the diagnosis of this condition. If HCG excretion is below the 95% confidence limit for the duration of pregnancy, the possibility of tubal pregnancy is enhanced.

5. Trophoblastic Disease

In the conditions of hydatidiform mole and choriocarcinoma, HCG levels are usually abnormally high and continue to rise. Following evacuation of the trophoblastic lesion, surveillance of the patient's HCG levels is mandatory for a period of 1 to 2 years. This follow-up is the basis of the British National Trophoblastic Tumor scheme whereby all patients with the disease are followed for 2 years.[6] Specimens of urine are assayed for HCG at weekly or fortnightly intervals until normal levels of HCG are obtained, and then monthly in the first year and 3-monthly in the second year. When

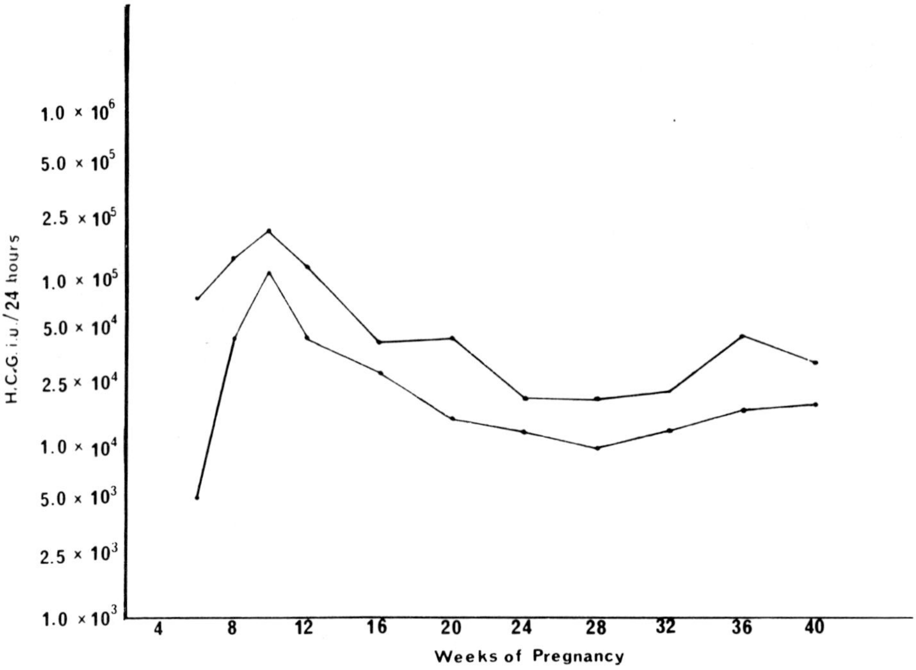

FIGURE 1. Output of HCG throughout pregnancy.

pregnancy is excluded, elevations of HCG level are indicative of recurrence of trophoblastic disease.

6. Fetoplacental Function

HCG assay has failed to provide a reliable index of fetoplacental function in late pregnancy. There was no correlation between maternal serum HCG and the outcome of pregnancy[7] nor between HCG levels and the outcome of pregnancy in patients with diabetes and toxemia.[8] Normal HCG levels have been reported immediately prior to loss of fetal viability.[9]

7. Actions of HCG

HCG appears to be luteotropic, functioning to preserve the corpus luteum.[10] However peak values of HCG occur at a time when the corpus luteum is no longer necessary. There is evidence that HCG is adrenocorticotropic in the fetus.[11] Dehydroepiandrosterone (DHEA) reduces the output of HCG if injected into a pregnant woman. It appears therefore that an autoregulatory feedback mechanism may be in operation, whereby a need for estrogen or its precursor DHEA causes a rise in HCG production, which in turn leads to increased production of DHEA, and vice versa. The secondary peak in HCG levels may therefore be caused by the fall off in estrogen production which occurs at the same time.

8. HCG β Subunit

It is possible to dissociate HCG into α and β subunits under in vitro conditions.[12] The α subunit is common to all four human glycoprotein hormones, HCG, LH, FSH, and TSH,[13] specificity being conferred by the β unit. Areas of homology exist between the β units of HCG and LH[14] suggesting a degree of cross reactivity by antisera. However, careful choice of reagents reduce this, making discrimination between the two hormones possible. With the elimination of fluctuating LH values, detection of very low levels of HCG can be achieved.

9. Radioimmunoassay of HCG[15]

Reagents

1. **Midgley's buffer, 0.01 *M* phosphate + additives** — 37.6 g disodium hydrogen phosphate · 2 H_2O; 6.0 g sodium dihydrogen phosphate · $2H_2O$; 186.0 g EDTA (disodium salt); 205.0 g NaCl; 25.0 g sodium azide (stored at 4°C); 1.25 ℓ 20% bovine serum albumin (BSA); 20 ℓ distilled water; pH to 7.5 with 5 *M* NaOH and make up volume to 25 ℓ.
2. **Antisera to HCG**
3. **Radioactive HCG ^{125}I** — The specific activity is in the range of 200 μCi/ug. For use a solution is prepared in Midgley's buffer containing 1 in 120 normal rabbit serum, to give a count of 50,000 cpm/0.1 mℓ.
4. **2nd antibody, donkey-antirabbit γ globulin** — This is used at a dilution of 1 in 10.
5. **HCG standard containing 53,000 IU/ℓ** — For use, a 3/1000 dilution is prepared to give 160 IU HCG/ℓ.

Apparatus: Selectronic γ Counter

Method *

1. Suitable dilutions of urine are prepared in Midgley's buffer. These vary from 1 in 2 for an expected level of less than 300 units to dilutions in excess of 1 in 2000 where values greater than 100,000 are expected.
2. Diluted urine (0.5 mℓ) is pipetted into the sample tubes.
3. To each tube 0.1 mℓ of 1 in 20,000 HCG antibody is added, immediately followed by addition of by 0.1 mℓ of radioactive HCG. The tubes are then vortex mixed and incubated at 30°C for 6 hr.
4. To each tube 0.1 mℓ of 1 in 12 dilution of 2nd antibody is added. The tubes are vortex mixed and incubated at 30°C overnight.
5. Next day the tubes are removed from the incubator and placed in a cold room at 4°C for 30 min.
6. The tubes, except the totals (see standards below), are centrifuged at 2000 r/min for 20 min.
7. The supernatent liquid is discarded and the precipitates are counted in a γ counter.

Standards

All standards, nonspecific binding tubes, and totals are set up in triplicate. A standard curve is prepared. Doubling dilutions in a range of 160 to 1.25 IU/ℓ of HCG standard are prepared and processed with the samples by the above method. Nonspecific binding tubes are prepared by the above method except that HCG antibody is omitted. Total tubes are prepared by the above method, omitting centrifugation.

* All sample tubes are set up in duplicate.

Calculation

The standard curve is calculated by using the four-parameter log logit method. The concentration of HCG in the unknown samples is calculated by reading from the graph.

Precision: Coefficient of variation = 15%.

10. Radioimmunoassay of β Subunit[16]

Reagents

1. **0.04 *M* phosphate buffer** — pH 7.0, containing 0.1% bovine serum albumin
2. **Antiserum to β subunit HCG**
3. **Radioactive HCG ^{125}I** — The specific activity is in the range of 200 μCi/ug. For use a solution is prepared in 0.04 *M* phosphate buffer containing 1 in 120 normal rabbit serum, to give a count of 30,000 cpm/25 μℓ.
4. **2nd antibody, donkey-antirabbit γ-globulin** — This is used at a dilution of 1 in 10.
5. **HCG standard containing 53,000 IU/ℓ** — For use a dilution is prepared to give 80 IU/ℓ.

Apparatus: Five-headed γ counter used for counting filtration discs from the Darias® filtration unit.

*Method**

1. Neat or suitable dilutions of plasma are prepared in 0.04 *M* phosphate buffer. These vary from 1 in 1 for an expected low level to greater than 1 in 2000 when grossly elevated levels are expected.
2. Diluted plasma (100 μℓ) is pipetted into the sample tubes together with 100 μℓ normal male plasma containing EDTA. To the undiluted (neat) plasma 100 μℓ of phosphate buffer added.
3. To each tube 25 μℓ of a suitable dilution of HCG antibody is added.
4. The tubes are incubated for 2 hr at 30°C.
5. 50 μℓ of radioactive HCG is added and the tubes are vortex mixed.
6. The tubes are incubated for 4 hr at 30°C.
7. 25 μℓ of 2nd antibody is added to each tube.
8. The tubes are incubated overnight at 30°C.
9. Next day the tubes are removed and placed in a cold room at 4°C for 30 min.
10. The tubes are then placed in the Darias® filtration unit and filtered through discs which are counted on the five-headed γ counter.

Standards

All standards and nonspecific binding tubes are set up in triplicate. A standard curve is prepared. Doubling dilutions in a range of 80 to 0.625 IU/ℓ of HCG are prepared and processed with the samples by the above method. Nonspecific binding tubes are prepared by the above method except that HCG antibody is omitted.

Calculation: as for HCG.

Precision: coefficient of variation = 15%.

* All sample tubes are set up in duplicate.

Notes: (1) All plasma samples should be collected in EDTA; (2) iodinated HCG should be freshly prepared.

B. Pregnancy-Specific β-Glycoprotein (SP_1)

1. General

There has recently been interest in a group of placental proteins which have the potential of providing specific markers of placental function. Prominent among these is a pregnancy-specific β-glycoprotein (SP_1). The compound is synthesized by the syncytiotrophoblast. It has a molecular weight of 90,000. The half-life of the protein is 30 to 40 hr and therefore the concentrations are fairly stable from hour to hour.

Pregnancy-specific β-glycoprotein may be detected in the plasma 7 days after fertilization and in the urine at 20 days.[17] In some cases the appearance of SP_1 in the plasma is delayed although there is usually a rapid increase to an upper level of 500 μg/ℓ within 20 days of ovulation. In normal women there is a skewed distribution of the excretion pattern: median levels rise progressively to reach a plateau in the last 4 weeks of pregnancy.[18] The results of assay in normal pregnancy and in intrauterine growth retardation are shown in Figure 2. In over 70% of women with growth retardation of the fetus, low concentrations of SP_1 have been noted. This indicates that the assay may prove to be a valuable index of fetal well-being.

Serial studies have shown that SP_1 concentrations move in parallel with HCG concentrations in patients with trophoblastic tumor and in some cases of gestational choriocarcinoma. These two substances were not related.[19] It has been postulated that SP_1 measurements may be useful in the detection of minimal residual tumor.

*2. Radioimmunoassay (Radioiodination)**

Material

1. **Antigen for labeling and standards** — SP_1, lyophilized (Dr. Bohn, Behringwerke, Marburg)
2. **First antibody** — SP1 antiserum from rabbit (Dr. Baudner, Behringwerke, Marburg)
3. **Second antibody** — anti-rabbit γ globulin serum "forte" from goat (Behringwerke, cat. no. ØTØP 14); rabbit serum, stabilized (Behringwerke, cat. no. ØTØR 04)
4. **Sodium iodide (^{125}I) for labeling, in alkaline solution** — (Behringwerke, cat. no. J 5006), 8 to 15 Ci ^{125}I per mg I, 500 mCi/mℓ
5. **Lactoperoxidase** — E. C. 1.11.1.7, supension in 3.2 *M* $(NH_4)_2SO_4$, 160 U/mg (Boehringer-Mannheim, cat. no. 15491)
6. **Hydrogen peroxide** — 30% H_2O_2, pro analysis (Merck, Darmstadt, cat. no. 7210)
7. **Phosphate buffered saline (PBS)** — pH 7.2, *M*/15 K-Na phosphate buffer according to Soerensen, prepared from NaH_2PO_4 and NaCl, p. a. quality (Merck, Darmstadt)
8. **Bovine serum albumin (BSA)** — pure (Behringwerke, cat. no. ØRHD04)
9. **Sodium azide** — p. a. quality (Merck, Darmstadt)

Preparations

All solutions have to be absolutely free of azide ions, thiocyanate ions, and other peroxidase inhibitors.

1. SP_1: Solution of 0.50 mg/mℓ in PBS, aliquots of 12 μℓ stored at −20°C; thawed immediately before use.

* Method of Lüben G. Behringwerke (Marburg). A homogeneous double antibody system is used.

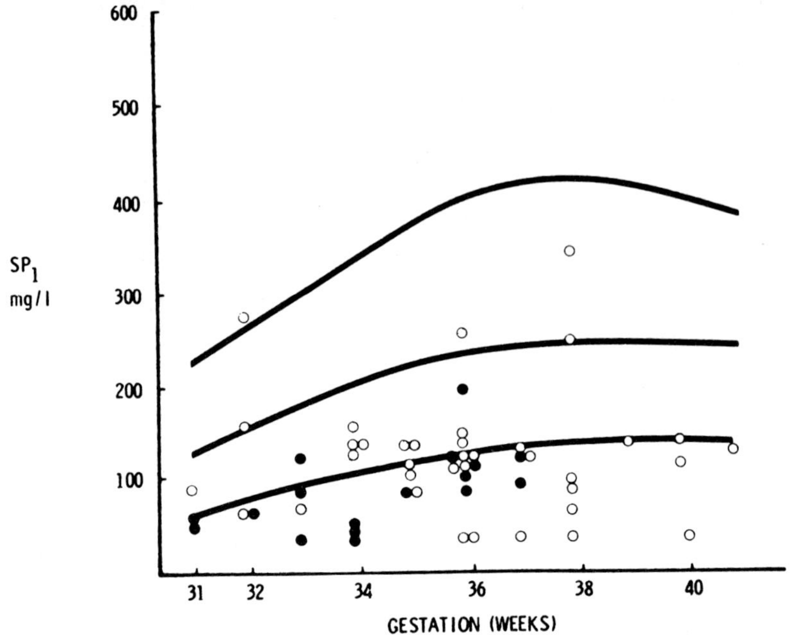

FIGURE 2. S.P.$_1$ concentrations are shown for pregnancies with (●) and without (○) maternal hypertension in which there was intrauterine growth retardation. Concentrations of pregnancy-specific β_1-glycoprotein in maternal blood in normal pregnancy and in intrauterine growth retardation. Solid lines represent median, 10th, and 90th centile of maternal plasma S.P.$_1$ after 30th week of normal pregnancy. (Figure reproduced from Gordon, Y. B., Grudzinskas, J. G., Jeffrey, D., and Chard, T., *Lancet*, 1, 331, 1977. With permission.)

2. Lactoperoxidase (LPO): 0.2 mℓ of crystalline ammonium sulfate suspension (1,0 mg LPO) is centrifuged and the pellet dissolved in 0.6 mℓ PBS to yield a stock solution of 1.66 mg/mℓ, which is stored in aliquots of 10 μℓ at −20°C. Immediately before use the contents of 1 vial are thawed, diluted with 90 μℓ of PBS, and homogenized by use of a vibromixer.
3. Hydrogen peroxide: A fresh solution (8.7 n*M*) is prepared by diluting 5 μℓ of perhydrol (30%) in 50 mℓ of PBS in a graduated flask. The dosage of perhydrol is preferably done in a 5 mℓ capillary pipette (e.g., Partigen-Dispenser, Behringwerke cat. no. ØTCKO2) the capillary of which is discarded after use. This avoids contamination of pipettes with high percentage H_2O_2 which might inhibit the enzyme reaction.
4. Stopping solution: PBS with 1% NaN_3, 0.2% NaCl, 0.2% NaI and 1% BSA
5. Gel chromatography column: Sephadex® G-200, gel bed 1 × 14 cm, elution with PBS containing 0.1% BSA, 0.025% NaN_3 and 0.9% NaCl.

Labeling procedure

A V-shaped plastic vial (1.5 mℓ AutoAnalyzer cup) is equipped with a 1- to 2-mm magnetic stirring bar, prepared by melting an iron thread into a suited glass capillary. In a fume cupboard under slow, but constant stirring, the following solutions are pipetted into the vial using the same 10 μℓ Hamilton syringe:

1. 5 μg of SP_1 in 10 μℓ of PBS

2. Undiluted Na ^{125}I-solution containing 500 μCi of radioactivity (normally) in 1 to 2 μℓ)
3. 1.0 μg of LPO in 6 μℓ of PBS
4. 10 μℓ of H_2O_2 solution (8.7 n*M*), 1 μℓ per min over a period of 10 min

After a further 10 min the reaction is finished by the addition of 0.2 mℓ stopping solution. After stirring for about 1 min a sample of 10 μℓ is taken preserved for calculation of the total amount of ^{125}I employed. The bulk of the reaction mixture is gel chromatographed, mainly to achieve the separation of protein bound and unbound ^{125}I.

The elution pattern of the radioactivity is established by measurement of the Sephadex® fractions after appropriate dilution. The amounts of radioactivity before and after gel chromatography are compared to give the total yield of ^{125}I. The radioactivity found in the protein fraction is taken to calculate the yield of iodination and the specific radioactivity of the labeled protein (in mCi/mg), assuming a homogeneous degree of substitution over the whole protein peak (approximation!).

The fractions to be pooled and further processed are selected by the following criteria: absence of free ^{125}I and homogeneity of labeled protein in SDS-PAGE (7.5% PAA, 0.1% SDS, pH 8.9), maximum immunoreactivity towards the antibody to be used in the radioimmunoassay. The pooled fractions are stored at −20°C until use after subdivision into aliquots.

Assay protocol

The incubates are composed in triplicates as follows:

Reagents (μℓ volumes)

	Assay buffer	First antibody	Tracer antigen	Sample or standards	Second antibody
Total activity (A)	—	—	200	—	—
Nonspecific binding (NB)	250	—	200	—	200
Zero-binding (B_o)	50	200	200	—	200
Sample or standards (B_x)	—	200	200	50	200

Working dilutions of reagents (dilution in assay buffer)

Assay-buffer:	0.02 *M* NaP pH 7.4 with 1% BSA and 0.1% NaN_3
First antibody:	1:150,000 (applies to lot no. 4134 A)
Tracer antigen:	250 ng/ℓ, specific activity ~ 60 Ci/g; with normal rabbit serum 1:700
Standards:	(0.5), 1, 2, 4, 8, 16, 32, and 64 μg/ℓ, respectively
Second antibody:	1:80, + $(NH_4)_2SO_4$(260 g/ℓ)

Reaction steps

Preincubation (without tracer-antigen): 5 hr at room temperature (r.t.)
First reaction (after addition of tracer antigen): 17 hr at r.t.
Second reaction: 2 hr at r.t.
Centrifugation: 30 min at 3000 g; 1 wash with 0.5-mℓ assay buffer

Evaluation

$$p\ (\%\ \text{bound}) = \frac{\overline{\text{Bj}}\ (\text{cpm}) - \overline{\text{NB}}\ (\text{cpm})}{\text{A (cpm)}} \cdot 100$$

Here $\overline{B}_i$ ($\equiv \overline{B}_o$ or $\overline{B}_x$), $\overline{NB}$ and $\overline{A}$: mean count rates of triplicates.

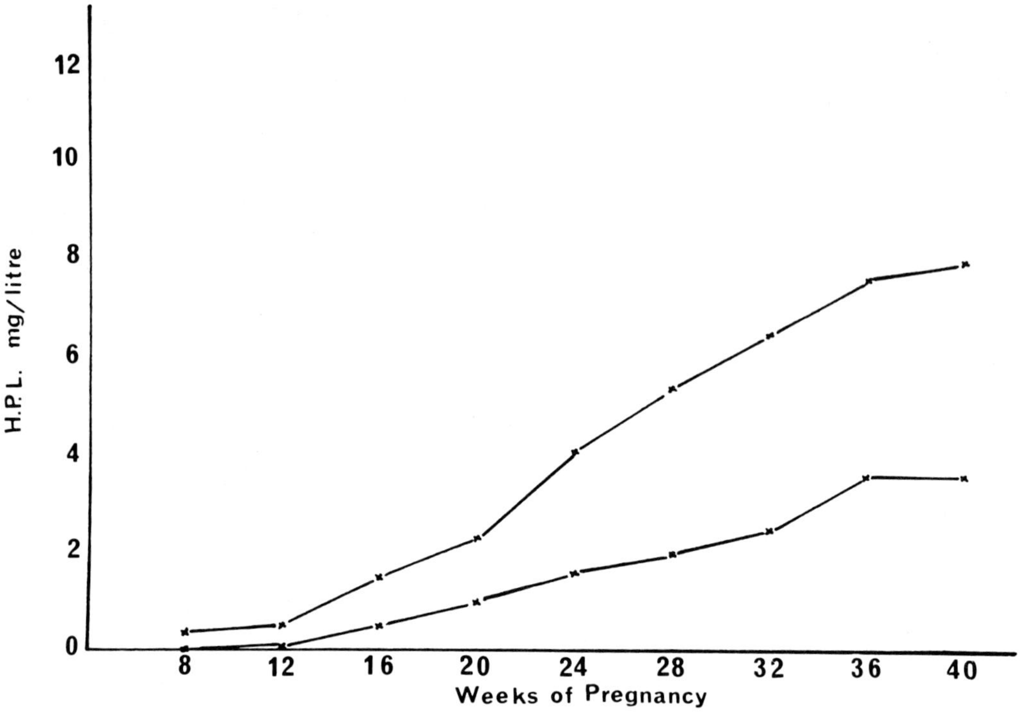

FIGURE 3. Serum HPL levels during normal pregnancy.

C. Human Placental Lactogen (HPL)

HPL is synthesized by the syncytiotrophoblast of the placenta during pregnancy.[20] The output increases during pregnancy but tends to remain constant during the last few weeks (Figure 3). HPL is first detectable in maternal serum at about 6 weeks gestation. In the last trimester the amount synthesized is in the order of 1 g per day.[21] The high rate of production coupled with a half-life of about 20 min explains the high circulating levels which are found at term. There is no circadian rhythm and its estimation is not affected by stress or metabolic changes.[22,23]

1. Threatened Abortion

In some cases the outcome of vaginal bleeding in early pregnancy is in little doubt, but some women are admitted with an intact pregnancy despite vaginal bleeding. It has been shown by several groups of workers that HPL assays are of value in predicting the outcome of a threatened abortion. Patients whose levels fell below the normal range or who had decreasing levels aborted,[24,25] and it appeared that HPL levels could be used to distinguish those patients whose pregnancy would go to term from those who would abort.[26]

2. Fetoplacental Function

HPL levels reflect the function of the placenta alone. In late pregnancy there appears to be little correlation between HPL levels and fetal distress.[25] HPL measurements were performed serially on a large number of women with various complications of pregnancy. It was concluded from the study that HPL assays did not help in the selection of patients who needed biophysical monitoring nor did they correlate with the infants' neurological development.[27] HPL assays appear to be of little value in monitoring diabetic pregnancies.[8,28] Raised levels have been noted,[29] probably reflecting an abnormally large placenta. In erythroblastosis, levels of HPL may be elevated above normal and again this is probably a reflection of the large placenta.

Low levels of HPL have been found in toxemic patients as a group[9,24,30] but the prognostic significance of HPL determinations in individual cases of pre-eclamptic toxemia is difficult to determine. There is also some controversy regarding the use of HPL assays as an indicator of retarded fetal growth. A positive correlation with fetal birth weight was demonstrated when HPL levels were assayed 10 days before birth[31] and when serial assays were performed after 36 weeks gestation.[32] Other workers have found no correlation between infant weight and HPL levels.[25]

3. Actions of Human Placental Lactogen

When HPL is given to normal people or to diabetics it impairs glucose tolerance.[33,34] It has been suggested that it is responsible for the diabetogenic effect of pregnancy, and that this function adjusts glucose and fat metabolism in favor of the fetus. However both estrogens and progesterone may have a similar effect and it is difficult to attribute a specific function to HPL. The mammotrophic and lactogenic effects of HPL are less than those of pituitary prolactin.

The absence of a well-defined function is accompanied by absence of control mechanisms. The high circulating levels together with lack of control suggests that synthesis and release may be autonomous. If this is so, circulating levels reflect the functional mass of the placenta.

*4. Radioimmunoassay of Human Placental Lactogen**
Reagents

1. **Antisera to HPL raised in rabbits** — This is used at a dilution of:

Dilution	Weeks of pregnancy
1 in 2500	6—11
1 in 600	12—21
1 in 126	22—term

2. **Iodinated ^{125}HPL** — specific activity 30 μCi/ug
3. **Phosphate buffered saline** — 0.05 *M* phosphate in 0.15 *M* sodium chloride, pH 7.4. To this is added 3 g/ℓ bovine serum albumin
4. **HPL-free diluent** — diluted horse serum
5. **Ethanol**

Apparatus: Packard Selectronic γ Counter

Method

Into 75 × 12 mm plastic tubes 0.1 mℓ plasma is pipetted. Standard HPL (0.1 mℓ) is pipetted into duplicate plastic tubes, the range used depending on the period of gestation.

Standard HPL range (μg/mℓ)	Weeks of pregnancy
0.025—0.4	6—11
0.1—1.6	12—21
0—16	22—term

* By Pharmacia Kit (supplied by Pharmacia Fine Chemicals AB, Uppsala, Sweden).

The different concentrations of standard are prepared in HPL-free diluent. To all tubes is added 0.2 mℓ iodinated HPL and 0.2 mℓ antiserum. The tubes are then incubated at room temperature for a time dependent on the period of gestation.

Incubation time (min)	Weeks of pregnancy
120	6—11
60	12—21
30	22—term

After incubation 1.0 mℓ ethanol is added to all tubes with thorough mixing. All tubes are then centrifuged at room temperature for 10 min at 2000 g. The supernatant is then aspirated and the tubes stoppered. The precipitate is counted in a γ counter.

Calculation

The standard curve is calculated by means of a spline function. The concentration of HPL in the unknowns is estimated by comparison with the standard curve.

III. PLACENTAL STEROID HORMONES

A. Progesterone

Initially progesterone is produced by the corpus luteum, but after the first 2 months the ovary plays no important part in human pregnancy. After implantation plasma progesterone levels rise steeply from the normal peak value and then they slowly decrease from the 5th to the 9th week. After the 9th week there is an increase in levels due to production by the syncitium of the placenta. High levels then continue for the remainder of pregnancy (Figure 4).

The half-life of progesterone in blood is between 3 and 5 min, suggesting a uniform pattern of production. Less than 10% of the circulating progesterone is in the free state.[35] Most is bound to albumin. Only very small amounts of progesterone are present in the urine — excretion rates of 0.5 to 3.0 μg/24 hours are found in pregnancy.[36]

1. Uses as a Test of Fetoplacental Function

Progesterone follows the trend of urinary estriol excretion but gives no warning of impending fetal death.[37] In early pregnancy significant changes in progesterone levels do not occur until after the placenta has separated.[38]

Although there is little experience in using progesterone as a test of placental function, evidence to date suggests that it is unlikely to provide useful information regarding fetal prognosis.

2. Actions of Progesterone

It is believed that progesterone reduces excitability of the muscle and high levels of the hormone have been found in the myometrium adjacent to the placenta.[39]

The acid-base characteristics of the extracellular fluid alter by the 50th day of pregnancy.[40] The standard bicarbonate of the arterial blood falls during pregnancy and the pCO_2 is reduced. These changes are thought to be due to progesterone as similar effects may be brought about in nonpregnant women by the administration of progesterone.[41]

B. Pregnanediol

1. General

There are several end products of progesterone metabolism. One of these is 5β-preg-

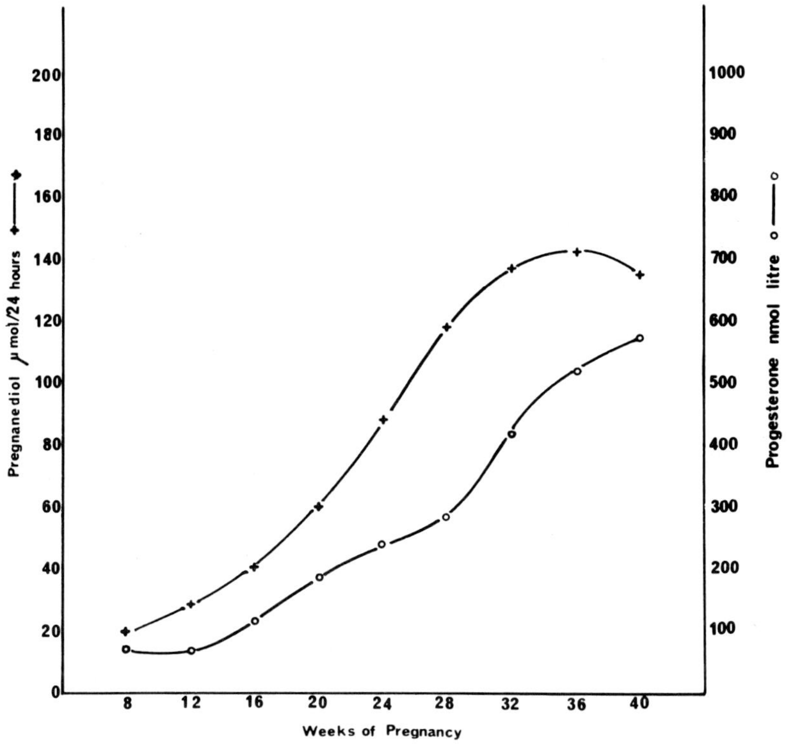

FIGURE 4. The urinary pregnanediol and plasma progesterone levels during normal pregnancy.

nane-3α, 20α-diol (pregnanediol). Pregnanediol is also derived from pregnenolone and deoxycorticosterone. The average conversion of progesterone to urinary pregnanediol was found to be 12.9%.[42] Therefore pregnanediol estimation can give only a crude indication of progesterone production.

The range of pregnanediol excretion during pregnancy is wide and shows considerable day-to-day variation.[43] The level is fairly constant during the first 12 weeks of pregnancy and then shows a steady rise until the 36th week when it plateaus. (Figure 4).

2. Uses as a Test of Fetoplacental Function

The measurement of urinary pregnanediol was the first widely used test of placental function, but due to the variability in the excretion of the hormone coupled with the fact that changes in excretion usually occur after the onset of placental malfunction, the test has proved to be of little value.

The results of serial assays in recurrent abortion showed that they had little predictive value.[44] In toxemia of pregnancy, pregnanediol excretion correctly predicted only 21% of cases with abnormal fetoplacental function.[45] Diabetes and rhesus isoimmunization appear to have no effect on pregnanediol excretion.[46] In hydatidiform mole the rates of excretion of pregnanediol tend to be low but are generally within normal limits.[46]

C. Estrogens

1. Urinary Excretion

The urinary excretion of estrogens in late pregnancy is about 1000 times greater than

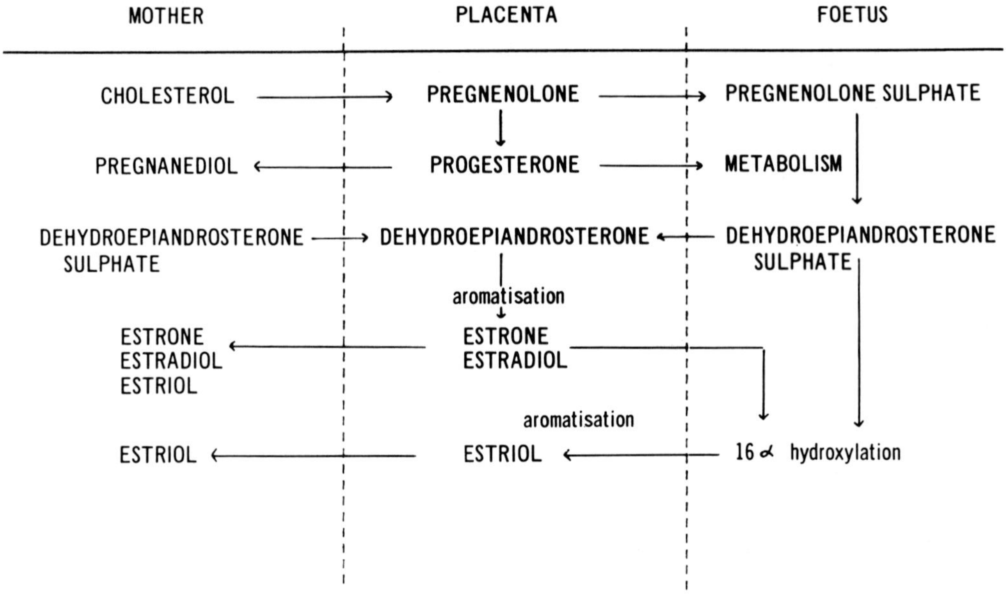

FIGURE 5. Diagramatic representation of the course of estrogen synthesis during pregnancy.

in nonpregnant women. The production of estrogens in pregnancy reflects the functional states of both the placenta and the fetus. A biological requirement for the relatively large amounts of estrogen formed has not been identified. In rare conditions it is possible for the fetus to develop normally in the absence of normal increases of estrogen production.

At least 27 estrogens have been isolated from pregnancy urine. The daily average production of the three "classical" estrogens is 10 mg estrone, 11 mg estradiol, and 222 mg estriol.[47] The estrogens found in pregnancy urine are the metabolic products from a complex set of interrelationships between the maternal, placental, and fetal compartments (Figure 5). The human placenta depends for its estrogen synthesis on neutral steroid precursors reaching it from the fetal and maternal circulations.

The principal estrogen precursors are the 3-hydroxy-androst-5-ene derivatives. The essential enzyme systems required for estrogen synthesis are distributed between the placenta and the fetus. Aryl sulfatase, 3β-hydroxysteroid dehydrogenase, and Δ^4- Δ^5-isomerase are present in the placenta, whereas 16 α-hydroxylating systems are present in the fetal liver. The aromatizing system is found mainly in the placenta and to a lesser extent in the fetus. Therefore, the fetus and the placenta together form a functional unit, carrying out the synthesis of the major part of estrogens excreted in pregnancy.

The placenta releases much more estrogen to the maternal than to the fetal compartment. Estrogen sulfates reaching the placenta with the fetal circulation are hydrolyzed by the placenta and transferred to the maternal compartment. Despite these processes considerable quantities of conjugated estrogens are accumulated in fetal tissues. Estrogen transfer from the maternal to the fetal compartment is limited.

Placental secretion of estriol to the mother is followed by a metabolism involving extensive conversion of unconjugated estriol, estriol 3-sulfate 16-glucosiduronate, and estriol-3-sulfate into estriol-16-glucosiduronate and then into estriol-3-glucosiduronate. Most of the dynamic changes in the pattern of conjugation take place in the form of repeated hydrolysis and reconjugation.

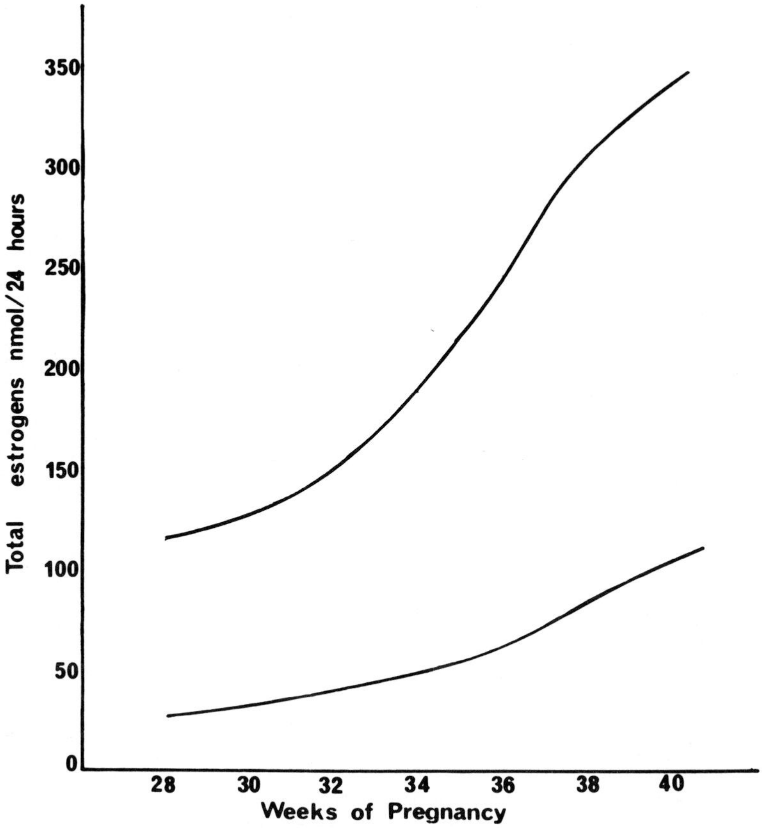

FIGURE 6. Excretion of total urinary estrogens from 30 weeks of pregnancy.

2. Methods of Estimation of Urinary Estrogen

Urinary estrogen excretion rises steadily throughout pregnancy but it is during the final trimester that the greatest increase in estrogen production occurs (Figure 6). Estrogen assays contribute little to the management of pregnancy prior to 30 weeks gestation. It has been suggested that only assays of the predominant estrogen, estriol, should be performed during pregnancy. However, total estrogen methods have proved to be as precise and as adequate as estriol determinations. The advantage of total estrogen methods is that specimens may be assayed quickly and that results are available daily. The daily variation (±18%) in estrogen excretion[48] must be considered when assessing the results of a single specimen. It is always preferable to rely on a series of assays. Falling values indicate a failure of estrogen production and premature delivery of the fetus may be indicated.

3. Automated Continuous Flow Method for the Estimation of Pregnancy Estrogens[49]
Reagents

1. **Kober reagent** — 60 g quinol is dissolved in 1 ℓ of concentrated sulfuric acid (solution A); 15 g ferrous sulfate is dissolved in 1 ℓ of distilled water to which is added 1 ℓ of concentrated sulfuric acid (solution B). Solution A is added to solution B.

2. **Ittrich reagent** — 1000 g chloral hydrate and 1000 g trichloracetic acid are dissolved in 3 ℓ of distilled water.
3. **Diluent solution** — 6 mℓ of concentrated sulfuric acid and 2 mℓ of Brij® 35 (30% w/v) are added to 2 ℓ of distilled water.
4. **Wash solution** — 2 mℓ of Brij® 35 is added to 2 ℓ of distilled water
5. **Standards** — A range of standards from 25 to 200 μmol /ℓ is prepared in 0.1 *M* NaOH from a stock solution containing 500 μmol /ℓ.

Fluorimetry

The heating block, fluorimeter, recorder, pump, and sampler are switched on. The wash solution is pumped through the system until the heating block equilibrates at 125°C. The Kober, Ittrich, and diluent solutions are pumped into the system until equilibrium is reached. This procedure takes about 20 min. A drift control consisting of a 25 μmol/ℓ standard is placed in the first cup. This is followed by 25, 50, 75, 100, 125, 150, and 200 μmol/ℓ standards. This series is followed by a urine control extract and another drift control. Eight sample extracts are placed in the following eight cups followed by a control extract and another drift control.

Calculation

From the recorder chart, peak heights are plotted derived from the standard solutions as a function of concentration. Peak heights derived from the urine samples are interpolated to obtain total estrogens.

Precision: Coefficient of variation = 4%.

Substances which may interfere with results

Glucose in the urine will give low results. It should be extracted by the following method:

A 10-cm column of XAD 2 suspended in water is prepared. 5 mℓ of urine is added to the column. The column is then washed with distilled water until the eluate is glucose free. Next 2 mℓ of methanol is added to the column and the eluate is discarded. 20 mℓ of methanol is added and the eluate is collected and evaporated to dryness. The residue is dissolved in 5 mℓ of distilled water and is used in the place of the original urine sample.

4. Factors Affecting Estrogen Output

Renal clearance — A change in renal clearance will cause a change in the excretion of steroids without their production being altered. A reduced renal clearance of estrogens was observed in pre-eclamptic patients who had high plasma estriol levels and low urinary estriol levels.[50] It has been shown that bed-rested supine patients in the last trimester of pregnancy had an increase in glomerular filtration rate and an increase in estrogen excretion.[51]

Urine collection — The variation in estrogen excretion has been shown to be inversely proportional to the length of the collection period.[48] The use of a 24-hr collection of urine reflects a compromise between short collection periods and the longer 48-hr collections. The main problem in 24-hr collections is to ensure that a complete collection of urine has been made. In an effort to overcome this, single specimens have been assayed for the estrogen-creatinine ratio.[52,53] Large discrepancies between the actual 24-hr collection and that calculated from the estrogen-creatinine ratio of a single specimen have been reported.[54]

Compounds which interfere with estrogen assay — The presence of glucose in the urine sample interferes with the assay. Treatment of the sample has been discussed

Table 1
APPARATUS[a]

Int. diameter (in.)	Color
Pump tubing in Tygon®	
0.040	white/white
0.065	blue/blue
0.073	green/green
0.045	red/red
0.090	purple/black
0.110	purple/white
0.020	orange/yellow
Pump tubing in Acidflex®	
0.073	green/green
0.060	yellow/blue

Item	Number
Glassware	
12-turn glass mixing coils	3
Connectors	
A10	1
DO	2
H1	1
C5	1 (used as de-bubbler)
Stream divider	
PT4	1
Fluorimeter: Perkin Elmer 1000	
Excitation wavelength 530 nm, selected by interference filter	
Emission wavelength 560 nm, selected by diffraction grating	

[a] Ismatec® proportioning pump and solid block heater at 125°C, with 2 28-turn mixing coils encapsulated in silicone rubber. See Figure 7.

previously under methodology. The laxatives cascara and senna, stilbestrol, and meprobamate have been reported to influence the Kober reaction.[55] Severe interference in assay procedure is observed in patients being treated with mandelamine (methenamine mandelate) for urinary tract infection.[56]

Fetal abnormality — ACTH is a major regulatory hormone for fetal adrenal C_{19} steroids and thus an important regulator of placental estrogen production. Fetal adrenal cortical atrophy is nearly always present in anencephalic fetuses. Lack of precursors is also found in primary congenital adrenal hypoplasia. Low excretion of estriol in the mother is associated with liver cirrhosis in the fetus. This is probably due to impairment of 16-α-hydroxylation in the fetal liver.

Placental enzyme activity — Placental sulfatase deficiency has been reported, in which the placenta lacks an enzyme crucial for estrogen biosynthesis.[57-59] This condition is associated with very low estriol output in the the mother. Despite this, healthy surviving fetuses may be produced.

Drug administration to the mother — Ingestion of penicillin reduces urinary estrogen excretion.[60] This may be due to an effect on the bacterial flora of the gastrointes-

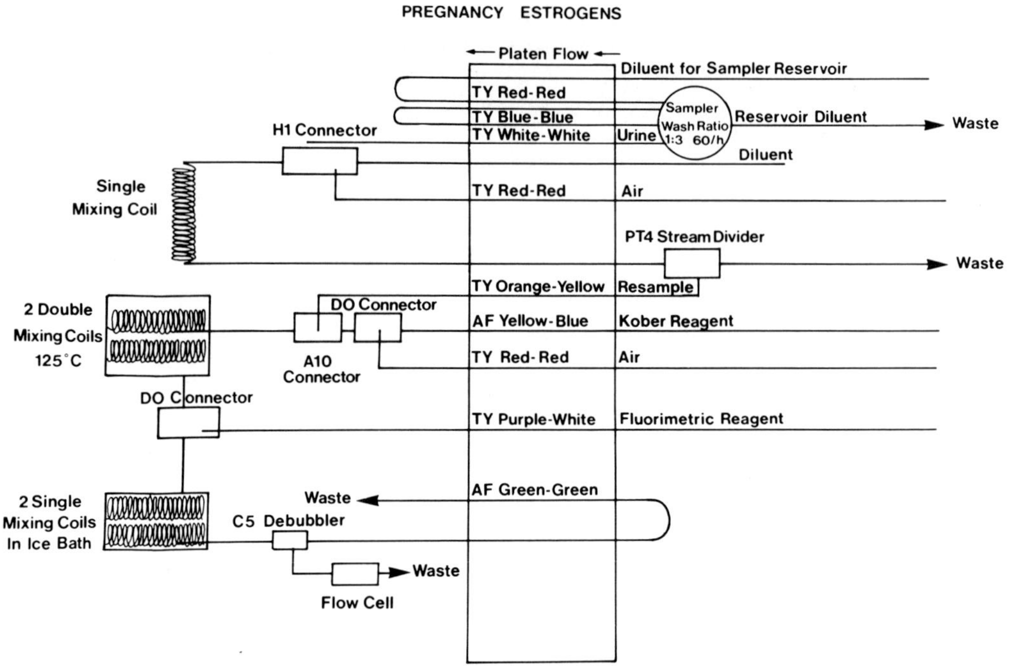

FIGURE 7. Diagram to show an automated continuous flow apparatus for the estimation of total estrogens during pregnancy.

tinal tract. Suppression of the fetal hypothalamic-pituitary-adrenal axis may occur when large doses of corticosteroids are administered to the mother.[61] In clinical assessments of urinary estrogen measurement it is not possible to distinguish between maternal, placental, or fetal causes for the abnormality in production.

5. Actions of Estrogens

The reason why the fetoplacental unit secretes such large quantities of estrogen during pregnancy remains obscure.

Estrogens alter the polymerization of the mucopolysaccharides, causing the ground substance to become hygroscopic. This accounts for the increase of body water and the common occurrence of edema during pregnancy. Softening of the ground substance in connective tissue allows it to become more stretchable, leading to laxness of joints and softening of the uterine cervix.

Estrogens may be responsible for some of the vascular changes which occur during pregnancy. Changes in the pattern of serum proteins including protein-binding capacity are caused by estrogens.

6. Uses of Pregnancy Estrogen Assay

Intrauterine growth retardation (IUGR) is known to be associated with an increased incidence of fetal death, neonatal death, and neurological sequelae. It affects about 1% of all pregnancies, but not all of these are detected prenatally.[62]

It is often difficult to identify the cause of IUGR. It has been demonstrated that neither fetal nor maternal growth hormone is necessary for normal fetal growth. Although growth factors as yet unidentified may be present in the fetus, it is thought that impairment of nutrients to the fetus combined with lack of elimination of toxic substances may be responsible for IUGR.

IUGR is associated with chronic renal disease, hypertension, and preeclampsia in the mother. Pregnancies complicated by bleeding in the second trimester also show an increased incidence of "light for date" infants and perinatal mortality.[63]

Urinary estriol excretion correlates well with fetal size.[64,65] Patients with IUGR show decreased urinary estrogen excretion when compared to normal patients.[66,67] It appears that the lower the urinary estrogen output the greater the chances that the fetus is in jeopardy.[68] It has been suggested that all pregnancies should have a routine 24-hr estriol estimation performed at 30 and 36 weeks of pregnancy,[69] as 50% of the infants associated with low levels showed evidence of IUGR. Serial assays should be used to follow the progress of any fetus suspected as being small for dates to help in the prediction of possible fetal deaths.

7. Toxemia of Pregnancy

Toxemia may occur with pre-existing essential hypertension or renal disease, and may present with different grades of severity. It has been found that in patients with hypertension the estrogen excretion was rarely low unless the fetus was small for dates or unless perinatal death occurred[70]. On the other hand in patients with severe toxemia the estrogen level was nearly always low.[70,71] Normal estrogen excretion is usually associated with live births. Subnormal excretion and falling levels coincide with deteriorating fetoplacental function.

8. Diabetes

Diabetes is a serious complication of pregnancy and the perinatal mortality rate is 5 to 10 times greater than that of a nondiabetic pregnancy.[72] Overt diabetic subjects have a normal or lower than normal excretion of estrogen during pregnancy,[73,74] and low and falling levels indicate fetal distress which will end in fetal death. It has been stressed that daily estrogen assays must be performed in order to detect significant falls in level.[75] It has been shown that daily serial assays are a good indicator of fetal well-being.[75,76]

9. Plasma Estrogens

The value of estimating plasma levels of estriol is the elimination of 24-hr collections, thereby obtaining an immediate sample. However this reflects estrogen production at a single point in time. It is not clear whether there is a significant variation in plasma estrogen concentration over a 24-hr period. No diurnal variation was noted by some,[77] but other workers have detected a significant diurnal variation.[78] Neither exercise nor rest had an effect on the values obtained.[79,80] Plasma estriol levels rise slowly until about 20 weeks of pregnancy and then more rapidly to term, with a surge between 35 and 36 weeks (Figure 8). This surge has been used to predict gestational age in the last trimester.[81]

10. Use as a Test of Fetoplacental Function

The usefulness of plasma estriol in high risk pregnancies is controversial. A comparative study of serum total estriol and urinary estrogens indicated that the use of serum estriol was not justified in high risk pregnancies.[82] A lack of correlation between plasma concentration of unconjugated estriol and urine content of estriol has been noted in uncomplicated pregnancies.[83] Other reports dispute these findings and have noted a close correlation between serum unconjugated estriol and urine estriol concentrations, in both normal and high risk pregnancies.[84] A reduction in plasma level has been found in patients with placental insufficiency.[85] The mean level was noted to be lower in IUGR.[86] No significant correlation was recorded between plasma estriol level

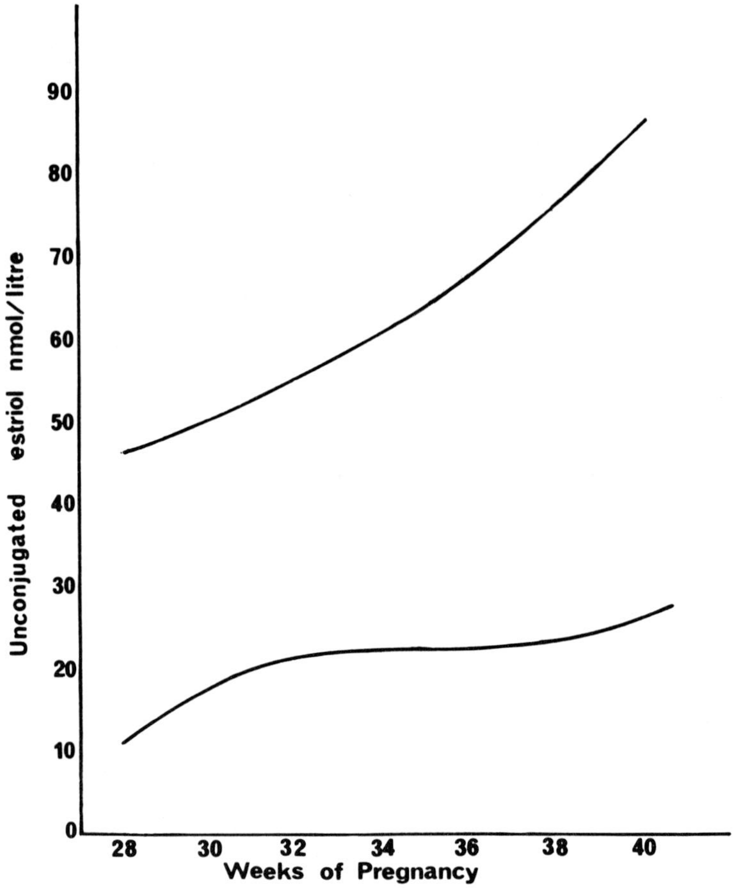

FIGURE 8. Plasma levels of unconjugated estriol from 30 weeks of pregnancy.

and the incidence of fetal distress.[87] Plasma unconjugated estriol was of value in predicting neonatal performance in pregnancies complicated by moderate to severe PET, chronic hypertension, and IUGR;[88] however, low plasma estriol values were not always ominous.

Plasma estrogen levels do not always provide an accurate prognostic guide to the outcome of pregnancy, and despite the fact that a same-day result is available, it is suggested that clinical indications and results of other tests for fetoplacental function should be considered along with plasma estrogen levels.

11. Radioimmunoassay of Plasma Estriol[89]
Reagents

1. **0.1 *M* Tris HCl buffer pH 7.0** — 15.8 g Tris HCl [*Tris* (hydroxymethyl)-aminomethane hydrochloride]; 0.975 g sodium azide; 800 mℓ distilled water. The pH is adjusted to 7.0 and the volume made up to 1 ℓ with distilled water. It is stored at 4°C.
2. **Tris HCl gelatin buffer pH 7.0** — 1 g gelatin is dissolved in 1 ℓ Tris HCl buffer. It is stored at 4°C.

3. **Estriol antiserum** — This is used at a dilution giving 30 to 40% binding of label in the zero standard tube.
4. **Labeled estriol** [2,4,6,9(n)^{3}H](Radiochemical Centre Amersham) — The specific activity is in the range of 70 to 110 Ci/ mmol. A stock solution is made in ethanol. For use the ethanolic solution is diluted in Tris HCl buffer to give a count of 15,000 cpm / 0.1 mℓ.
5. **Dextran-coated charcoal** — 25 mg Dextran T-70; 250 mg charcoal Norit® A; 100 mℓ Tris HCl gelatin buffer. This solution is stirred at 4°C for at least 1 hr before use. During use it should be stirred continuously.
6. **Standard estriol** — The stock solution is 1 g /ℓ in ethanol and this is stored at 4°C. For a working standard 500 μℓ is evaporated to dryness. The residue is taken up in 100 mℓ of buffer. Of this 400 μℓ is further diluted to 50 mℓ to give an estriol concentration of 139 nmol / ℓ. This is stored at 4°C.

Apparatus: Liquid scintillation counter, Packard 3380, using a PPO *bis*-MSB counting fluid.

*Method**

1. 50 μℓ of sample, 100 μℓ of antiserum, and 100 μℓ of label are pipetted into plastic test tubes. They are incubated at room temperature overnight.
2. Next day the samples are placed in an ice bath for 15 min.
3. 0.5 mℓ of dextran-charcoal is added to each tube and the tubes are vortex mixed and immediately replaced in the ice bath for 15 min.
4. The tubes are centrifuged at 2000 r/min for 10 min at 4°C.
5. 0.5 mℓ of supernatent is removed for counting.

Standards

All standards, nonspecific binding tubes, and totals are set up in triplicate. A standard curve is prepared. Doubling dilutions in a range of 139- to 4.35 nmol/ℓ of estriol standard are prepared and processed with the samples by the above method. Total and blank tubes are prepared.

12. 15α-Hydroxyestriol

It has been suggested that any steroid originating solely in the fetus would be an accurate indicator of fetal well-being. Under normal circumstances 15-hydroxylation appears to be a reaction occurring in the fetal liver.

In normal pregnancies the levels of estriol and 15α-hydroxyestriol in maternal blood and urine run closely parallel.[90, 91] Coefficients of variation for consecutive 24-hr collections of urine were found to be similar to those of estriol.[90] No regular pattern of diurnal variation was noted in plasma levels.[91] At term the urinary levels were shown to correlate well with the birth weight.

In complicated pregnancies a retrospective study failed to indicate a useful role for 15α-hydroxyestriol in patients with hypertension, rhesus isoimmunization, intrauterine fetal death, or twin pregnancy.[92] It has been shown to be of some value in patients with severe toxemia and fetal distress in that concentrations decreased before fetal death.[93,94] Levels of 15α-hydroxyestriol in plasma and urine do not differ significantly from normal or correlate with the severity of the disease in diabetes mellitus.[91,93]

As dissociation between fetal and placental pathology is rare in abnormalities of fetoplacental function, purely fetal steroids may be of limited use in monitoring pathological pregnancies.

* All sample tubes are set up in duplicate.

IV. GENERAL CONCLUSIONS

Acute functional failure affecting the fetus in labor present as changes in the fetal heart rate, passage of meconium, or changes in the fetal blood pH. During pregnancy the fetoplacental function test should be used to determine whether the fetus is in jeopardy and to find the optimum time for delivery, balancing the dangers of prematurity against the hostile maternal environment.

Total estrogen or estriol assays performed on a 24-hr sample of urine are the most widely used of all tests of fetoplacental function. They are simple to perform and results may be made available on the same day. However, there may be problems in collecting an accurate 24-hr sample of urine and there is an inevitable delay during the collection period. A single index may not give a true picture of fetoplacental function and a combination of tests may be of more value. The combination of urinary total estrogen or estriol with serial serum HPL assays has found wide acceptance and seems to provide a good prognostic index.

A single reading from any test should not carry much credence. Serial estimations are usually necessary to detect any trend, especially in monitoring high-risk pregnancies. In all tests of fetoplacental function there is an overlap between normal and abnormal values and due to biological variation a fairly wide range of normal values is found.

A. Early Pregnancy

Urinary chorionic gonadotropin assay is a valuable indicator of placental function in very early pregnancy. It is used routinely in the diagnosis of pregnancy and in the diagnosis and follow up of trophoblastic disease and choriocarcinoma.

The sensitive assay for the estimation of HPL has proved of value in cases of threatened abortion,[26] to differentiate those patients in danger of imminent abortion from those whose pregnancies are not in immediate danger.

Estrogen assay is of no value in early pregnancy.

B. Antepartum Hemorrhage

The main risk to the fetus in this condition is prematurity. Low estriol levels have been noted at the time of bleeding. These levels return to normal after bleeding ceases.[95] In placental abruption, estrogen levels may be normal until after fetal death has occurred. Placenta previa is not associated with abnormal estrogen excretion.[96] High levels of HPL have been reported in placenta previa where there is necrotic placental tissue, although no definite pattern of levels has been found.

C. Prolonged Pregnancy

Prolonged pregnancy by itself is probably not inevitably associated with high perinatal mortality. Postmaturity syndrome is associated with an increased incidence of placental lesions, fetal hypoxia, IUGR, perinatal mortality, and neonatal morbidity.[97] In uncomplicated prolonged pregnancies estrogen excretion is maintained at a constant or slightly rising level. Infants with the postmaturity syndrome are sometimes delivered by women whose estrogen excretion is normal, but usually the mothers have had low estrogen excretion prior to the birth. However, there is overlap between levels in the normal prolonged pregnancy and those with postmaturity. Because of this, estrogen excretion alone is of limited value in monitoring these cases. There are variable opinions regarding the use of HPL assays in prolonged pregnancy. Some workers have stated that HPL levels are of limited prognostic value,[98] while others have stated that prediction rates for postmature infants are good.[99-101]

D. Diabetes Mellitus

HPL levels reflect placental states and have proved of little value in the management of diabetes.[102, 103] Low normal or subnormal levels are associated with increased fetal risk[104] but as elevated values have also been reported in this condition[25,105] considerable care is needed in the interpretation of results. Estrogen assays are useful in monitoring diabetic pregnancies. As fetal distress can occur rapidly it is essential to monitor estrogen output daily. While serial estrogen assays are satisfactory delivery may be safely postponed.

E. Toxemia of Pregnancy

The average excretion of estrogens falls with increasing severity of the disease but no particular level of output may be taken as indicating acute danger to the fetus. Normal excretion is usually associated with live births; perinatal deaths are usually preceded by subnormal excretion of estrogen. HPL levels are often lower in this group of patients but they are of limited value in predicing fetal distress.

F. Intrauterine Growth Retardation (IUGR)

HPL levels may be lower than those of normal subjects[106] and in hypertensive subjects with IUGR were shown to detect growth retardation better than urinary estriol levels.[101] On the other hand, as HPL levels correlate well with placental but not fetal size[107] and as not all problems of IUGR are related to placental problems, other reports have indicated normal HPL levels in IUGR.[28] There is general agreement that estrogen excretion is lower when fetal growth is retarded but overlap with normal values does occur.[108] Usually the lower the urinary estrogen excretion the greater the chance that the fetus is in danger.

G. Rhesus Incompatibility

The levels of estrogen excretion do not reflect the condition of the erythroblastic fetus. Changes in steroid metabolism may not occur until after severe fetal damage. HPL levels are frequently elevated and high levels prior to the 26th week of pregnancy may be used as a guide to the severity of the disease.[109]

H. Lecithin Sphingomyelin Ratio (L/S Ratio)

Respiratory distress syndrome occurs in babies born prematurely or after early induction of labor performed because of obstetric complications, particularly diabetes, and rhesus sensitivity.

It was found that fetal lung secretions accumulate in the amniotic fluid[110] and that measurement of phospholipids in the liquor could be used as a means of assessing fetal lung maturity.[111] Amniotic fluid lecithin levels rise gradually from 26 weeks of pregnancy and then rapidly from 36 weeks until term. Sphingomyelin levels increase gradually until 26 weeks and then they decrease. Therefore the L/S ratio is less than unity in early pregnancy and starts to increase from the 33rd week. It is generally agreed that the L/S ratio is a useful indicator of fetal lung maturity, and ratios greater than 2 are not associated with development of respiratory distress syndrome in the newborn whereas ratios of less than 1.5 have a high incidence of respiratory distress.[112] In diabetes mellitus a fall in L/S ratio may follow the initial rise[113] and therefore serial measurements of ratio were advocated. However, it has recently been suggested that ratios of 2 or more are a reliable index of maturity in diabetes.[114] The L/S ratio may be accelerated in severe diabetes and in pre-eclampsia, chronic hypertension, severe hemoglobinopathies, and prolonged rupture of the membranes. Conversely, in mild diabetes and hepatitis the L/S ratio may be delayed.[115]

1. Determination of L/S Ratio[116]

Reagents

1. Chloroform-methanol mixture (2:1)
2. Acetone
3. Chloroform-methanol-water mixture (16.5:6.5:1.0)
4. 10% phosphomolybdic acid in ethanol

Apparatus

1. Thin layer plates (TLC) 2.5 × 10.0; plastic backing coated with 0.25 mm silica gel 60
2. Hot air oven 150 to 160°C
3. Gelman® DCD 16 transmission densitometer

Method

Extract 2 mℓ centrifuged amniotic fluid with 6 mℓ chloroform-methanol mixture by vortex mixing for 30 sec. Centrifuge at 1000 g for 5 min. Immediately aspirate the aqueous and protein layers and evaporate the organic phase to dryness at 50°C in a stream of air. Add 5 mℓ cold acetone to the residue, mix, and decant the acetone. Evaporate the residual acetone to dryness in air. To the residue add 20 μℓ chloroform and shake to dissolve. On a TLC plate, 2 cm from one end, spot (1) 1.5 μℓ chloroform extract; (2) 2.5 μℓ 2:1 mixture lecithin/sphingomyelin; and (3) 3.5 μℓ chloroform extract. Dry the plate in a hot air oven for 1 min. Develop the chromatogram for 45 min by ascending chromatography in chloroform-methanol-water mixture. Remove plate and dry in a hot air oven for 2 min.

Spray the plate with 10% phosphomolybdic acid in ethanol, then develop the color by heating in a hot air oven at 150°-160°C for 5 min. The phospholipids appear as blue spots on a yellow background. It is essential that the conditions for the color development of the spots are strictly followed. Density of the spots is read on a densitometer at a wavelength of 605 nm. The ratio of the lecithin and sphingomyelin spots may then be calculated.

The results from blood-stained samples should be interpreted with care since a 3% contamination of red blood cells will halve the L:S ratio.[117]

I. Screening Tests of Fetoplacental Function

Laboratory tests of placental function are now part of the routine care of the high-risk antenatal patient. Screening tests for all pregnant women have been advocated, as the purely clinical approach will not detect every compromised fetus. The use of HPL has been suggested for this purpose. Values of less than 4 μg/mℓ after the 35th week may predict fetal distress during labor and subsequent neonatal asphyxia.[118]

Early morning specimens of urine for estrogen:creatinine ratio have also been suggested as a screening test. With a normal ratio the perinatal loss was 2/1000 live births. When the estrogen-creatinine ratio was below the 5th percentile the fetal loss was 303/1000 live births.[119]

Routine screening of all pregnant patients at 32 to 33 and 35 to 37 weeks by utilizing urinary estriol assay has been advocated.[120]

Any screening test may cause false alarm in those cases where low values are not associated with fetal distress but it will also help in identifying unsuspected cases of IUGR and other complications of pregnancy.

REFERENCES

1. **Rhodes, P.**, Obstetric prevention of mental retardation, *Br. Med. J.*, 1, 399, 1973.
2. **Jones, G. S.**, in *Intra-Uterine Development*, Barnes, A. C., (Ed.), Lea and Febiger, Philadelphia, 1968, 68.
3. **Thiede, H. A. and Choate, J. W.**, Chorionic gonadotropin localization in the human placenta by immunofluorescent staining. 11. Demonstration of HCG in the trophoblast and amnion epithelium of immature and mature placentas, *Obstet. Gynecol.*, 22, 433, 1963.
4. **Rosal, T. P., Saxena, B. N., and Landesman, R.**, Application of a radioreceptorassay of human chorionic gonadotropin in the diagnosis of early abortion, *Fertil. Steril.*, 26, 1105, 1975.
5. **Hughes, H. E., Loraine, J. A., Bell, E. T., and Layton, R.**, Cytological observations, cervical mucus 'ferning' and hormone assays in early pregnancy, *Amer. J. Obstet. Gynecol.*, 90, 1297, 1964.
6. **Anon.**, Better results with choriocarcinoma, *Br. Med. J.*, 3, 543, 1974.
7. **Carlsson, M. G.**, The use of haemagglutination inhibition reaction for qualitative and quantitative determination of HCG in normal and pathological pregnancies, *Acta Endocrinol.*, 46, 142, 1964.
8. **Samaan, N. A., Bradbury, J. T., and Goplerud, C. P.**, Serial hormone studies in normal and abnormal pregnancy, *Amer. J. Obstet. Gynecol.*, 104, 781, 1969.
9. **Spona, J. and Janisch, H.**, Serum placental lactogen (HPL) as index of placental function, *Acta Endocrinol.*, 68, 401, 1971.
10. **Palmer, A.**, Chorionic gonadotrophin: its place in the treatment of infertility, *Fertil. Steril.*, 8, 220, 1957.
11. **Lauritzen, C. H. and Lehmann, W. D.**, Levels of chorionic gonadotrophin in the newborn infant and their relationship to adrenal dehydroepiandrosterone, *J. Endocrinol.*, 39, 173, 1967.
12. **Canfield, R. E., Morgan, F. J., Kammerman, S., Bell, J. J., and Agosto, G. M.**, Studies of human chorionic gonadotropin, *Rec. Prog. Horm. Res.*, 27, 121, 1971.
13. **Morgan, F. J. and Canfield, R. E.**, Nature of the subunits of human chorionic gonadotrophin, *Endocrinology*, 88, 1045, 1971.
14. **Carlsen, R. B., Bahl, O. P., and Swaminathan, N.**, Chorionic gonadotrophin; linear amino acid sequence of the subunit, *J. Biol. Chem.*, 248, 6810, 1973.
15. **Wilde, C. E., Orr, A. H., and Bagshawe, K. D.**, A sensitive radioimmunoassay for human chorionic gonadotrophin and luteinising hormone, *J. Endocrinol.*, 37, 23, 1967.
16. **Kardana, A. and Bagshawe, K. D.**, A rapid, sensitive and specific radioimmunoassay for human chorionic gonadotrophin, *J. Immunol. Methods*, 9, 297, 1976.
17. **Grudzinskas, J. G., Gordon, Y. B., Jeffrey, D., and Chard, T.**, Specific and sensitive determination of pregnancy-specific glycoprotein by radioimmunoassay. A new pregnancy test, *Lancet*, 1, 333, 1977.
18. **Gordon, Y. B., Grudzinskas, J. G., Jeffrey, D., and Chard, T.**, Concentrations of pregnancy-specific β_1 glycoprotein in maternal blood in normal pregnancy and in intrauterine growth retardation, *Lancet*, 1, 331, 1977.
19. **Searle, F., Leake, B. A., Bagshawe, K. D., and Dent, J.**, Serum SP_1 pregnancy-specific-β-glycoprotein in choriocarcinoma and other neoplastic disease, *Lancet*, 1, 579, 1978.
20. **Sciarra, J. J., Kaplan, S. L., and Grumbach, M. M.**, Localisation of anti-human growth hormone serum within the human placenta: evidence for a human chorionic growth hormone-prolactin, *Nature (London)*, 199, 1005, 1963.
21. **Kaplan, S. L., Gurpide, E., Sciarra, J. J., and Grumbach, M. M.**, Metabolic clearance rate and production rate of chorionic growth hormone-prolactin in late pregnancy, *J. Clin. Endocrinol. Metab.*, 28, 1450, 1968.
22. **Teoh, E. S., Spellacy, W. N., and Buhi, W. C.**, Human chorionic somatomammotrophin (HCS): a new index of placental function, *J. Obstet. Gynaecol. Brit. Commonw.*, 78, 673, 1971.
23. **Tyson, J. E., Jones, G. S., Huth, J., and Thomas, P.**, Patterns of insulin, growth hormone, and placental lactogen release after protein and glucose-protein ingestion in pregnancy, *Amer. J. Obstet. Gynecol.*, 110, 934, 1971.
24. **Genazzani, A. R., Casoli, M., Aubert, M. L., Fioretti, P., and Felber, J. P.**, Use of human placental lactogen radioimmunoassay to predict outcome in cases of threatened abortion, *Lancet*, 2, 1385, 1969.
25. **Singer, W., Desjardins, P., and Friesen, H. G.**, Human placental lactogen: an index of placental function, *Obstet. Gynecol.*, 36, 222, 1970.
26. **Niven, P. A. R., Landon, J., and Chard, T.**, Placental lactogen levels as guide to outcome of threatened abortion, *Br. Med. J.*, 3, 799, 1972.
27. **Spellacy, W. N., Buhi, W. C., Birk, S. A., and Holsinger, K. K.**, Human placental lactogen levels and intrapartum fetal distress: meconium stained amniotic fluid, fetal heart rate patterns and Apgar scores, *Amer. J. Obstet. Gynecol.*, 114, 803, 1972.

27. **Spellacy, W. N., Buhi, W. C., Birk, S. A., and Holsinger, K. K.,** Human placental lactogen levels and intrapartum fetal distress: meconium stained amniotic fluid, fetal heart rate patterns and Apgar scores, *Amer. J. Obstet. Gynecol.,* 114, 803, 1972.
28. **Josimovich, J. B., Kosor, B., Boccella, L., Mintz, D. H., and Hutchinson, D. L.,** Placental lactogen in maternal serum as an index of fetal health, *Obstet. Gynecol.,* 36, 244, 1970.
29. **Ursell, W., Brudenell, M., and Chard, T.,** Placental lactogen levels in diabetic pregnancy, *Br. Med. J.,* 2, 80, 1973.
30. **Letchworth, A. T. and Chard, T.,** Human placental lactogen levels in pre-eclampsia, *J. Obstet. Gynaecol. Br. Commonw.,* 79, 680, 1972.
31. **Seppala, M. and Ruoslahti, E.,** Serum concentration of human placental lactogenic hormone (HPL) in pregnancy complications, *Acta Obstet. Gynecol. Scand.,* 49, 143, 1970.
32. **Letchworth, A. T., Boardman, R. J., Bristow, C., Landon, J., and Chard, T.,** A rapid semi-automated method for the measurement of human chorionic somatomammotrophin. The normal range in the third trimester and its relation to fetal weight, *J. Obstet. Gynaecol. Br. Commonw.,* 78, 542, 1971.
33. **Beck, P. and Daughaday, W. H.,** Human placental lactogen: studies of its acute metabolic effects and disposition in normal man, *J. Clin. Invest.,* 46, 103, 1967.
34. **Samaan, N., Yen, S. C. C., Gonzalez, D., and Pearson, O. H.,** Metabolic effects of placental lactogen (HPL) in man, *J. Clin. Endocrinol.,* 28, 485, 1968.
35. **Yannone, M. E., Mueller, J. R., and Osborn, R. H.,** Protein binding of progesterone in the peripheral plasma during pregnancy and labour, *Steroids,* 13, 773, 1969.
36. **Van der Molen, H. J. and Corpechot, C.,** Isolation and identification of progesterone from urine of nonpregnant women, *J. Clin. Endocrinol.,* 28, 1361, 1968.
37. **Coyle, M. G., Greig, M., and Walker, J.,** Blood progesterone and urinary pregnanediol and oestrogens in foetal death from severe pre-eclampsia, *Lancet,* 2, 275, 1962.
38. **Lurie, A. O., Reid, D. E., and Villee, C. A.,** The role of the foetus and placenta on maintenance of plasma progesterone, *Amer. J. Obstet. Gynecol.,* 96, 670, 1966.
39. **Wiest, W. G.,** Estimation of progesterone in biological tissues and fluids from pregnant women by double isotope derivative assay, *Steroids,* 10, 279, 1967.
40. **Prystowsky, H., Helleger, S. A. E., and Bruns, P. D.,** A comparative study of the alkali reserve of normal and pregnant women, *Amer. J. Obstet. Gynecol.,* 82, 1295, 1961.
41. **Tyler, J. M.,** The effect of progesterone on the respiration of patients with emphysema and hypercapnia, *J. Clin. Invest.,* 39, 24, 1960.
42. **Klopper, A. and Michie, E. A.,** The excretion of urinary pregnanediol after the administration of progesterone, *J. Endocrinol.,* 13, 360, 1956.
43. **Klopper, A.,** Variability of urinary sex steroid hormone output in pregnancy, *Res. Steroids,* 1, 119, 1964.
44. **MacNaughton, M. C. and Michie, E. M.,** Some observations on the excretion of pregnanediol in the urine of women with a bad obstetric history, *Adv. Abstr. of Short Communications, 1st Int. Cong. Endocrinology,* Fuchs, F., Ed., Periodica, Copenhagen, 1960, 669.
45. **Keller, P. J., Baertschi, U., Bader, P., Gerber, C., Schmid, J., Soltermann, R., and Kopper, E.,** Biochemical detection of fetoplacental distress in risk pregnancies, *Lancet,* 2, 729, 1971.
46. **Russell, C. S., Paine, C. G., Coyle, M. G., and Dewhurst, C. J.,** Pregnanediol excretion in normal and abnormal pregnancy; together with Paine, C. G., Observations on placental histology in normal and abnormal pregnancy, *J. Obstet. Gynaecol. Br. Emp.,* 64, 649, 1957.
47. **Fishman, J., Brown, J. B., Hellman, L., Zumoff, B., and Gallagher, T. F.,** Estrogen metabolism in normal and pregnant women, *J. Biol. Chem.,* 237, 1489, 1962.
48. **Klopper, A., Wilson, G., and Cooke, I.,** Studies on the variability of urinary oestriol and pregnanediol output during pregnancy, *J. Endocrinol.,* 43, 295, 1969.
49. **Lever, M., Powell, J. C., and Peace, S. M.,** Improved estriol determination in a continuous flow system, *Biochem. Med.,* 8, 188, 1973.
50. **Roy, E. J., Harkness, R. A., and Kerr, M. G.,** Concentration of oestrogens in blood and urine of patients suffering from pre-eclampsia, *J. Obstet. Gynaecol. Br. Commonw.,* 70, 597, 1963.
51. **Dickey, R. P., Carter, W. T., Besch, P. K., and Ullery, J. C.,** Effect of posture on oestrogen excretion during pregnancy, *Amer. J. Obstet. Gynecol.,* 96, 127, 1966.
52. **Siddiqui, S. A. and Watson, D.,** Urine oestriol measurement from a 12 hour specimen, *Lancet,* 2, 659, 1971.
53. **Salvadori, B., Vadora, E., Coppola, F.,** Diurnal variation in the oestrogen-creatinine ratio in pregnancy, *Lancet,* 2, 659, 1971.
54. **Shelley, T. F., Cummings, R. V., Rourke, J. E., and Marshall, L. D.,** Estrogen creatinine ratios. Clinical application and significance, *Obstet. Gynecol.,* 35, 184, 1970.
55. **Diczfalusy, E., Lauritzen, C.,** *Oestrogene beim Menschen,* Springer-Verlag, Berlin, 1961, 258.

56. **Eraz, J. and Hausknecht, R. V.**, Diminished urinary estriol due to mandelamine administration during pregnancy, *Amer. J. Obstet. Gynecol.*, 104, 924, 1969.
57. **France, J. T. and Liggins, G. C.**, Placental sulfatase deficiency, *J. Clin. Endocrinol.*, 29, 138, 1969.
58. **France, J. T., Seddon, R. J., and Liggins, G. C.**, A study of a pregnancy with low oestrogen production due to placental sulfatase deficiency, *J. Clin. Endocrinol. Metab.*, 36, 1, 1973.
59. **Oakey, R. E., Cawood, M. L., and MacDonald, R. R.**, Biochemical and clinical observations in a pregnancy with placental sulphatase and other enzyme deficiencies, *Clin. Endocrinol.*, 3, 131, 1974.
60. **Pulkkinen, M. C. and Willman, K.**, Maternal oestrogen levels during penicillin treatment, *Br. Med. J.*, 4, 48, 1971.
61. **Oakey, R. E.**, The interpretation of urinary oestrogen and pregnanediol excretion in pregnant women receiving corticosteroids, *J. Obstet. Gynaecol. Br. Commonw.*, 77, 922, 1970.
62. **Campbell, S. and Kurjak, A.**, Comparison between urinary oestrogen assay and serial ultrasonic cephalometry in assessment of fetal growth retardation, *Br. Med. J.*, 4, 336, 1972.
63. **South, J. and Naldrett, J.**, The effect of vaginal bleeding in early pregnancy of the infant born after the 28th week of pregnancy, *J. Obstet. Gynaecol. Br. Commonw.*, 80, 236, 1973.
64. **Bergsjø, D., Bakke, T., Salamonsen, L. A., Støa, K. F., and Thorson, T.**, Urinary oestriol in pregnancy, daily fluctuation and correlation with foetal growth, *J. Obstet. Gynaecol. Br. Commonw.*, 80, 305, 1973.
65. **Martin, J. D., Hahnel, R., Kean, B. P., and Troy, U. G.**, Urinary oestrogen excretion in women with intrauterine foetal growth retardation, *Aust. N. Z. J. Obstet. Gynaecol.*, 12, 102, 1972.
66. **Galbraith, R. S., Low, J. A., and Boston, R. W.**, Maternal urinary oestriol excretion pattern in patients with chronic foetal insufficiency, *Am. J. Obstet. Gynecol.*, 106, 352, 1970.
67. **Certulo, C. L. and Freeman, R.**, Bioelectric evaluation in intrauterine growth retardation, *Clin. Obstet. Gynecol.*, 20, 979, 1977.
68. **Low, J. A., Galbraith, R. S., and Boston, R. W.**, Maternal urinary estrogen pattern in intrauterine growth retardation, *Obstet. Gynecol.*, 42, 325, 1973.
69. **Beischer, N. A. and Brown, J. B.**, Current status of oestrogen assays in obstetrics and gynecology. II. Estrogen assays in late pregnancy, *Obstet. Gynaecol. Surv.*, 27, 303, 1972.
70. **Michie, E. A.**, Urinary oestriol excretion in pregnancies complicated by suspected retarded intrauterine foetal growth, toxaemia or essential hypertension, *J. Obstet Gynaecol. Br. Commonw.*, 74, 893, 1967.
71. **Heys, R. F., Scott, J. S., Oakey, R. E., and Stitch, S. R.**, Estriol excretion in abnormal pregnancy, *Obstet. Gynecol.*, 33, 390, 1969.
72. **Felig, P.**, Diabetes mellitus, in *Medical Complications during Pregnancy,* Burrow, G. N. and Ferris, T. F., Eds., W. B. Saunders, Philadelphia, 1975, 176.
73. **Easterling, W. E. and Talbert, L. M.**, Estriol excretion in normal and complicated pregnancies, *Amer. J. Obstet. Gynecol.*, 107, 417, 1970.
74. **Evans, J. H., Taft, H. P., Rome, R. M., and Brown, J. B.**, Oestriol excretion in pregnancy complicated by diabetes mellitus, *Aust. N. Z. J. Obstet. Gynaecol.*, 12, 95, 1972.
75. **Goebelsmann, U. T., Freeman, R. K., Mestman, J. H., Nakamura, R. M., and Woodling, B. A.**, Estriol in pregnancy 11. Daily urinary estriol in the management of the pregnant diabetic woman, *Am. J. Obstet. Gynecol.*, 115, 795, 1973.
76. **Gabbe, S. G., Mestman, J. H., Freeman, R. K., Goebelsmann, U. T., Lowensohn, R. I., Nochimson, D., Cetrulo, C., and Quilligan, E. J.**, Management and outcome of pregnancy in diabetes mellitus Classes B to R, *Am. J. Obstet. Gynecol.*, 129, 723, 1977.
77. **Levitz, M., Slyper, A. J., and Selinger, M.**, On the lack of periodicity in plasma estriol in human pregnancy, *J. Clin. Endocrinol.*, 38, 698, 1974.
78. **Townsley, J. D., Dubin, N. H., Grannis, G. F., Gartman, L. J., and Crystle, C. D.**, Circadian rhythms of serum and urinary estrogens in pregnancy, *J. Clin. Endocrinol.*, 36, 289, 1973.
79. **Macourt, D., Corker, C. S., and Naftolin, F.**, Plasma oestriol in pregnancy, *J. Obstet. Gynaecol. Br. Commonw.*, 78, 335, 1971.
80. **Masson, G. M. and Wilson, G. R.**, Variability of total plasma oestriol in late human pregnancy, *J. Endocrinol.*, 54, 245, 1972.
81. **Sakakani, J., Buster, J. E., and Killam, A. P.**, Serum unconjugated estriol levels in the third trimester and their relationship to gestational age, 11, *Am. J. Obstet. Gynecol.*, 127, 452, 1977.
82. **Dubin, N. H., Crystle, C. D., Grannis, C. F., and Townsley, J. D.**, Comparison of maternal serum estriol and urinary estrogen determinations as indices of fetal health, *Amer. J. Obstet. Gynecol.*, 115, 835, 1973.
83. **Lindberg, B. S. and Carlstrom, K.**, Plasma and urinary estriol during late uncomplicated pregnancy, *Acta Obstet. Gynaecol. Scand.*, 55, 163, 1976.
84. **Miller, C. A., Fetter, M. C., Boguslaski, R. C., and Heiser, E. W.**, Maternal serum unconjugated estriol and urine estriol concentration in normal and high-risk pregnancy, *Obstet. Gynecol.*, 49, 287, 1977.

85. **Tulchinsky, D., Hobel, C. J., and Korenman, S. G.,** A radioligand assay for plasma unconjugated estriol in normal and abnormal pregnancies, *Amer. J. Obstet. Gynecol.*, 111, 311, 1971.
86. **Sarda, I. R. and Gorwill, R. H.,** Hormonal studies in pregnancy. 111 Unconjugated estrone and estradiol in mother and fetus at delivery in IUGR, *Obstet. Gynecol.*, 49, 546, 1977.
87. **Masson, G. M.,** Plasma oestriol in retarded intrauterine foetal growth, *J. Obstet. Gynaecol. Br. Commonw.*, 80, 423, 1973.
88. **Bashore, R. A. and Westlake, J. R.,** Plasma unconjugated estriol values in high-risk pregnancy, *Am. J. Obstet. Gynecol.*, 128, 371, 1977.
89. **Stafford, J. E. H.,** A versatile radioimmunoassay for the determination of serum oestriol in pregnancy, *Ann. Clin. Biochem.*, 10, 159, 1973.
90. **Heikkila, J.,** Excretion of 15α-hydroxyestriol and estriol in maternal urine during normal pregnancy, *J. Steroid Biochem.*, 2, 83, 1971.
91. **Tulchinsky, D., Frigoletto, F. D., Jr., Ryan, K. J., and Fishman, J.,** Plasma estetrol as an index of fetal well-being, *J. Clin. Endocrinol. and Metab.*, 40, 560, 1975.
92. **Notation, A. D. and Tagatz, G. E.,** Unconjugated estriol and 15α-hydroxyestriol in complicated pregnancies, *Am. J. Obstet. Gynecol.*, 128, 74, 1977.
93. **Heikkila, J. and Luukkainen, T.,** Urinary excretion of estriol and 15 α-hydroxyestriol in complicated pregnancies, *Am. J. Obstet. Gynecol.*, 110, 509, 1971.
94. **Kundu, N. and Grant, M.,** Radioimmunoassay of 15 α-hydroxyoestriol (estetrol) in pregnancy serum, *Steroids*, 27, 785, 1976.
95. **Muir, K. C.,** Urinary estriol measurement in management of antepartum haemorrhage, *Br. J. Obstet. Gynaecol.*, 83, 425, 1976.
96. **Beischer, N. A., Brown, J. B., MacLeod, S. C., Smith, M. A.,** The value of urinary oestriol estimation in patients with antepartum vaginal bleeding, *J. Obstet. Gynaecol. Br. Commonw.*, 74, 51, 1967.
97. **Vorherr, H.,** Placental insufficiency in relation to post term pregnancy and foetal postmaturity, *Am. J. Obstet. Gynecol.*, 123, 67, 1975.
98. **Berkowitz, R. L. and Hobbins, J. C.,** A re-evaluation of the value of HCS determination in the management of prolonged pregnancy, *Obstet. Gynecol.*, 49, 156, 1977.
99. **Hobbins, J. C., Goldstein, L., and Hofschild, J.,** Value of HCS determinations in management of prolonged pregnancy, *Obstet. Gynecol.*, 44, 802, 1974.
100. **Genazzani, A. R., Cocola, F., Casoli, M., Mello, G., Scarselli, E. G., Neri, P., and Fioretti, P.,** Human chorionic somatomammotrophin radioimmunoassay in evaluation of placental function, *J. Obstet. Gynaecol. Br. Commonw.*, 78, 577, 1971.
101. **Granat, M., Sharf, M., Diengott, D., Spindel, A., Kahana, L., and Elrad, H.,** Further investigation on the predictive value of human placental lactogen in high-risk pregnancies, *Am. J. Obstet. Gynecol.*, 129, 647, 1977.
102. **Beard, R. W., Brudenell, J. M.,** Fetal monitoring in diabetic pregnancy, in *Early Diabetes in Early Life*, Camerini-Davalos, R. A. and Cole, H. S., Eds., Academic Press, New York, 1975, 523.
103. **Soler, N. G., Nicholson, H. O., and Malins, J. M.,** Serial determinations of human placental lactogen in the management of diabetic pregnancy, *Lancet*, 2, 54, 1975.
104. **Ursell, W., Brudenell, M., and Chard, T.,** Placental lactogen levels in diabetic pregnancy, *Br. Med. J.*, 2, 80, 1973.
105. **Saxena, B. N., Emerson, K., and Selenkow, H. A.,** Serum placental lactogen (HPL) levels as an index of placental function, *New Engl. J. Med.*, 281, 225, 1969.
106. **Spellacy, W. N.,** Monitoring of high-risk pregnancies with human placental lactogen, in *Management of the High Risk Pregnancy*, Spellacy, W. N., Ed., University Park Press, Baltimore, 1976, 107.
107. **Spellacy, W. N., Usategui-Gomez, M., and Fernandez-Decastro, A.,** Plasma human placental lactogen, oxytocinase and placental phosphatase in normal and toxemic pregnancies, *Am. J. Obstet. Gynecol.*, 127, 10, 1977.
108. **Bjoro, K.,** Oestriol assay in obstetric practice, *Acta Endocrinol.*, 68 (Suppl.), 161, 1972.
109. **Ward, R. H. T., Letchworth, A. T., Niven, P. A. R., and Chard, T.,** Placental lactogen levels in rhesus isoimmunisation. *Brit. Med. J.*, 1, 347, 1974.
110. **Biggs, J. S. G., Gaffney, T. G., and McGeary, H. M.,** Evidence that fetal lung fluid and phospholipids pass into amniotic fluid in late human pregnancy, *J. Obstet. Gynaecol. Br. Commonw.*, 80, 125, 1973.
111. **Gluck, L., Kulovich, M. V., Borer, R. C., Brenner, P. H., Anderson, G. G., and Spellacy, W. N.,** Diagnosis of the respiratory distress syndrome by amniocentesis, *Amer. J. Obstet. Gynecol.*, 109, 440, 1971.
112. **Whitfield, C. R., Chan, W. H., Sproule, W. B., and Stewart, A. D.,** Amniotic fluid lecithin:sphingomyelin ratio and fetal lung development, *Br. Med. J.*, 2, 85, 1972.
113. **Whitfield, C. R. and Sproule, W. B.,** Fetal lung maturation, *Br. J. Hosp. Med.*, 12, 678, 1974.

114. **Gabbe, S. C., Lowensohn, R. I., Mestman, J. H., Freeman, R. K., and Goebelsmann, U. T.**, Lecithin/sphingomyelin ratio in pregnancies complicated by diabetes mellitus, *Amer. J. Obstet. Gynecol.*, 128, 757, 1977.

115. **Morrison, J. C., Whybrew, W. D., Bucovaz, W. L., Wiser, W. L., and Fish, S. A.**, The lecithin/sphingomyelin ratio in cases associated with feto-maternal disease, *Amer. J. Obstet. Gynecol.*, 127, 363, 1977.

116. **Armstrong, D. and Van Wormer, D. E.**, Rapid determination of pulmonary surfactant, *Am. J. Obstet. Gynecol.*, 114, 1083, 1972.

117. **Stein, S. M. and Monaghan, J. M.**, Prediction of respiratory distress syndrome, *Lancet*, 2, 378, 1973.

118. **Letchworth, A. T. and Chard, T.**, Placental lactogen levels as a screening test for fetal distress and neonatal asphyxia, *Lancet*, 1, 704, 1972.

119. **Rao, L. G. S.**, Predicting fetal death by measuring oestrogen:creatinine ratios in early morning samples of urine, *Br. Med. J.*, 2, 874, 1977.

120. **Tulchinsky, D.**, Endocrine evaluation in the diagnosis of intrauterine growth retardation, *Clin. Obstet. Gynecol.*, 20, 969, 1977.

Chapter 6

HORMONAL EXCRETION IN CHILDHOOD AND OLD AGE*

George W. Pennington, Sandra Naik, and R. Hall

TABLE OF CONTENTS

* A table of conversion factors for traditional and SI units (tables 2 and 4 and Figures 2, 3, and 7) is given on page 177.

I. INTRODUCTION

In this chapter an assessment is made of the changes in hormonal secretion at the extremes of life — namely, in childhood and old age. Until recently, comparatively little had been written about the hormonal secretion during these periods, particularly when compared to the enormous number of publications devoted to the subject in the adult.

II. HORMONAL EXCRETION IN CHILDHOOD

A. Hypothalamus and Pituitary Gland

It is now accepted that the hypothalamic control of the pituitary gland is mediated by nervous impulses acting on the median eminence to produce neurosecretions called releasing factors (RF). These have been described elsewhere. It is of interest to note, however, that the maturity of the individual is of importance if a maximal response is to be elicited. Roth et al.[1] have demonstrated that the intravenous injection of LHRH has a marked effect on the testosterone concentration, a peak level being reached in 4 hr in the adult and pubertal male, but not in the prepubertal male. This suggests that there may be ordered sequential maturation of the hypothalamic-pituitary-gonadal axis preceding the onset of puberty.

B. Anterior Pituitary Hormones

Total gonadotropin excretion in children was studied by Fitschen and Clayton,[2] who also summarized the findings in 22 previous papers on this subject published since 1931. With the advent of radioimmunoassays, and the consequent improvement in quality control which has resulted in more precise assays being developed, only data obtained using these techniques will be discussed.

Several groups of workers[3-10] have reported ranges of values for the urinary excretion of FSH and LH. Typical patterns are shown in Figure 1. It will be observed that the mean levels of both FSH and LH remain low during the first 10 years of life, but with the suggestion of a slow continuing rise. Subsequently with the onset of puberty the output increases substantially. Gonadotropins can be detected in the serum and urine of the vast majority of children, but it should be emphasized that little reliance can be placed on the results obtained from a single sample. The normal range cannot be considered other than approximate as, in addition to the daily variations in serum LH in individuals, levels will also vary according to the stage of sexual development. In girls the onset of menstruation heralds the change to adult patterns of FSH and LH secretion. This is discussed elsewhere. It does appear, however, that an increase in gonadotropic activity is the main stimulus for the onset of puberty, although it is unlikely to be the only stimulus.

FSH and LH cause maturation of the testes, the former to stimulate spermatogenesis and the latter to stimulate the Leydig cells with the subsequent production of androgens. Androgens are also produced in the adrenal cortex, and it is the hormones from this source which are probably responsible for some of the growth of the pubic and axillary hair.

The maturation of the ovary seems dependent on the cyclical release of FSH and LH. Winter and Faiman,[11] however, were unable to demonstrate any hormonal rhythms prior to the onset of puberty although random episodic fluctuations in FSH and other hormones were observed in early puberty.

In the investigation of the integrity of the hypothalamic-pituitary-gonadal axis in cases of delayed puberty, the one-bolus LHRH test has proved of great use[12,13] and

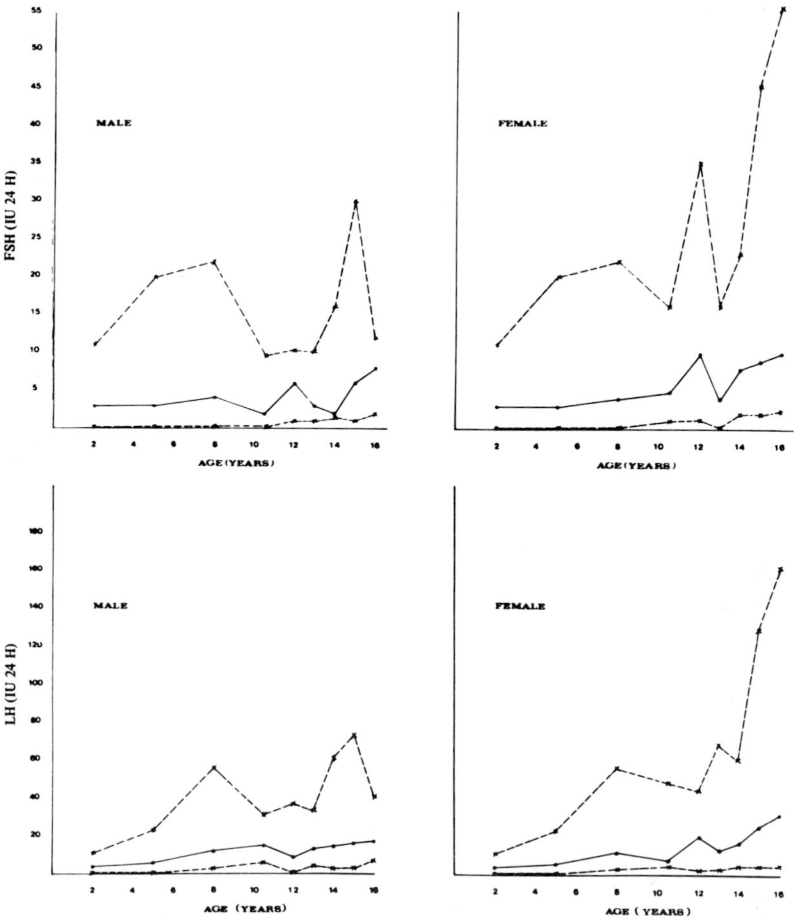

FIGURE 1. The output of FSH and LH in male and female children. The mean and 95% confidence limits are shown. (From Pennington, G. W., *Clin. Obstet. Gynecol.*, 1(3), 513, 1974. With permission.)

makes it possible to establish the diagnosis of isolated gonadotropin deficiency in a selective pituitary failure.

Isolated deficiencies of both ACTH and TSH have been described but are extremely rare, the former usually being incompatible with life. In addition to a low or absent secretion from the pituitary gland, end-organ failure is usually observed. The syndrome of growth retardation, obesity, and small genitalia (Frolich's syndrome) arises from the development of a suprasella craniopharyngioma. Clinical differentiation is very difficult from the case of the obese child where the genitalia may be embedded in fatty tissue and thus appear to be small. In the latter case FSH and LH values will be normal for age.

It is assumed that most cases of idiopathic pituitary deficiency are due to intrauterine or perinatal damage. In any progressive pituitary disorder the gonadotropins are often the first to disappear and this should be detectable if looked for at an early age. It must be remembered, however, that the clinical manifestations of such an absence would not be apparent until puberty. Lack of ACTH may have a direct effect on the reproductive organs leading to defective sexual development due to a lack of adrenal androgens.

Craniopharyngiomas are the most common pituitary tumors encountered in childhood.[14] Dependent upon the location of the tumor, a failure of pituitary secretion occurs at an early stage. The clinical signs and symptoms resulting from the absence of trophic hormones other than FSH and LH, plus pressure on surrounding structures, are likely to be the salient presenting features. Other tumors arising primarily from the basophil cells of the anterior pituitary may give rise to the signs and symptoms of Cushing's disease, consequent upon the excessive release of ACTH.

Elevated levels of FSH and LH production have been demonstrated in precocious puberty by Buckler and Clayton,[15] although Pennington[8] was unable to demonstrate a rise in LH despite observing elevations in estrogens, 17-oxosteroids and 17-oxogenic steroids.

Growth hormone (GH), thyroid stimulating hormone (TSH), and prolactin first appear during intrauterine life at the 9th, 11th, and 18th weeks of pregnancy.[16] Serum prolactin at term is lower in the neonate than in the mother (4000 μu/mℓ). It is, however, much higher than in the normal nonpregnant adult, and remains so until 3 to 6 months of age. No changes have been found in the prolactin levels of prepubertal girls but rises are found at the end of puberty.[17,18] These appear to be related to the simultaneous increases in plasma estrone levels.[19,20]

Typical reported values for pituitary and other hormones in childhood are shown in Tables 1 and 2.

C. Ovarian Function

A review of estrogen excretion in childhood was undertaken by Loraine and Bell[21] while, more recently, Pennington and Dewhurst[5] and Pennington[8,9] have reported on the output of individual estrogens in children between the ages of 1 and 15 years, together with an assessment of daily excretion as revealed by a study of two girls aged 10 and 11 years with early secondary sexual development (stage 3 according to the criteria of Tanner[22]).

A representation of the output of estrogens is shown in Figure 2. It will be observed that there is a steadily increasing excretion of estrogens which accelerates at the time of puberty. Figure 3 shows the day-by-day excretion in two girls, and represents a reasonable assessment of the fluctuations that occur. It is evident that it is possible to detect estrogens in the urine of all young girls, although the precise extent of the ovarian and adrenal contributions is not known. The amount excreted appears to be more directly correlated to physical maturity than to chronological age.

Levels of plasma estrone in prepuburtal girls of 6 to 8 years of age are constant at around 110 pmol/ℓ.[23] A progressive rise to adult levels has been described by Augsusingha and his group,[24] Ducharme et al.,[23] and by Gupta and his co-workers.[25]

Only small quantities of estrogen are secreted by boys. There is little increase at puberty and little evidence of a cyclical fluctuation.

D. Androgenic Function

The two sources of androgens are the testis (testosterone) and the adrenal cortex (dehydroepiandrosterone-DHA). The ovary will make a small contribution to the total androgens in the female. The classical group determination for these C-19 steroids is the estimation of 17-oxosteroids. The output of this group of steroids in normal infants has been reported to be as high as 8.75 μmol in 24 hr during the first week of life,[26] with a fall thereafter to 1.75 μmol/24 hr throughout the first year. There is little appreciable difference in childhood between males and females and it is only following puberty that the excretion in the male child exceeds that in the female (Figure 4). The results as shown[9] are essentially similar to those previously reported by Knorr.[27] There

Table 1
HORMONAL SURVEY IN CHILDHOOD AND ADOLESCENCE[a]

F.S.H. i.u./24 h

	1–3 y M & F	4–6 y M & F	7–9 y M & F	10–11 y M	10–11 y F	12 y M	12 y F	13 y M	13 y F	14 y M	14 y F	15 y M	15 y F	16 y M	16 y F
Mean	3	3	4	2	5	6	10	3	4	2	8	6	9	8	10
Range	0 11	0 20	0-22	0 9	1 16	1 10	1 35	1-10	0 16	1·5 16	2 23	1 30	2·45	2 12	2·5 55
Mean	3	3	4	2	5	6	10	3	4	2	8	6	9	8	10
Range	0 11	0 20	0 22	0·9	1·16	1·10	1 35	1 10	0-16	1·5·16	2 23	1 30	2 45	2·12	2·5 55
No. in group	9	25	13	9	11	6	9	8	9	13	10	21	18	14	20

L.H. i.u./24 h

	1–3 y M & F	4–6 y M & F	7–9 y M & F	10–11 y M	10–11 y F	12 y M	12 y F	13 y M	13 y F	14 y M	14 y F	15 y M	15 y F	16 y M	16 y F
Mean	4	6	12	15	8	9	20	13	13	14	17	16	25	17	32
Range	0-11	0 23	3 56	6 31	5-48	0 37	3-44	4 28	3 68	3 61	5 60	3 73	5 128	7 40	5 160
Mean	4	6	12	15	8	9	20	13	13	14	17	16	25	17	32
Range	0-11	0-23	3-56	6 31	5-48	0 37	3 44	4 28	3·68	3 61	5-60	3 73	5 128	7 40	5 160
No. in group	10	24	17	11	11	10	8	9	10	10	10	25	18	13	25

Total oestrogens µmol/24 h

	1–3 y F	4–6 y F	7–9 y F	10–11 y F.	12 y F	13–14 y F	15 y F	16 y F
Mean	7	9	14	21	35	18	48	38
Range	0·21	0–42	0–83	4·111	0–104	0 225	10·256	10 173
Mean µg/24 h	2	2·5	4	6	10	5	14	11
Range	0–6	0·12	0·24	1 32	0·30	0·65	3 74	3 50
No. in group	9	11	17	9	10	11	21	16

17 Oxosteroids µmol/24 h

	0–3 mth M & F	4 mth–1 y M & F	1–3 y M	1–3 y F	4–6 y M	4–6 y F	7–9 y M	7–9 y F	10 y M	10 y •F	11 y •M	11 y F	12 y M	12 y F	13 y M	13 y F	14 y M	14 y F	15 y M	15 y F	16 y M	16 y F
Mean	1·5	1·5	4·5	2·5	7	4	12	7	14	10	14	12	14	10	12	14	14	14	16	17	19	19
Range	0·3–5·5	0·3–5·0	1–21	0·3–12	3–25	2–17	6–28	3·5 22	5–40	3 22	5 48	3–41	3·52	3·28	4–27	7 29	3·43	5 38	9–36	6·36	7–52	7·49
Mean mg/24 h	0·4	0·4	1·5	0·7	2·1	1·2	3·5	2·0	4·0	3·0	4·0	3·5	4·0	3·0	3·5	4·0	4·0	4·0	4·5	5·0	5·5	5·5
Range	0·1–2·0	0·1–1·5	0·5–6·0	0·1–3·5	1·0–7·0	0·5–5·0	2·0–8·0	1·0–6·5	1·5–11·5	1 6·5	1·5 14·0	1·12·0	1·0–15·0	1·0–8·0	1·0–8·0	2·0–8·0	1·0–12·5	1·5 11·0	2·5–10·5	1·5 10·5	2·0–15·0	2·0–14·0
No. in group	40	11	26	20	17	39	20	29	13	14	15	10	21	7	16	14	12	14	14	15	11	24

17 Oxogenic steroids µmol/24 h

	0–3 mth M & F	4 mth–1 y M & F	1–3 y M & F	4–6 y M & F	7–9 y M & F	10 y M & F	11 y M & F	12 y M & F	13 y M & F	14 y M & F	15 y M & F	16 y M & F
Mean	3·5	5	7	17	20	21	26	28	28	24	24	31
Range	1 7	0·7–19	1–24	5 44	7–45	10–40	6–46	10·69	13–72	10 69	7 69	14 73
Mean mg/24 h	1·0	1·5	2·0	4·9	5·8	6·0	7·4	8·0	8·0	7·0	7·0	9·0
Range	0·3–2·0	0·2–5·5	0·3–7·0	1·5 13·0	2·0 13·0	3·0–11·5	2·0–13·5	3·0–20·0	4·0–21·9	3·0 20·0	2·0 20·0	4·0 21·0
No. in group	40	12	46	43	54	24	25	28	32	28	33	38

Androsterone µmol/24 h

	0–3 mth to 4–6 y M & F	7–9 y to 15 y M	7–9 y to 15 y F
Mean	0·2	1·7	1·7
Range	0–2·8	0·15–5·0	0·07 9·0
Mean mg/24 h	0·06	0·5	0·5
Range	0–0·8	0·04–1·5	0·02 2·5
No. in group	10	4	7

Aetiocholanolone µmol/24 h

	0–3 mth to 4–6 y M & F	7–9 y to 16 y M	7–9 y to 16 y F
Mean	0·2	1·0	1·0
Range	0·2·1	0·1–3·8	0·3–9·0
Mean mg/24 h	0·07	0·3	0·3
Range	0–0·6	0·03 1·1	0·09 2·5
No. in group	10	4	7

Dehydroepiandrosterone µmol/24 h

	0–3 mth to 4–6 y M & F	7–9 y to 16 y M	7–9 y to 16 y F
Mean	0·07	0·7	0·2
Range	0–1·7	0·025 10·0	0·07 4·5
Mean mg/24 h	0·02	0·2	0·06
Range	0–0·5	0·07 3·0	0·02 1·5
No. in group	7	4	7

Pregnanetriol µmol/24 h

	0–3 mth M & F	1–3 y M & F	4–6 y M & F	7–9 y M & F	13–16 y F
Mean	0·3	0·3	0·9	1·0	1·8
Range	0–5	0·1 1·0	0·3 7·0	0·3 5·0	0·6 7·0
Mean mg/24 h	0·1	0·1	0·3	0·4	0·6
Range	0·1·5	0·03·0·4	0·08 2·0	0·1 2·0	0·2 2·0
No. in group	16	18	14	30	6

Pregnanediol µmol/24 h

	12–16 y F
Mean	1·5
Range	0·3 9·0
Mean mg/24 h	0·5
Range	0·1 3·0
No. in group	11

Plasma Cortisol nmol/l

	1–3 y M & F a.m.	4–6 y M & F a.m.	4–6 y M & F p.m.	10–12 y M & F a.m.	13–14 y M & F a.m.	13–14 y M & F p.m.	15–16 y M & F a.m.	15–16 y M & F p.m.
Mean	193	331	220	276	276	138	386	221
Range	77–410	138–772	83–689	28–673	130–533	55–345	138·706	33·519
Mean µg/100 ml	7	12	8	10	10	5	14	8
Range	3·15	5–28	3–25	1·0–24·5	4·7·19·0	2·0 12·5	5·0–25·5	1 19
No. in group	5	6	5	8	9	9	11	8

[a] In SI and traditional units. Male and female as indicated.

From Pennington, G. W., *Clin. Obstet. Gynecol.*, 1(3), 509, 1974. With permission.

is general agreement that 17-oxosteroid excretion seldom exceeds 7 µmol/24 hr up to the age of 8 years and that there is a substantial increase after this age.

The three main components of the 17-oxosteroid group are androsterone, etiocholanolone, and DHA. There are in addition small amounts of oxygenated products of these three compounds thought to be exclusively produced by the adrenal cortex. Some doubt has recently been expressed about this. DHA is present in the urine and blood of normal children in only small amounts.[28] In prepubertal girls Hopper and Yen,[29] Sizonenko and Paunier,[30] and Ducharme et al.[23] all found that DHA levels increase slightly from 6 to 8 years until the first stage of puberty (Tanner[22]). The same authors, and also Korth-Schutz et al.,[31] reported further progressive rises reaching the adult levels at the fourth to fifth stages of puberty.

Table 2
PLASMA STEROID LEVELS IN PREPUBERTAL AND PUBERTAL GIRLS

Prepubertal girls of 1–4 years: LH, FSH, Prl and steroids plasma levels.

Name	Chron. Age	LH mU/ml	FSH mU/ml	Prl ng/ml	Cortisol ng/ml	DHA-S ng/ml	DHA pg/ml	Δ_5-P pg/ml	P pg/ml	17-P pg/ml	A pg/ml	T pg/ml	DHT pg/ml	E_2 pg/ml
F.S.	17 m	2.9	1.6	2.3		15.5	384	151	73	351	307	55	26.7	17
P.E.	17 m		2.4	4.4	110	11	135	277	32	367	312	51	29	18
D.L.	2 yrs	3.5	3.5	4.6	140	27	375	152	54	135	120		13	63
A.R.	2 yrs	2.0	1.1			17				365	181		18.8	19
M.G.	2½ yrs	4.5	1.75		140	28.5	395	135	142			47	24	19
F.M.	3 yrs	3.2	1.0		170		245	346	65	195	101	139	12.8	68
D.B.	3 yrs	3.0	1.75	6.7		28.5	435	131		271		90	27	
O.M.	4 yrs		1.0	8.7	160	15	409	314	57	341			17	48
P.S.	4 yrs	3.2	1.75			25	640		35		155	53	23.2	21
S.S.	4 yrs	4.2	2.1	13.8	80	60	477	207		414	272		21	27.5
Mean		3.31.	1.79	6.75	133	25.2	388.3	214.1	65.4	304.8	206.8	72.5	21.2	33.4
± Sem		0.27	0.23	1.8	15	5.1	49.8	32.7	15.0	36.4	36.3	16.1	1.9	7.3
N		8	10	6	6	9	9	8	7	8	7	6	10	9

Prepubertal girls of 5–6 years: LH, FSH, Prl and steroid plasma levels.

Name	Chron. Age	LH mU/ml	FSH mU/ml	Prl ng/ml	Cortisol ng/ml	DHA-S ng/ml	DHA pg/ml	Δ_5-P pg/ml	P pg/ml	17-P pg/ml	A pg/ml	T pg/ml	DHT pg/ml	E_2 pg/ml
A.M.	5 yrs	2.6	2.5			17	392	721		299	308			
S.F.	5 yrs			10.6		35	272	709		490	347			52
M.G.	5 yrs	5.7	3.5	8.7		42.5	342	480	155	274		126	17	68
B.S.	5 yrs	5.2	2	5		37.5	293	582	194	304	212	146	28	
S.M.T.	5 yrs	2.2	2	10.8	60	180	858		162	102	114	83	26	58
D.K.	5 yrs	3.2	2.4	5	105	180	904		163	360	239	56	56	63
P.O.	5 yrs				80	130			215	154	205	84		
C.G.	6 yrs			3.8			684	830	41	380	397	101		84
L.M.A.	6 yrs	3.2	2.4		140		780	753		227		180	14	
P.A.	6 yrs			6.9	200	175	364	229	67	452			33	65.5
P.M.	6 yrs	3.1	5.9	12.5		20	923	429	120	501	206		26	
S.M.	6 yrs			4.6	120		545		180					
N.P.	6 yrs	3.1	5		130	105	939		202	524		61	58	
Mean		3.53	3.21	749	119.2	76.4	608.0	591.6	149.9	338.9	253.0	104.6	32.2	65.1
± Sem		0.43	0.51	1	18	22.1	80.6	76.1	19.1	41.4	34.5	16.3	6.2	4.9
N		8	8	10	7	10	12	8	10	12	8	8	8	6

Prepubertal girls of 7–9 years: LH, FSH, Prl and steroid plasma levels.

Name	Chron. Age	LH mU/ml	FSH mU/ml	Prl ng/ml	Cortisol ng/ml	DHA-S ng/ml	DHA pg/ml	Δ_5-P pg/ml	P pg/ml	17-P pg/ml	A pg/ml	T pg/ml	DHT pg/ml	E_2 pg/ml
S.E.	7 yrs	3.9	3		160	108	1274	960	80	349	244	201	–	60
S.M.R.	7 yrs	3.3	4.5	5		115	647	540	92	579	241	64	25	47.5
R.P.	7 yrs	2.3	2	6.3	160	70	431	650	223		285	50	55	30
S.R.	7 yrs			5.5	80	75	508		150	719		89	43	52
D.M.E.	8 yrs	3.2	2	7.5			441	655	103	250	229		16	465
C.S.	8 yrs	3.85	3.7	10	130	460	1295	720	278	620	307	101	66	87
S.D.	9 yrs	5.9	3.9	8.5		180			210	758			62	
T.L.	9 yrs	3.8	3.7	8.9	100	130	785				153	64	36	45
M.S.	9 yrs	3.1	3.6		80	105	115	830	180	362			96	
Mean		3.66	3.30	7.38	118.5	155	812	725.8	164.5	519.6	243.2	94.8	49.9	52.6
± Sem		0.39	0.34	0.71	16.5	48	138.6	66.6	26.7	81.2	23.8	24.7	9 .6	7.2
N		8	8	7	6	8	8	6	8	7	6	6	8	7

From Pintor, C. et al., in *Rec. Prog. Paediatric Endocrinology,* Chiumello, G. and Laron, Z., Eds., Academic Press, London. 1977, 162. With permission. Copyright by Academic Press, Inc. (London), Ltd.

Androstenedione does not appear to show any particular variation in girls up to the age of 8 years.[32] Values then increase progressively in relation both to chronological age[22] and to the stage of puberty.[31]

Testosterone levels have been reported to be significantly higher in peripheral than in cord blood at birth[33] and these values decrease progressively in the female during the first week of life[32-34] and then remain unmodified throughout the prepubertal period.[23,30,33,35] At puberty a significant and progressive rise has been demonstrated by Sizonenko and Paunier,[30] Ducharme et al.,[23] and Korth-Schultz et al.,[31] that occurs between the first and third stage of puberty (Tanner[22]).

The excretion of androsterone in both boys and girls is similar between the ages of 8 and 12 years,[36] with ranges varying between 0.34 and 0.68 μmol/24 hr at the age of 8 to 1.03 to 3.26 μmol/24 hr at skeletal age 12 years.

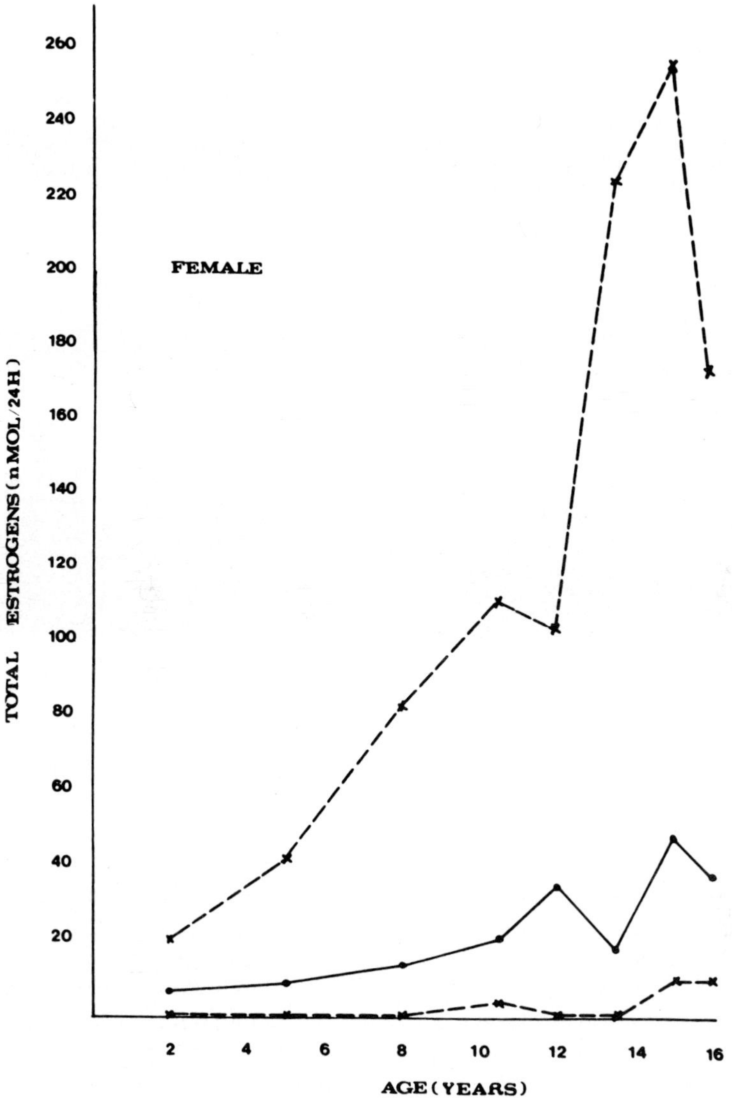

FIGURE 2. Estrogen excretion in female children. (From Pennington, G. W., *Clin. Obstet. Gynecol.* 1(3), 517, 1974. With permission.)

The stable secretion of sex steroids of primarily gonadal origin (testosterone and estrogens) contrasts markedly with the increased output of the androgens of adrenal origin (DHA and androstenedione) which occurs long before any change in secondary sexual characteristics. As cortisol and aldosterone secretion rates (per m^2 of body surface area) do not change throughout life, this rise in blood levels of adrenal androgens must represent a change in adrenal biosynthesis that is termed adrenal puberty.

E. Adrenal Steroids

The androgenic component of the adrenal has already been discussed. The output of hormones from the adrenal cortex is controlled by a complex interrelationship involving the hypothalamus, the pituitary and the gland itself. The major components

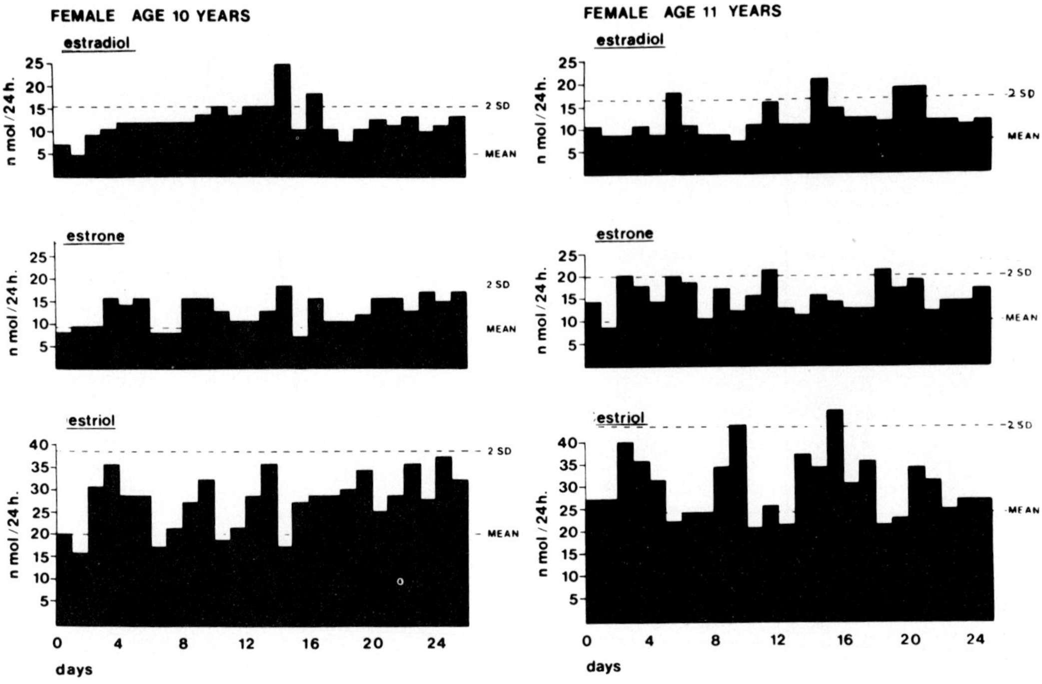

FIGURE 3. Daily urinary estrogen output in two girls aged 10 and 11 with early secondary sexual development. (From Pennington, G. W. and Dewhurst, C. J., *Arch. Dis. Child.*, 44, 629, 1969. With permission.)

arising from the adrenal gland are discussed elsewhere, together with their anabolism from cholesterol and subsequent metabolism to water soluble derivatives.

Cortisol is the main secretory product of the adrenal cortex, and it has been demonstrated[37,38] that cortisol production is high in babies under 5 days old and then falls between 5 and 20 days. Subsequently cortisol levels rise slowly until adult values are reached at about 15 years. The normally occurring diurnal rhythm of plasma cortisol is present throughout childhood. Barnes and his group[39] in a study of 70 children demonstrated the existence of this diurnal rhythm with mean levels of 477 ± 215 nmol/ℓ in the morning and 85.5 ± 3.7 nmol/ℓ at midnight. Ducharme et al.[23] and Pintor[10] have recently suggested that there is little if any variation or elevation in values throughout the prepubertal years.

The main urinary assessment of cortisol-like compounds is the measure of 17-oxogenic steroids. Most workers agree that in childhood there is considerable scatter of results. This is well illustrated by the work of Pennington[8] and Knorr.[27] The mean excretion between the ages of 1½ and 15 years is shown in Figure 5. It will be observed that levels vary between 3.5 and 30 μmol/24 hr according to age. A similar range of values has been reported by Natoli and Natoli[40] who found a mean output during the first year of life of 1.9 μmol/24 hr which then increased with age.

III. HORMONAL SECRETION IN OLD AGE

The usefulness of hormonal investigation in old age should be emphasized because endocrine disease is common and at this time of life many patients are unable to give a helpful clinical history; physical examination may be more difficult and the physical

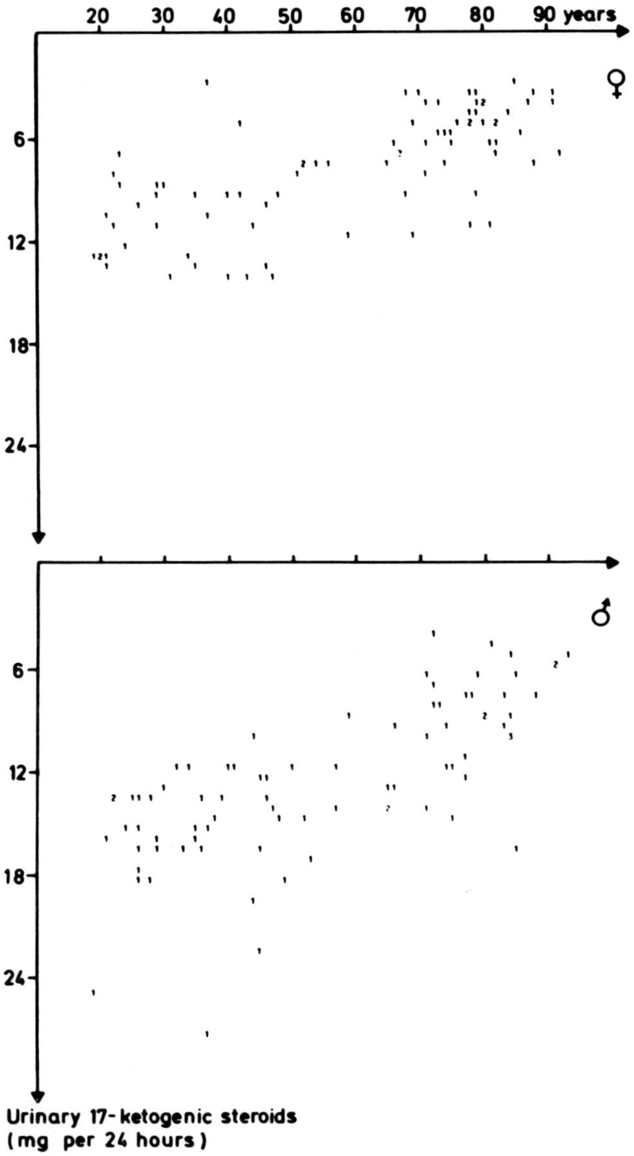

FIGURE 6. Urinary 17-oxogenic steroid excretion in females aged between 20 and 90 years. (From Blichert-Toft, M., in *Geriatric Endocrinology,* Vol. 5, Greenblatt, R. B., Ed., Raven Press, New York, 1978, 85. With permission.)

4. Mineralocorticoid Secretion

The secretion rate of aldosterone has been found to be significantly lowered in healthy elderly patients, while the metabolic clearance rate and the circulating level decrease with age. The observation of Weidmann et al.[62] of lowered plasma renin activity in the elderly may be at least one of the causative factors.

C. Pituitary Function in the Elderly

It seems likely that changes in the output of some pituitary hormones do occur with

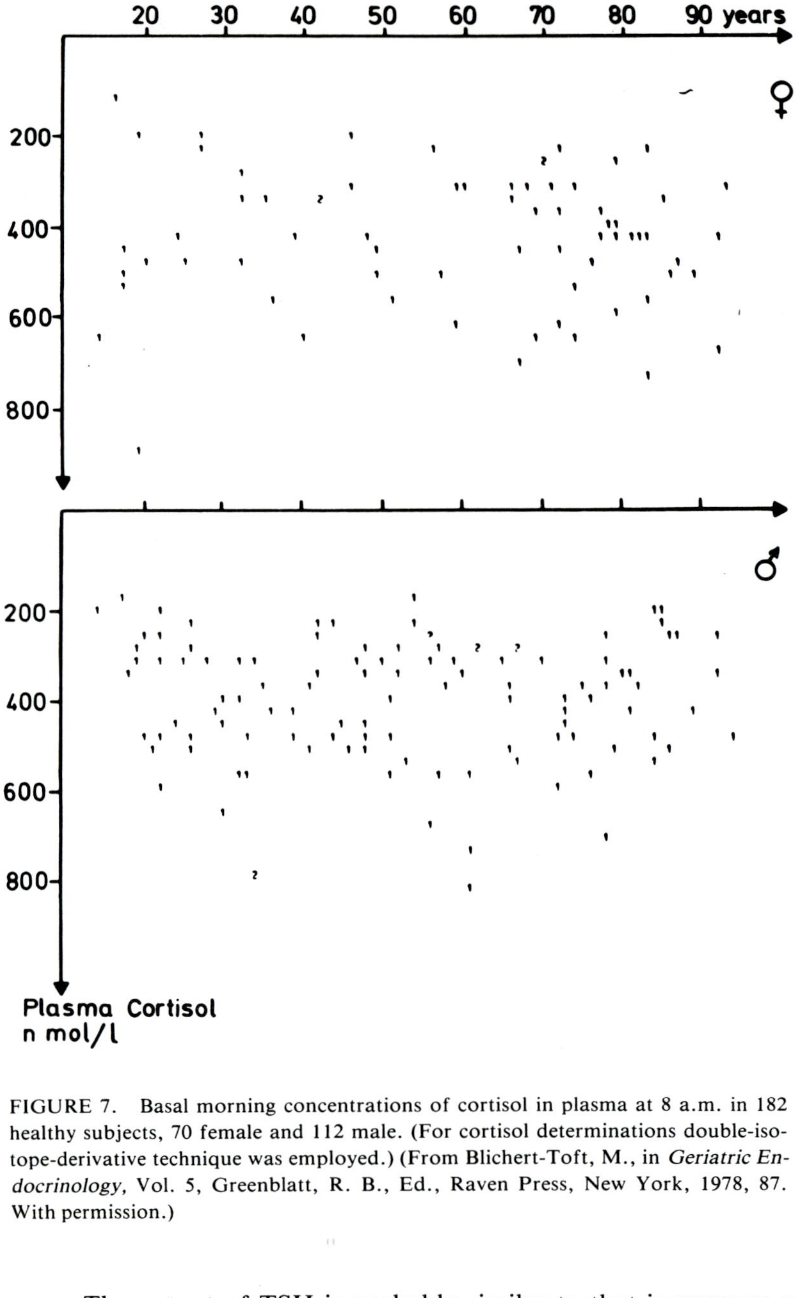

FIGURE 7. Basal morning concentrations of cortisol in plasma at 8 a.m. in 182 healthy subjects, 70 female and 112 male. (For cortisol determinations double-isotope-derivative technique was employed.) (From Blichert-Toft, M., in *Geriatric Endocrinology*, Vol. 5, Greenblatt, R. B., Ed., Raven Press, New York, 1978, 87. With permission.)

increasing age. The output of TSH is probably similar to that in younger people, although some controversy exists about this. Ingbar[68] reported that differences could not be detected, whereas the earlier findings of Cuttelod[69] indicated an elevation in secretion in old age. There would appear to be an unaltered response to TRH in the female, although a progressive decline in response in the male has been reported.[70,71]

Fasting levels of serum growth hormone appear to be higher in the old when compared with young males.[72] However, inexplicably, serum levels in the aged female are lower than those found in young women.[72,73] Serum prolactin concentrations show no change in the male, although a decline has been reported in the female coincident with the onset of the menopause.[74,75]

Table 3
EXCRETION OF HORMONES IN THE POSTMENOPAUSAL PERIOD COMPARED WITH EXCRETION DURING THE MENSTRUAL CYCLE

		Levels during menstrual cycle	
Hormone	Postmenopausal	Follicular phase	Maximum
FSH (IU/24 hr)	78—258	5—36	10—70
LH (IU/24 hr)	86—198	5—60	34—160
Total estrogens (nmol/24 hr)	8—56	20—195	80—300
Pregnanediol (μmol/24 hr)	0.4—2.8	1—4.5	6—23

As previously indicated, the response to stress in the elderly, as demonstrated by the response to ACTH, is not impaired when compared with that in the young.

A gradual increase in serum FSH and LH with age has been reported in men by Isurugi,[76] although this is nothing like as dramatic as that observed in the female at the menopause. At this time in the female there is a decline in the function of the ovary and a concomitant increase in pituitary gonadotropin secretion. Blood levels can rise to extremely high values with LH in the range of 60 to 90 mIU/mℓ and FSH of 75 to 200 mIU/mℓ.[77-83] These changes are reflected in urinary studies. It has been reported that urinary gonadotropins are also elevated in the perimenopausal years.

D. Ovarian Function

The output of estrogens in the elderly female is well shown in Table 3. These data are derived from samples submitted to the Sheffield and Region Endocrine Investigation Center for analysis. It may be observed that the steroid production and secretion from the postmenopausal ovary is markedly altered from the reproductive years. This alteration is chiefly due to the loss of production of estradiol from the ovary, although androgen production apparently continues. The major origin of estrogens during the menopause is from the peripheral conversion of androgens.[85] The actual level of estrogens throughout this period does not change significantly, but after a further ten years again decreases markedly.[86] Mean levels of serum estradiol, together with those for androstenedione and testosterone, as reported by Asch and Greenblat[87] are shown in Table 4.

E. Androgenic Function

In the elderly male the testicles usually remain normal in size. There is a significant decline in the mean levels of free testosterone, starting in the fifth decade,[88] with a fall in total testosterone in the sixth decade. Despite this, there are considerable variations, the levels found being usually in the normal range for adult men. This is in marked contrast to the decline in function observed in elderly women. In the male, even when the testosterone levels are low, the plasma FSH and LH values fail to rise significantly. This phenomenon has been attributed to the action of inhibin, a substance secreted by the Sertoli cells of the testis. It is a heat labile protein, not as yet isolated, which seems to have an inhibitory effect on the secretion of the pituitary gonadotropins.

The change in testosterone levels does not always parallel the decrease in sexual activity that occurs with increasing age. The response of the Leydig cells to HCG stimulation is impaired with changes in the estrogen-androgen ratio.

Plasma estrogen in the elderly male is elevated. This appears to be due to the increased peripheral conversion of androgens. Peripheral estradiol originates in nearly

Table 4

MEAN ± VALUES OF SERUM ESTRADIOL (E_2), Δ^4-ANDROSTENEDIONE (Δ^4-A), AND TESTOSTERONE (T) LEVELS IN 11 MENOPAUSAL AND 10 NORMAL WOMEN

	Peripheral			Adrenal			Ovarian		
	E_2 (pg/mℓ)	Δ^4-A (ng/mℓ)	T (ng/mℓ)	E_2 (pg/mℓ)	Δ^4-A (ng/mℓ)	T (ng/mℓ)	E_2 (pg/mℓ)	Δ^4-A (ng/mℓ)	T (ng/mℓ)
Normal	41 ± 15[a] 58 ± 11[b]	1.47	0.28 ± 0.4	—	—	—	83.1	1.72	0.87
Menopausal	21.26 ± 2.18	1.09 ± 0.10	0.53 ± 0.06	21.44 ± 1.92	1.85 ± 0.15	0.85 ± 0.11	30.52 ± 2.49	2.12 ± 0.17	0.91 ± 0.13

[a] Follicular phase.
[b] Luteal phase.

From Asch, R. H. and Greenblatt, R. B., in *Geriatric Endocrinology*, Vol. 5, Greenblatt, R. B., Ed., Raven Press, New York, 1978, 141. With permission.

equal amounts from direct testicular secretion and peripheral conversion of testosterone.[89]

CONVERSION FACTORS

Table No.	Compound	Traditional units	SI units	Factor (multiply ×)
Table 2	Cortisol	ng/mℓ	nmol/ℓ	2.76
	DHAS	ng/mℓ	nmol/ℓ	2.48
	DHA	pg/mℓ	pmol/ℓ	3.47
	Δ_5P	pg/mℓ	pmol/ℓ	3.15
	P	pg/mℓ	pmol/ℓ	3.15
	17P	pg/mℓ	pmol/ℓ	3.0
	A	pg/mℓ	pmol/ℓ	3.47
	T	pg/mℓ	pmol/ℓ	3.47
	DHT	pg/mℓ	pmol/ℓ	3.47
	E_2	pg/mℓ	pmol/ℓ	3.68
Table 4	Estradiol	pg/mℓ	pmol/ℓ	3.68
	Androstenedione	ng/mℓ	nmol/ℓ	3.47
	Testosterone	ng/mℓ	nmol/ℓ	3.47

REFERENCES

1. **Roth, J. C., Grumbach, M. M., and Kaplan, S. C.,** Effect of synthetic luteinising hormone releasing factor on serum testosterone and gonadotrophins in prepubertal, pubertal and adult males, *J. Clin. Endocrinol. Metab.,* 37, 680, 1973.
2. **Fitschen, W. and Clayton, B. E.,** Urinary excretion of gonadotrophins with particular reference to children, *Arch. Dis. Child.,* 40, 16, 1965.
3. **Kulin, H. E., Rifkind, A. B., and Ross, G. T.,** Human luteinizing hormone (LH) activity in processed and unprocessed urine measured by radioimmunoassay and bioassay, *J. Clin. Endocrinol. Metab.,* 28, 543, 1968.
4. **Laiman, C. and Ryan, R. F.,** Radioimmunoassay for human follicle stimulating hormone, *J. Clin. Endocrinol. Metab.,* 27, 444, 1967.
5. **Pennington, G. W. and Dewhurst, C. J.,** Hormonal excretion in premenarchal girls, *Arch. Dis. Child.,* 44, 629, 1969.
6. **Bagshawe, K. D., Wilde, C. E., and Orr, A. H.,** Radioimmunoassay for human chorionic gonadotrophin and luteinizing hormone, *Lancet,* 1, 1118, 1966.
7. **Blizzard, R. M., Johanson, A., Guyda, H., Baghdas-Savian, A., Raiti, S., and Migeon, C. J.,** Recent developments in the study of gonadotrophin-secretion in adolescence, in *Adolescence Endocrinology,* Butterworths, London, 1970, 1.
8. **Pennington, G. W.,** Hormonal variation in childhood and adolescence, *Proc. Int. Symp. Adolescentology,* Dewhurst, C. J. and De Negri, M., Eds., Carlo Erba Foundation, Milan, 1973, 45.
9. **Pennington, G. W.,** The reproductive endocrinology of childhood and adolescence, in *Clinics in Obstetrics and Gynecology,* Vol. 3(1), Dewhurst, C. L., Ed., W. B. Saunders, London, 1974, 509.
10. **Pintor, C., Genozzani, A. R., Facchinetti, F., Romagnino, S., Corda, R., and Fioretti, P.,** Plasma steroid levels in prepubertal and pubertal girls and in cases of delayed puberty, in *Rec. Prog. Ped. Endocrinol.,* Chiumello, G. and Laron, Z., Eds., Academic Press, London, 1977, 157.
11. **Winter, J. S. D. and Faiman, C.,** The development of cyclical pituitary-gonadal function in adolescent females, *J. Clin. Endocrinol. Metab.,* 37, 714, 1973.
12. **Dickerman, Z., Prager-Lewin, R., and Laron, Z.,** Response of plasma LH and FSH to synthetic LH-RH in children at various pubertal stages, *Amer. J. Dis. Child.,* 130, 634, 1976.

13. **Dickerman, Z., Prager-Lewin, R., and Laron, Z.**, The effect of synthetic luteinizing hormone-releasing hormone on the response of plasma luteinizing hormone and follicle-stimulating hormone in young hypogonadotropic-hypogonadal patients, *Fertil. Steril.*, 27, 162, 1976.
14. **Lambertz, J.**, Cranio-pharyngiomes de l'enfant. *Arch. Française de Pédiatrie.*, 24, 561, 1967.
15. **Buckler, J. M. H. and Clayton, B. E.** The output of luteinizing hormone in the urine of normal children and in those with advanced sexual development, *Arch. Dis. Child.*, 45, 478, 1970.
16. **Mussa, G. C., Bona, G., Madon, E., and Rapetti, G.**, Prolactin (PRL), GH and TSH response to TRH in the newborn, in *Research Progress in Pediatric Endocrinology,* Chiumello, G. and Laron, Z., Eds., Academic Press, London, 1977, 47.
17. **Enharra, Y., Yen, S. S. C., and Siler, T. M.**, Serum prolactin levels during puberty, *Amer. J. Obstet. Gynecol.*, 121, 995, 1975.
18. **Aubert, M. L., Sizonenko, P. C., Kaplan, S. L., and Grumbach, M. M.**, in *Prolactin and Human Reproduction,* Crosignani, P. G. and Robyn, C., Eds., Academic Press, London, 1976, 9.
19. **Del Pozo, E., Hiba, J., Lancranian, I., and Künzig, H. J.**, in *Prolactin and Human Reproduction,* Crosignani, P. G., and Robyn, C., Eds., Academic Press, London, 1976, 61.
20. **Robyn, C., Delvoye, P., Exter, C., Vebemans, M., Cantriez, A., De Nayer, P., Delogne-Desnoeck, J., and L'Hermit, M.**, in *Prolactin and Human Reproduction,* Crosignani, P. G. and Robyn, C., Eds., Academic Press, London, 1976, 71.
21. **Loraine, J. A. and Bell, J. E.**, *Hormone Assays and Their Clinical Interpretations,* Livingstone, Edinburgh, 1966.
22. **Tanner, J. M.**, *Growth and Adolescence,* Blackwell Scientific, Oxford, 1962.
23. **Ducharme, J. R., Forest, M. G., Deperetti, E., Sempe, M., Collu, R., and Bertrand, J.**, Plasma adrenal and gonadal sex steroids in human pubertal development, *J. Clin. Endocrinol. Metab.*, 42, 468, 1976.
24. **Augsusingha, K., Kenny, F. M., Nankin, H. R., and Taylor, F. H.**, Unconjugated estrone, estradiol and FSH and LH in prepubertal and pubertal males and females, *J. Clin. Endocrinol. Metab.*, 39, 63, 1974.
25. **Gupta, D., Attanasio, A., and Raar, S.**, Plasma estrogen and androgen concentrations in children during adolescence, *J. Clin. Endocrinol. Metab.*, 40, 636, 1975.
26. **Bongiovanni, A. M. and Root, A. W.**, The adrenogenital syndrome, *N. Engl. J. Med.*, 268, 1342, 1963.
27. **Knorr, D.**, Untersuchungen zur Altersabhähgigkeit der Ausscheidung einzelner chromatographisch getnemter Steroids während des Kindes und Refungsallers, in *Fortschritte der Pädologie Bal.*, Springer, Berlin, 1965, 109.
28. **Cathro, D. M.**, Adrenal cortex and medulla, in *Paediatric Endocrinology,* Hubble, D., Ed., Blackwell Scientific, Oxford, 1969, 187.
29. **Hopper, B. R. and Yen, S. S. C.**, Circulating concentrations of dehydroepiandrosterone and dehydroepiandrosterone sulphate during puberty, *J. Clin. Endocrinol. Metab.*, 40, 458, 1975.
30. **Sizonenko, P. C. and Paunier, L.**, Hormonal changes in puberty. III. Correlation of plasma dehydroepiandrosterone, testosterone, FSH, and LH with stages of puberty and bone age in normal boys and girls and in patients with Addison's disease or hypogonadism or with premature or late adrenarche, *J. Clin. Endocrinol. Metab.*, 41, 894, 1975.
31. **Korth-Schutz, S., Levine, L. S., and New, M. I.**, Serum androgens in normal prepubertal and pubertal children and in children with precocious adrenarche, *J. Clin. Endocrinol. Metab.*, 42, 117, 1976.
32. **Winter, J. S. D., Hughes, I. A., and Faiman, C.**, Pituitary-gonadal relations in infancy. II. Patterns of serum gonadal steroid concentrations in man from birth to two years of age, *J. Clin. Endocrinol. Metab.*, 42, 679, 1976.
33. **Forest, M. G. and Cathiard, A. M.**, Patterns of plasma testosterone and Δ^4-androstenedione in normal newborns: evidence for testicular activity at birth, *J. Clin. Endocrinol. Metab.*, 41, 977, 1975.
34. **Forest, M. G., Sizonenko, P. C., Cathiard, A. M., and Bertrand, J.**, Hyphophysogonadal function in humans during the first year of life, *J. Clin. Invest.*, 53, 819, 1974.
35. **Gupta, D.**, Changes in the gonadal and adrenal steroid patterns during puberty, *J. Clin. Endocrinol. Metab.*, 4, 27, 1975.
36. **Tanner, J. M. and Gupta, D. A.**, A logitudinal study of the urinary excretion of individual steroids in children from 8-12 years old, *J. Endocrinol.*, 41, 139, 1968.
37. **Kenny, F. M., Malvaux, P., and Migeon, C. J.**, Cortisol production rate in newborn babies, older infants and children, *Pediatrics,* 31, 360, 1963.
38. **Kenny, F. M., Preeyambombat, C., and Migeon, C. J.**, Cortisol production rate. II. Normal infants and adults, *Pediatrics,* 37, 34, 1966.
39. **Barnes, W. D., Joseph, J. M., Atherden, S. M., and Clayton, B. E.**, Functional tests of adrenal axis in children with measurement of plasma cortisol by competitive protein binding, *Arch. Dis. Child.*, 47, 66, 1972.

40. **Natoli, G. and Natoli, V.**, Studio dell'eliminazione urinaria degli steroidi 17 chetogeneci nell infanzia (secondo la methodica di Norymberski). 2. Ricerche in bambini normali appartenìnti alla prima infanzia, *Archiv. Ital. Pediatr. Pueric.*, 21, 380, 1961.
41. **Denham, M. J., Hodkinson, H. M., and Fisher, M.**, Glomerular filtration rate in sick elderly inpatients, *Age Ageing*, 4, 32, 1975.
42. **Jeffreys, P. M., Farran, H. E. A., Hoffenberg, R., Fraser, P. M., and Hodkinson, H. M.**, Thyroid function tests in the elderly, *Lancet*, 1, 926, 1972.
43. **Jeffreys, P. M.**, Prevalence of thyroid disease in patients admitted to a geriatric hospital, *Age Ageing*, 1, 33, 1972.
44. **Bahemuka, M. and Hodkinson, H. M.**, Screening for hypothyroidism in the elderly healthy patient, *Br. Med. J.*, 2, 601, 1975.
45. **Hodkinson, H. M. and Denham, M. J.**, Thyroid function tests in the elderly in the community, *Age Ageing*, 6, 67, 1977.
46. **Britton, K. E., Quinn, V., Brown, B. L., and Ekins, R. P.**, A strategy for thyroid function tests, *Br. Med. J.*, 3, 350, 1975.
47. **Britton, K. E., Quinn, V., Ellis, S. M., Cayley, A. D. C., Miralles, J. M., Brown, B. L., and Ekins, R. P.**, Is T4-toxicosis a normal biochemical finding in elderly women?, *Lancet*, 2, 141, 1975.
48. **Burrows, A. W., Shakespear, R. A., Hesch, R. D., Cooper, E., Aickin, C. M., and Burke, C. W.**, Thyroid hormones in the elderly sick: 'T4 euthyroidism', *Br. Med. J.*, 4, 437, 1975.
49. **Hodkinson, H. M.**, *Biochemical Diagnosis of the Elderly*, Chapman and Hall, London, 1977, 71.
50. **Baruch, A. L. H., Davis, C., and Hodkinson, H. M.**, Causes of high free-thyroxine index values in sick euthyroid elderly patients, *Age Ageing*, 5, 224, 1976.
51. **Burger, A., Nicod, P., Suter, P., Valotton, M. B., Vagenkais, A., and Braverman, A.**, Reduced active thyroid hormone levels in acute illness, *Lancet*, 1, 653, 1976.
52. **Bray, G. A., Fisher, D. A., and Chopra, I. J.**, Relation of thyroid hormones to body weight, *Lancet*, 1, 1206, 1976.
53. **Taylor, B. B., Thompson, J. A., and Caird, F. I.**, Further studies of thyroid function tests in the elderly at home, *Age Ageing*, 3, 122, 1974.
54. **Kind, P. R. N. and Ghosh, S.**, Observations on thyroid function tests in the elderly, *Age Ageing*, 5, 141, 1976.
55. **Harvey, R. F.**, Serum thyroxine and thyroxine-binding globulin in seriously ill patients, *Lancet*, 1, 208, 1971.
56. **Hodkinson, H. M.**, Diagnostic and prognostic aspects of routine laboratory screening of the geriatric inpatient, D. M. thesis, University of Oxford, 1975.
57. **Shalet, S. M., Beardwell, C. G., Lamb, A. M., and Gowland, E.**, Value of routine serum triiodothyronine estimations in the diagnosis of thyrotoxicosis, *Lancet*, 2, 1008, 1975.
58. **Ingbar, S. H.**, The influence of ageing on the human thyroid economy, in *Geriatric Endocrinology*, Vol. 5, *Ageing*, Greenblatt, R. B., Ed., Raven Press, New York, 1978, 13.
59. **Galloway, N. O., Foley, C. F., and Lagerbloom, P.**, Uncertainties in geriatric data. 2. Organ size, *J. Am. Geriatric Soc.*, 13, 20, 1965.
60. **Haughen, D. A.**, The adrenal glands of elderly men in relation to abnormal prostatic growth, *Acta Pathol. Microbiol. Scand.*, 81, 831, 1973.
61. **Dobbie, J. W.**, Adrenocortical nodular hyperplasia: the ageing adrenal, *J. Pathol.*, 99, 1, 1969.
62. **Weidmann, P., Myttenaere-Bursztein, S., Maxwell, M. H., and Lima, J.**, Effect of ageing on plasma renin and aldosterone in normal man, *Kidney Int.*, 8, 325, 1975.
63. **Romanoff, L. P., Morris, C. W., Welch, P., Rodriguez, R. M., and Pincus, G.**, The metabolism of cortisol-4-C^{14} in young and elderly men, *J. Clin. Endocrinol. Metab.*, 21, 1413, 1961.
64. **Blichert-Toft, M.**, The adrenal glands in old age, in *Geriatric Endocrinology*, Vol. 5, *Ageing*, Greenblatt, R. B., Ed., Raven Press, New York, 1978, 81.
65. **West, C. D., Brown, H., Simons, E. C., Carter, D. B., Kumagai, L. F., and Englert, E.**, Adrenocortical function and cortisol metabolism in old age, *J. Clin. Endocrinol. Metab.*, 21, 1197, 1961.
66. **Migeon, C., Keller, A. R., Lawrence, B., and Shepard, T. H.**, Dehydroepiandrosterone and androsterone levels in human plasma. Effect of age and sex, day to day and diurnal variations, *J. Clin. Endocrinol. Metab.*, 17, 1051, 1957.
67. **Vihko, R.**, Gas chromatographic-mass spectrometric studies on solvolyzable steroids in human peripheral plasma, *Acta Endocrinol. (Copenhagen)*, Suppl. 109, 1966.
68. **Ingbar, S. H.** Effect of ageing on thyroid economy in man, *J. Am. Geriatric Soc.*, 24, 49, 1976.
69. **Cuttelod, S., Lemarchand-Beraud, T., Magnenat, P., Perret, C., Poli, S., and Vanotti, A.**, Effect of age and role of kidneys and liver on thyrotrophin hormone in man, *Metabolism*, 23, 101, 1974.
70. **Azizi, F., Vagenakis, A. G., Portnay, G. I., Rapoport, B., Ingbar, S. H., and Braverman, L. E.**, Pituitary-thyroid responsiveness to intra-muscular TRH, based on the analysis of serum thyroxine, triiodothyronine and thyrotrophin concentrations, *N. Engl. J. Med.*, 292, 273, 1975.

71. **Snyder, P. J. and Utiger, R. D.**, Thyrotrophin response to TRH in normal females over forty, *J. Clin. Endocrinol. Metab.*, 34, 1096, 1972.
72. **Vidalon, C., Khurana, R. C., Chae, S., Gegick, C. G., Stephan, T., Nolan, S., and Danowski, T. S.**, Age related changes in growth hormone in non-diabetic women, *J. Am. Geriatric Soc.*, 21, 253, 1973.
73. **Sandberg, H., Yoshimire, N., Maeda, S., Symonds, D., and Zarodnick, J.**, Effects of an oral glucose load on serum immunoreactive insulin, free fatty acids, growth hormone and blood sugar levels in young and elderly subjects, *J. Am. Geriatric Soc.*, 21, 433, 1973.
74. **Ben-David, M.**, Prolactin and menopause, in *Consensus on Menopause Research,* Van Keep, P. A., Greenblatt, R. B., and Albeaux-Fernet, M., Eds., M.T.P. Press, Lancaster, England, 1976, 19.
75. **Yamaji, T., Shimamoto, K., Ishibashi, M., Kosaka, K., and Ormino, H.**, Effect of age and sex on circulating and pituitary prolactin levels in humans, *Acta Endocrinol. (Copenhagen),* 83, 711, 1976.
76. **Isurugi, K., Fukutani, K., Tabayasu, H., Wakabayshi, K., and Tamoki, B.**, Age related changes in serum luteinizing hormone and follicle stimulating hormone in normal men, *J. Clin. Endocrinol. Metab.*, 39, 955, 1974.
77. **Czygan, P. J. and Reich, W.**, Der akute Ruckkoppelungseffekt exogen zugeführter Oestrogene auf die Serum. Gonadotropinspiegel in der Prä und Post-menopause, *Arch. Gynaekol.*, 215, 17, 1973.
78. **Odell, W. D. and Swerdloff, R. S.**, Progesterone-induced luteinizing and follicle stimulating hormone surge in post-menopausal women — a stimulated ovulatory peak, *Proc. Natl. Acad. Sci. U.S.A.*, 61, 529, 1968.
79. **Root, A., De Cherney, A., Russ, D., Duckett, G., Garcia, C. R., and Wallach, E.**, Episodic secretion of luteinizing and follicle stimulating hormones in agonadal and hypogonadal adolescents and adults, *J. Clin. Endocrinol. Metab.*, 35, 700, 1972.
80. **Wise, A. J., Gross, M. A., and Schlach, D. S.**, Quantitative relationships of the pituitary-gonadal axis in post menopausal women, *J. Lab. Clin. Med.*, 81, 28, 1973.
81. **Yen, S. S. C., Tsai, C. C., Naftolin, F., Vandenberg, G., and Ajabor, L.**, Pulsatile patterns of gonadotrophin release in subjects with and without ovarian function, *J. Clin. Endocrinol. Metab.*, 34, 671, 1972.
82. **Yen, S. S. C., Vandenberg, G., and Silar, T. M.**, Modulation of pituitary responsiveness to LRF by oestrogen, *J. Clin. Endocrinol. Metab.*, 39, 170, 1974.
83. **Yen, S. S. C., Martin, P. L., Burnier, A. M., Czekala, N. M., Greavey, M. D., and Callantine, M. R.**, Circulating estradiol, estrone and gonadotrophin levels following the administration of orally active 17β-estradiol in post menopausal women, *J. Clin. Endocrinol. Metab.*, 40, 518, 1975.
84. **Adamopoulos, D. A., Loraine, J. A., and Dove, G. A.**, Endocrinological studies in women approaching the menopause, *J. Obstet. Gynaecol. Br. Commonw.*, 78, 62, 1975.
85. **Poortman, J., Thijssen, J. H. H., and Schwarz, F.**, Androgen production and conversion to oestrogens in normal menopausal women and in selected breast cancer patients, *J. Clin. Endocrinol. Metab.*, 37, 101, 1973.
86. **Grattarola, R., Secreto, G., and Recchione, C.**, Correlation between urinary testosterone and interstitial cell-stimulating hormone concentrations in normal menopausal women, *Am. J. Obstet. Gynecol.*, 121, 380, 1975.
87. **Asch, R. H. and Greenblatt, R. B.**, The ageing ovary: morphologic and endocrine correlations, in *Geriatric Endocrinology,* Vol. 5, *Ageing,* Greenblatt, R. B., Ed., Raven Press, New York, 1978, 141.
88. **Vermulen, A., Reubens, R., and Verdenck, L.**, Testosterone secretion and metabolism in male senescence, *J. Clin. Endocrinol. Metab.*, 34, 730, 1972.
89. **Albeaux-Fernet, M., Bellot, L., Deribreux, J., and Gelinet, M.**, Appreciation de l'androgenicité chez homme, *Ann. Endocrinol. (Paris),* 24, 105, 1972.

Chapter 7

TUMOR MARKERS

K. D. Bagshawe

TABLE OF CONTENTS

I. INTRODUCTION

For many years workers have sought biochemical changes in the serum which would in some way characterize the patient with malignant disease. Three broad classes of potentially useful information have been identified. The first class are changes in various biochemical indexes which result from the presence of the tumor reacting on host tissues. In general such changes as those in C-reactive protein, β_2 microglobulin, and serum glycoproteins are less than specific but they may nevertheless be of some clinical value, particularly in multivariate analysis. The second class of information concerns the presence of changes in macromolecular structure in the cell membrane and where the macromolecules concerned are not secreted into the body fluids in sufficient concentration to be detected by present methods. Such antigenic markers have, at present, little application in serodiagnosis but the possibility exists, at least in theory, that if such markers are autoantigenic then sensitization to them by the patient's own lymphocyte populations may be detectable by in vitro tests. Although high specificity has been claimed for such methods as the MEM test[1] and the SCM test[2] their usefulness in clinical application has not yet been demonstrated. The third class of information relates to macromolecules which are secretory products of tumor cells. It is these substances which are our principle concern in this chapter.

A. Diagnosis and Screening

Although a number of substances have been found to be produced by a substantial proportion of patients with malignant disease it does not follow that measurement of such substances is necessarily a useful exercise. Some recent studies have shown that the incidence of false positives when attempting to apply such measurements is so high that the financial consequences they would incur would be prohibitive.[3] So far biochemical screening for cancer has been largely restricted to well-defined high population risk groups such as those who have recently had hydatidiform mole and are therefore at risk to choriocarcinoma.[4] On such a limited scale screening has proved both practicable and economically viable, for in this case the cancer concerned can be eliminated.

One of the main advantages of measuring tumor products compared with other methods of tumor detection is the promptness of the observed response. Tumor masses are complex ecological systems and tumor volume changes only slowly with respect to changes in the size of the viable tumor cell component. Secretion products from tumors however tend to change much more promptly in response to therapy. Since time is an important factor in the manipulation of cancer chemotherapy the prompt recognition of resistance to a drug regimen is critically important.

If the marker for a particular tumor is sufficiently sensitive to detect a smaller mass than alternative methods, then of course the marker provides the basis for defining "remission status". The rate of decrease of concentration of a tumor marker can also be used as a guide to the duration of treatment required to achieve cure. This is a complex concept depending on many variables, but one of the most important of these is the minimal viable mass of tumor which can be detected by the monitoring system. Even with the most sensitive systems a substantial number of cells remain in the patient when the limit of detection is reached, and it is necessary for treatment to be planned to continue well beyond this time if this minimal residual mass is to be eliminated.

Substances that are suitable for monitoring the course of a tumor are not necessarily suitable for diagnostic purposes. A substance, for instance, produced by a benign tumor of the breast as well as by carcinoma of the breast would have little or no value in diagnosis but may still be valuable in monitoring the response to therapy.

B. Classification of Secreted Tumor Markers

The substances produced by tumors include hormones, enzymes, antibodies, and substances of unknown biological function.[5] In addition to "intact" or "authentic" products, the precursors and degradation products, or subunits of such products, may be produced. The secreted products may exhibit species, individual, tissue, or tumor specificity. However, no truly tumor specific secretory products have yet been identified and for the most part we depend on detecting these substances in excess of the concentrations found in comparable subjects without malignant disease.

Tumor proteins may be adult or embryonic in type. A variety of molecular forms for various substances are known to be produced during ontogeny and these may be detectable in normal adult body fluids or present only in low concentrations. The best recognized biochemical aberration of the cancer cell is the frequent expression of synthesizing activity uncharacteristic of the cell line from which the tumor is derived. The mechanism responsible for the production of such substances is not understood but is widely supposed to result from derepression of genes coded for the production of embryonic substances and allelic forms. Embryonic substances may be of placental or fetal type.

A further classification of tumor products distinguishes them according to whether they are "appropriate" or "eutopic" to the tissue of origin of the tumor or whether they are "inappropriate" or "ectopic". Although "ectopic" synthesis was first defined in relation to hormones it should be recognized that it also includes enzymes and antigens of unknown biological function.

Wide recognition of the "ectopic" hormone syndrome has been achieved largely because of the bizarre syndromes associated with some tumors. These include Cushing's syndrome, with corticotropin-producing tumors; galactorrhea associated with prolactin production; nonmetastatic hypercalcemia associated with calcitonin, prostaglandins, and parathyrin production; malabsorption associated with glucagon; hyponatremia associated with vasopressin, and gynecomastia associated with gonadotropins and placental lactogen.[5] Ectopic production of nonhormone proteins may be no less common.

C. Differences between Tumor and Normal Products

Various differences have been reported between tumor polypeptides and those produced by normal tissues. Some of the differences may be phenotypic variants and others may be due to differing degrees of sialation of glycoproteins. Polymeric forms also occur in many instances and fragments of the product, such as the "C" and "N" terminal ends of corticotropin, or subunits of chorionic gonadotropin, may be produced.

D. Relationship of Serum Concentrations to Tumor Mass

When a hormone is synthesized by tumor and when the hormone is indistinguishable from the normal product, values are of diagnostic significance only if the total concentration exceeds the normal physiological range. In the case of hormones, feedback mechanisms ensure that small contributions from tumors inhibit physiological synthesis within the normal range so that blood concentrations are unaltered or remain within the normal physiological range.

The most useful tumor products are those whose concentration in body fluids closely reflects the total body burden of tumor cells. Such substances are likely to cover a substantial range of concentrations in the body fluids of patients with malignant disease. A patient with advanced malignant disease has a total body burden of tumor of the order of 10^{11} to 10^{12} cells and the ideal tumor marker would reflect the range 10^0

to 10^{12}. The markers which approach nearest to this ideal are human chorionic gonadotropin and α-fetoprotein, both of which cover a 10^7-fold range of concentration in the serum of appropriate tumor patients. When the concentration of a tumor product in the serum shows a demonstrable relationship with the tumor cell mass, it follows that serial measurements reflect the growth or regression of the tumor. It is, however, necessary to take account of the clearance rate of such substances since this determines the rate of fall in serum concentration after reduction in tumor mass has occurred.

II. PLACENTAL AND FETAL PRODUCTS

A. Human Choriogonadotropin

This glycoprotein is synthesized predominantly by the syncytiotrophoblast and to a lesser extent by the cytotrophoblast. It is not detected in serum or urine of normal subjects except during pregnancy although small amounts of HCG-like material have been identified in the testes, pituitary, and possibly at other sites.[6] It has a urinary clearance rate of 1.0 to 1.5 mℓ/min so that serum and urine concentrations are of similar magnitude.

The molecule consists of α and β subunits which are noncovalently bound.[7] The α subunit has a molecular weight of 14,900 and a similar sequence homology to the α subunits of lutropin, follitropin, and thyrotropin. The β subunit, molecular weight of 23,000, is larger by some 30 amino acid residues at the "C"-terminal end than lutropin. Both subunits have a high content of sialic acid. The majority of antisera raised to intact human choriogonadotropin cross-react with lutropin. Antisera raised to the β subunit may or may not discriminate between HCG and LH. Some antisera are about 100 times more sensitive to HCG than to LH. Antisera raised to the tail fragment of HCG-β are said not to cross-react with LH to a detectable extent. Standard assays with antisera to β-HCG measure both intact HCG and free HCG-β. In normal non-pregnant subjects values less than 1 mIU/mℓ (0.5 μg/ℓ) are observed. With assays using antisera to intact HCG the normal range is determined by the subject's physiological status with respect to lutropin or to LH.[8]

1. Hydatidiform Mole

After the evacuation of hydatidiform mole, HCG excretion tends to persist much longer than after normal pregnancy or nonmolar abortion.[4] Following an initial fall, HCG values may continue to fall progressively to normal and reach undetectable levels by 15 to 20 days postevacuation, or alternatively it may persist for up to several months. Persisting detectability of HCG defines the presence of persisting trophoblastic elements. In 90 to 95% of patients these trophoblastic elements die out spontaneously within 6 months. Of the remaining 5 to 10% of cases about one half develop choriocarcinoma and the remainder have invasive moles. HCG measurement can be used advantageously to define those patients who require treatment. The indications include any level of continued HCG production 5 months after evacuation of the mole, progressive increase in HCG excretion at any time after evacuation of the mole, or persisting high levels of HCG not showing an inclination to fall. About 0.2% of all mole patients develop choriocarcinoma after a period during which HCG values have been persistently normal. It is therefore advisable for HCG estimations to be done every 2 weeks after evacuation of the mole until values in, or close to, the normal range for the method are obtained. After this it is satisfactory to perform assays monthly up to 1 year postevacuation and then 3-monthly during the second year of follow-up.

2. Invasive Mole and Choriocarcinoma

Patients undergoing treatment for a trophoblastic tumor should have their HCG values monitored on a regular, twice weekly basis.[9] The limit of sensitivity of HCG-β assay corresponds to a rate of production of approximately 10^4 to 10^5 viable choriocarcinoma cells. Serial measurements are a valuable guide to the response of the tumor to the particular cytotoxic regimen in use. Drug resistance is readily detected and indicates the need for changing treatment.[10]

In the absence of brain metastases the plasma/cerebrospinal fluid ratio for HCG exceeds 60; 1 and values below this indicate the presence of brain metastases, provided sampling is performed during a period of relative stability in the plasma concentration. In patients where metastatic disease is present predominantly within the central nervous system, cerebrospinal fluid concentrations may exceed plasma values.[11] Serial measurements of plasma cerebrospinal fluid ratios provide a means of monitoring the response of intracerebral metastases to therapy.

Patients successfully treated for gestational choriocarcinoma require regular follow-up. Although the risk of relapse is highest in the first few months following completion of therapy occasional patients may relapse as long as 3 or even 7 years later, after intervening values have been persistently normal.[9] It is also important that any patient who has a pregnancy subsequent to hydatidiform mole or choriocarcinoma should have further assays carried out after the end of such pregnancy, since these patients have a somewhat increased risk of choriocarcinoma compared with patients who have never had a trophoblastic lesion.

3. Malignant Teratoma

Reliable estimates of the incidence of HCG production in malignant teratoma are difficult to obtain. In our series over 85% of patients produce HCG, a similar percentage of that producing α-fetoprotein.[12,13] This is in contrast to the low incidence of trophoblast identified histologically in primary testicular teratoma. HCG is a less complete marker for teratomas than for gestational choriocarcinoma since the hormone reflects the activity of only one cell line within a tumor which may be multiclonal. However with "pure" trophoblastic tumors the course of the disease is reliably reflected in HCG measurements. Occasional malignant teratomas, in addition to producing HCG and α-fetoprotein, may produce human placental lactogen, placental alkaline phosphatase, pregnancy specific B_1SP_1, carcinoembryonic antigen, and casein.

Any patient complaining of testicular pain or swelling should have HCG and AFP measurements. Similar measurements are appropriate in patients with anterior mediastinal masses.

4. Nontrophoblastic Tumors

HCG is also produced by some dysgerminomas and the literature records occasional hepatomas producing comparatively large amounts of HCG. A variety of other tumors are also associated with detectable HCG values.[14] In the majority of patients with ectopic production of HCG, values are under 100 mIU/mℓ although occasional patients produce much larger amounts. Where extensive disease is seen clinically or radiologically and the amount of excess HCG is quite small, serial measurements are of little value in monitoring the course of the disease. Occasional tumors produce either HCG-α or HCG-β as ectopic products.[15] At present the incidence of this would appear too low to merit the routine screening of tumor patients for these antigens.

5. Methodology for HCG Assay

Intradermal injection of 80 μg of HCG-β in complete Freund's adjuvant is made at multiple sites on the backs of New Zealand white rabbits and this is repeated after intervals of 4 weeks to 4 months, after which the rabbits are bled. Guinea pig-antirabbit-gamma-globulin precipitating sera are obtained after intradermal injections of 1 mg of rabbit-gamma-globulin in complete Freund's adjuvant, followed by further 1-mg injections at 6- and 9-week intervals. The guinea pigs are bled out 10 to 14 days after the last immunization. Sheep can be used instead of guinea pigs.

6. Iodination

Iodination is performed by the chloramine-T method of Greenwood, Hunter, and Glover.[15a] Carrier-free sodium (^{125}I) iodide (ISM-3) obtained from the Radiochemical Center, Amersham, England, is used in the concentration of 5 mCi/10 μg of intact HCG, giving specific activities in excess of 200 μCi/ng.

Optimal dilutions of the rabbit anti-HCG-β and the guinea pig-antirabbit-gamma-globulin are defined. Equal quantities of the sera at their optimized dilutions are mixed and incubated at 4°C for a minimum of 3 days. Aliquots are lyophilized and vacuum sealed in vials.

Average concentrations of the antisera are 1:72,000 for the HCG-β antiserum and 1:900 for the guinea pig-antirabbit-gamma-globulin when diluted to the final assay volume. The antisera are reconstituted in 0.04 *M* phosphate buffer, pH 7.0, containing 0.1% bovine albumin.

7. Assay Procedure

To 100 μℓ of the serum or diluted serum to be assayed is added 50 μℓ of the preincubated antiserum. If the serum is to be assayed undiluted, 100 μℓ of 0.04 *M* phosphate buffer (pH 7.0) containing 0.1% albumin, is added to the tube. When diluted serum is used, 100 μℓ of normal male serum is added, so that the reaction volume is constant and protein content remains approximately equal. The addition of normal serum is necessary to avoid nonspecific effects from plasma proteins observed with other assay systems. In addition, 100 μℓ of normal male serum is added to tubes containing reference standards and the zero antigen controls. All the tubes are incubated at 37°C for 1.5 hr. Then 50 μℓ of labeled antigen is added to every tube. All tubes are then subjected to a further incubation at 37°C for a minimum of 2 hr.

Alternatively, ^{125}I HCG is added at the same time as the antiserum and incubation is then allowed to proceed at 4°C for 16 hr.

The HCG-antibody complex is separated from the free labeled HCG by vacuum filtration on either glass fiber (Whatman® GF/F) or cellulose acetate (Oxoid®) discs. In routine operations these are performed on an automated analyzer (KEMTEK® 3000) which automatically performs the inputting and dilution operations, addition of reagents, separation, counting, and calculations at a rate of up to 300 reactions per hour.[17] Calculations are based on the logit transform of the response variant versus the log dose of the antigen. A value of 2 mIU/mℓ is used as the lower cut-off for routine operations.

For HCG assay on urine the procedure is essentially similar except that protein is not added to the diluted samples nor to the reference standards and controls.

In our experience the use of an HCG-β antiserum has provided some additional specificity when compared with an antiserum raised to intact HCG in urine assays. Urine assays should always be based on timed collections of either 12 or 24 hr and the results expressed in excretion rate per 24 hr.[18] In normal nonpregnant subjects values in the range 5 to 30 IU/24 hr are obtained and may be somewhat higher in oophorectomized or menopausal subjects.

B. Human Placental Lactogen

Although this hormone has been found in the serum of patients with gestational choriocarcinoma and malignant teratoma and as a eutopic product in 8% of patients with a variety of cancers,[19] there is little evidence that it is a valuable tumor product in the clinical context except for a few rare patients.

C. PSBG (Pregnancy Specific β_1 Globulin, β_1SP_1)

This glycoprotein was identified independently by several groups of workers in the serum of pregnant women. It is produced by the syncytial trophoblast and can be localized in that site by histochemical methods. It is also detectable in the serum of most patients with trophoblastic tumors before treatment.[20] PSBG concentrations in the serum of these patients tends to parallel that of human chorionic gonadotropin and although its molecular weight is 90,000 it appears to have a similar clearance rate to HCG. Although PSBG parallels HCB, its concentration is generally substantially lower by an order of 10 to 100-fold.[21] It is therefore a less effective marker than HCG for these tumors. It is possible that in a few patients with low levels of marker activity, particularly in patients with malignant teratoma, PSBG values may provide additional information to that provided by HCG but further study is required before this can be confirmed. The finding of this antigen by histochemical means in a large proportion of breast tumors has so far not been confirmed and even in the presence of extensive metastatic disease it is rarely detectable in the serum.

1. Assay Methods

Pregnancy-specific PSBG glycoprotein and rabbit antisera (Batch No. 2998B, Behringwerke) are used for the assay in this laboratory. Precipitating sheep antirabbit-γ-globulin antiserum (782) was raised by injection of 20 μg of rabbit-γ-globulin intramuscularly in Freund's complete adjuvant at day 1, and boosting injection of 10 mg on days 45 and 75. The antigen is labeled with iodine ^{125}I (Amersham IMS-30) by a modification of the method of Hunter, Greenwood, and Glover to a specific activity of 60 to 90 $\mu ci/\mu g$, separation from unreacted iodine being achieved by passage through Sephadex® G-100 (Pharmacia K 9/50 column). Dilution buffers consist of 0.0375 *M* phosphate, pH 7.5, containing 0.0375 *M* sodium chloride, merthiolate 0.01%, bovine serum albumin 0.1%, and EDTA 0.2%. First and second antisera are preincubated and used at final dilutions of 1/96,000 and 1/33,600, respectively. After incubation for 18 hr at 37°C 30% of the radioactivity is recovered in zero antigen tubes. Standards, in doubling dilution from 128 $\mu g/\ell$ are made up in pooled normal serum, the assay being performed on 100 $\mu\ell$ aliquots of sample in triplicate. The within-assay coefficient of variation is 5%; the between-assay cumulative variation is 11%.

D. Placental Alkaline Phosphatase

This isoenzyme produced by the placenta exists as several phenotypic variants and they were initially characterized as heat-stable and L-phenylalanine-sensitive.[22] It was first recognized in the serum and tumor of a patient (Regan) with carcinoma of the lung and has since been identified in association with tumors at various sites and occasionally in large amounts but more often in low concentration. Studies with sensitive immunoenzymatic methods have demonstrated some activity in all normal sera and in a somewhat higher proportion of patients with cancer.[23] Apart from the occasional patients in whom large amounts of placental alkaline phosphatase may be produced by cancers, measurements of this isoenzyme have so far little utility in clinical practice.[24]

E. α-Fetoprotein (AFP)

α-Fetoprotein is a glycoprotein containing some 4% of sugar residues and has a molecular weight of 70,000.[25] It is synthesized in the yolk sac and fetal liver and also by the hepatocyte. Concentrations are high in the fetus and decrease rapidly after birth.

α-Fetoprotein has been isolated from fetal cord serum, fetal serum, hepatoma tissue, and from the serum of patients with hepatoma.

Preparations derived from hepatomas have sometimes shown multiple components which can be decreased by neuraminidase treatment. However, not all the microheterogeneity identified in α-fetoprotein resides in sialic acid constituents. The question whether specific variants are associated with malignant disease has not yet been fully resolved but it seems unlikely that a sharp distinction between physiological and pathological variants exists.

α-Fetoprotein is an important marker for both hepatocellular carcinoma and for malignant teratoma.[26,27] In addition some gastrointestinal tract tumors produce α-fetoprotein with or without known liver involvement. Nonmalignant conditions associated with modest elevations in the concentration of AFP in adult sera include hepatic cirrhosis, hepatic coma, acute hepatitis, and in the child, ataxia, telangiectasia and congenital tyrosinemia have been reported to give increased values.

The presence of α-fetoprotein in malignant teratomas appears to correlate well with the presence in the tumor tissue of identifiable yolk sac elements. The proportion of such elements which constitute the entire tumor is highly variable but pure yolk sac tumors (Teilum's tumor) are well recognized. It is therefore appropriate that all known or suspected cases of malignant teratoma, whether arising in the testis, ovary, mediastinum, or other site, should be tested regularly for both α-fetoprotein and human chorionic gonadotropin.[5]

The clearance rate of α-fetoprotein is lower than that of HCG and therefore values of α-fetoprotein tend to fall more slowly than those of HCG when comparable reductions in tumor bulk are achieved by therapy.

1. Assay Methods

The early studies with α-fetoprotein were based on immunodiffusion and counterimmunoelectrophoresis but radioimmunoassay is necessary to detect the concentration present in normal human serum. Double-antibody systems have been devised by Ruoslahti and Seppala,[28] Chayvialle and Ganguli[29] and Purves.[30] The method used in this laboratory is as follows.

α-Fetoprotein,* derived from the serum of a patient with hepatoma, is labeled with iodine-^{125}I (IMS-30, Amersham) to a specific activity of 180 μCi/μg by the chloramine-T method, separation from unreacted iodine being achieved by passage through Sephadex® G-200. Dilution buffers and sample volumes are as for the serum HCG-assay. Rabbit anti-α-fetoprotein antiserum (raised to α-fetoprotein from fetal serum and absorbed with 10 mg/mℓ of pooled normal human serum) is preincubated in the proportion 1:25 for 3 days with guinea-pig antirabbit-γ-globulin and used in the assay at a final dilution of 1° antiserum of 1/50,000. There is 40% recovery of the radioactivity in the zero antigen tubes after incubation for 18 hr at 37°C. Standards covering the range from 666 to 2.0 MRC** units/mℓ are made up in pooled normal serum. The within-assay coefficient of variation is 5%; the between-assay coefficient of variation is 9%.

Methods relying on polyethylene glycol at the separation stage have also been used for α-fetoprotein assay.

* Prepared by Dr. Melica Wass in this department.

** MRC unit = Medical Research Council unit.

F. Carcinoembryonic Antigen (CEA)

This glycoprotein, which has a molecular weight of 200,000, was first obtained from colonic adenocarcinoma or liver metastases from such tumors.[31] It is defined immunologically since its biological activity is unknown.

CEA has been localized to the striated border of the normal columnar cell of the colon and the membrane of certain cancer cells.

Preparation of the antigen has been performed by the use of perchloric acid extraction of the homogenized tissue, followed by separation on Sepharose® 4B and Sephadex® G-200. The homogeneity of preparations has been investigated by ultracentrifugation, polyacrylamide-gel electrophoresis, electrofocusing, and epichlorohydrin chromatography.[32,33] Claims to have produced species of carcinoembryonic antigen with improved specificity compared with standard preparations have not been substantiated to date.[34]

Conventional preparations have been achieved that are relatively consistent in amino acid content but show heterogeneity in carbohydrates. The CEA molecule can be closely associated with blood group determinants and some of these may be linked to the CEA molecules.

Further problems in the purification of CEA resulted from the presence of closely related antigens in both normal and malignant tissues. These have been designated NCA_1 and NCA_2.[35] Antisera of three types have been defined with respect to these cross-reactions.[36] One gives an immunoprecipitin line with carcinoembryonic antigen that is not shared with NCA. The second cross-reacts wth NCA but this can be absorbed with normal tissue extracts. The third type of antiserum does not discriminate between NCA and CEA.

The evidence suggests that the immunological activity of CEA is associated with a glycoprotein containing N-terminal lysine. Loss of immunological activity occurs with treatments that would be expected to rupture disulfide bonds. The immunological activity of the protein is unaltered by trypsin, chymotrypsin, thermolysin, ficin, pronase, and subtilisin though it is rapidly degraded by pepsin. Although stable to temperature and acid treatment, the molecule is vulnerable to mild alkali.

1. Clinical Application

Various studies have shown that screening of the population for elevated CEA values is not justified. High levels of false positives and false negatives have been obtained in most series.

In monitoring the response of a tumor to chemotherapy or irradiation the concentration of CEA approximately reflects the tumor mass although deviations from this relationship are probably not uncommon. The main application of CEA measurements would appear to be in patients who have had apparently successful resections of colorectal cancer.[37,38] Patients with raised CEA values would be expected to fall to the normal range following successful surgery and subsequent increases in CEA values have been shown to herald clinical and radiological recurrence by several months in some patients. In one trial, elevated CEA values were seen in 16 of a total of 18 patients with unequivocal tumor recurrence.[38] However, in 106 patients without definite evidence of recurrence, elevated concentrations were seen in 29 patients on at least one occasion. In another study of 220 patients, 36 of 53 who developed local recurrences or metastases had sustained abnormal CEA values.[39] However it has to be recognized that increases in CEA concentrations tend to occur most commonly with the presence of hepatic metastases and this tends to negate the clinical value of the observation in the absence of highly effective therapy for metastases at this site. Evidence that CEA values may be of value in the identification of a malignant cause for pleural effusions and ascites has recently been presented[40] and there is also the possibility that grossly elevated CEA values may be used to avoid more expensive and distressing methods of investigation for old people presenting a picture of advanced malignant disease.

2. CEA Values

The early work suggested that the normal range of serum CEA was less than 2.5 μg/ℓ. Subsequent studies, however, showing that CEA values may be increased in smokers and various other conditions such as chronic pulmonary infection, has led to caution in the interpretation of results below 20 μg/ℓ. Above this value the probability of a malignant cause for the elevated CEA is high.

Some discrepancy in CEA values has resulted from differences in methodology. Thus some of the groups using double antibody methods have reported much higher values than those quoted elsewhere in the literature. Numerical differences between these normal ranges are largely accounted for by inclusion or noninclusion of background serum in standards and not by double antibody methods per se.

3. Assay Methods

The original CEA assay was developed from the modified Farr technique and subsequently a system of separation based on zirconyl phosphate gel was employed. Latterly double antibody methods on nonextracted serum have been preferred although some techniques still make use of perchloric acid extracted serum. Valid comparisons between assays in the same hands have shown little evidence to suggest that one method has a particular advantage over the others in specificity.[41] The choice of assay therefore depends largely on convenience. In this laboratory we have found that the double antibody system with preprecipited antiserum used on unextracted serum provides a convenient methodology.

CEA -2B,* prepared by affinity chromatography on concanavalin-A Sepharose® of a conventional CEA preparation, is labeled with iodine-^{125}I (IMS-30, Amersham) by a modification of the chloramine-T method to a specific activity of 160 μc/μg, and separated from unreacted iodine by passage through Sephadex® G-200. Rabbit anti-CEA antiserum, absorbed with 20 mg/mℓ each of perchloric acid extracts of normal colon, normal spleen, normal liver, and 20 ng/mℓ of freeze-dried human plasma is preincubated for 3 days with sheep antirabbit-γ-globulin (in the proportion 1:70) and used in the assay at a final dilution of 1/23,000. Dilution buffers and sample volumes are as for the HCG-serum assay. In the zero antigen tubes, 35% of the radioactivity is recovered after incubation for 18 hr at 37°C. Standards, in doubling dilution in normal serum, cover the range 174 to 1 MRC units/mℓ. The within-assay coefficient of variation is 10%, between-assay coefficient of variation is 15%.

III. NONFETAL PRODUCTS

A. Calcitonin

This hormone is produced by the parafollicular or C-cells of the thyroid and by medullary carcinoma of the thyroid that arises from these cells. The tumor tends to be familial and to be associated with parathyroid hyperplasia or adenoma, pheochromocytoma, and Cushing's syndrome. A raised serum calcitonin value in a patient with a familial syndrome, with or without mucosal neuromas is suggestive of one of these tumors. In some of these patients both CEA and calcitonin are increased but in

* Prepared by Dr. G. T. Rogers in this department.

others an increase in calcitonin concentration is detected only after an infusion of calcium ions or after stimulation by gastrin or whiskey.[42]

Calcitonin has recently been identified as an ectopic product of some tumors including carcinoma of the breast and carcinoma of the bronchus.[43] The elevation in concentration, however, is again small in most instances and it remains to be seen whether such ectopic production of calcitonin is likely to have any useful clinical application.

B. Casein

Immunologically detectable kappa casein is present in the serum of lactating women and is not normally detectable at concentrations greater than 100 $\mu g/\ell$ in the serum of nonlactating persons. It was reported that serum kappa casein levels were increased in patients with breast cancer and that there was a correlation with the extent of disease.[44] Further studies have confirmed that patients with breast cancer may have elevated levels of serum casein but elevated values have also been found in patients with benign breast disease and the correlation between casein values and total body burden has proved to be an unreliable guide to response to therapy.[45] It therefore seems unlikely that serum casein values will find an established place in the management of this tumor.

IV. SOME OTHER POTENTIAL TUMOR MARKERS

A. Polyamines (Putrescine, Spermidine, Spermine, and Cadaverine)

Many amino acids undergo decarboxylation resulting in short-chain-aliphatic amines and some of these have vasopressor activity. Polyamines are present in all nucleated cells and it has been suggested that they have an important function in regulating nucleic acid synthesis. Increased urinary excretion of polyamine has been reported in patients with cancer and it was suggested that one of these, spermidine, might serve as a marker of tumor cell kill, whereas putrescine reflects the proliferative behavior or "growth fraction" of the tumor.[46] Measurements have been made by adaptation of a standard amino acid analyzer[47] but although meriting further study the place of these substances as tumor markers in clinical practice also remains to be established.

B. Hydroxyproline

This amino acid is excreted in the urine bound to peptide and is derived from collagen metabolism so that the amount excreted is increased in bone disorders, malabsorption states, finger clubbing, and rheumatoid arthritis. It is also increased in patients with bone metastases and occasionally in those with only soft tissue metastases. The hydroxyproline/creatinine ratio may be increased before bone metastases are demonstrable by other methods.[48] Clinical opinions appear to be divided on the value of this marker but the improvement in scintillation techniques or bone scanning has tended to render it superfluous.

REFERENCES

1. **Pritchard, J. A. V., Moore, J. L., Sutherland, W. H., and Joslin, C. A. F.,** Macrophage-electrophoretic-mobility (MEM) test for malignant disease, *Lancet,* 2, 627, 1972.
2. **Cercek, L. and Cercek, B.,** Application of the phenomenon of changes in the structuredness of cytoplasmic matrix (SCM) in the diagnosis of malignant disorders. A review, *Eur. J. Cancer,* 13, 903, 1977.
3. **Williams, R. R., McIntire, K. R., Waldmann, T. A., Feinleib, M., Go, V. L. W., Kannel, W. B., Dawber, T. R., Castelli, W. P., and McNamara, P. M.,** Tumor-associated antigen levels (carcinoembryonic antigen, human chorionic gonadotropin and alpha-fetoprotein) antedating the diagnosis of cancer in the Framingham Study, *J. Nat. Cancer Inst.,* 58, 1547, 1977.
4. **Bagshawe, K. D., Wilson, H., Dublon, P., Smith, A., Baldwin, M., and Kardana, A.,** Follow up after hydatidiform mole. Studies using radioimmunoassay for urinary human chorionic gonadotrophin (hCG), *J. Obstet. Gynaecol. Br. Commonw.,* 80, 461, 1973.
5. **Bagshawe, K. D. and Searle, F.,** Tumor markers, *Essays Med. Biochem.,* 3, 25, 1977.
6. **Braunstein, G. D., Rasor, T., and Wade, M. E.,** Presence of chorionic gonadotrophin-like substance in normal testes, *N. Engl. J. Med.,* 293, 1339, 1975.
7. **Morgan, F. J. and Canfield, R. E.,** Nature of the sub-unit of human chorionic gonadotrophin, *Endocrinology,* 88, 1045, 1971.
8. **Bagshawe, K. D., Wilde, C. E., and Orr, A. H.,** Radioimmunoassay for human chorionic gonadotrophin and luteinising hormone, *Lancet,* 1, 1118, 1966.
9. **Bagshawe, K. D.,** Choriocarcinoma. The clinical biology of the trophoblast and its tumors, Edward Arnold, London, 1969.
10. **Bagshawe, K. D.,** Treatment of trophoblastic tumors, *Recent Results Cancer Res.,* 62, 192, 1977.
11. **Bagshawe, K. D. and Harland, S.,** Immunodiagnosis and monitoring of gonadotrophin-producing metastases in the central nervous system, *Cancer,* 38, 112, 1976.
12. **Newlands, E. S., Dent, J., Kardana, A., Searle, F., and Bagshawe, K. D.,** Serum α_1 fetoprotein and HCG in patients with testicular tumors, *Lancet,* 1, 744, 1976.
13. **Waldemann, T. A. and McIntire, K. R.,** The use of a radioimmunoassay for α fetoprotein in the diagnosis of malignancy, *Cancer,* 34, 1510, 1974.
14. **Muggia, F. M., Rosen, S. W., Weintraub, B. D., and Hansen, H. H.,** Ectopic placental proteins in non-trophoblastic tumors. Serial measurements following chemotherapy, *Cancer,* 36, 1327, 1975.
15. **Vaitukaitis, J.,** Immunologic and physical characterisation of human chorionic gonadotrophin (hCG) secreted by tumors, *J. Clin. Endocrinol. Metab.,* 37, 505, 1973.

15a. **Greenwood, F. C., Hunter, W. M., and Glover, J. S.,** The preparation of I-131-labelled human growth hormone of high specific radioactivity, *Biochem. J.,* 89, 114, 1963.

16. **Kardana, A. and Bagshawe, K. D.,** A rapid, sensitive and specific radioimmunoassay for human chorionic gonadotrophin, *J. Immunol. Methods,* 9, 297, 1976.
17. **Bagshawe, K. D.,** Computer controlled automated radioimmunoassay, *Lab. Pract.,* 573, 1975.
18. **Wilde, C. E., Orr, A. H., and Bagshawe, K. D.,** A sensitive radioimmunoassay for chorionic gonadotrophin and luteinising hormone, *J. Endocrinol.,* 37, 23, 1967.
19. **Weintraub, B. D. and Rosen, S. W.,** Ectopic production of human chorionic somatomammatrophin by non-trophoblastic cancers, *J. Clin. Endocrinol. Metab.,* 32, 94, 1971.
20. **Tatarinov, Y. S., Mesnyanaina, N. V., Nikoulina, D. M., Novikova, L. A., Toloknov, B. O., and Falaleeva, D. M.,** Immunochemical identification of β globulin of the pregnancy zone in serum of patients with trophoblastic tumor, *Int. J. Cancer,* 14, 548, 1974.
21. **Bagshawe, K. D., Searle, F., Leake, B. A., and Dent, J.,** Serum-SP_1-pregnancy-specific-β-glycoprotein in choriocarcinoma and other neoplastic disease, *Lancet,* 1, 579, 1978.
22. **Fishman, W. H.,** Immunologic and biochemical approaches to alkaline phosphatase isoenzyme analysis. The Regan isoenzyme, *Ann. N. Y. Acad. Sci.,* 166, 745, 1969.
23. **Cadeau, B. J., Blackstin, M. E., and Malkin, A.,** Increased incidence of placental-like alkaline phosphatase activity in breast and genitourinary cancer, *Cancer Res.,* 34, 729, 1974.
24. **Jacoby, B. and Bagshawe, K. D.,** A radioimmunoassay of placental type alkaline phosphatase, *Cancer Res.,* 32, 2413, 1972.
25. **Ruoslahti, E. and Seppala, M.,** Studies of carcinofetal proteins: physical and chemical properties of human α fetoprotein, *Int. J. Cancer,* 7, 218, 1971.
26. **Waldemann, T. A. and McIntire, K. R.,** The use of a radioimmunoassay for α fetoprotein in the diagnosis of malignancy, *Cancer,* 34, 1510, 1974.
27. **Matsumoto, Y., Suzuki, T., Ono, H., Nakaso, A., and Honjo, I.,** Response of α fetoprotein to chemotherapy in patients with hepatomas, *Cancer,* 34, 1602, 1974.
28. **Ruoslahti, E. and Seppala, M.,** Studies of carcinofetal proteins. III. Development of a radioimmunoassay for α fetoprotein in the serum of healthy adults, *Int. J. Cancer,* 8, 374, 1971.

29. **Chayvialle, J. A. P. and Ganguli, P. C.,** Radioimmunoassay for α fetoprotein in human plasma, *Lancet,* 1, 1355, 1973.
30. **Purves, L. R. and Purves, M.,** Serum α fetoprotein, *S. Afr. Med. J.,* 46, 1290, 1972.
31. **Gold, P. and Freedman, S. O.,** Demonstration of tumor specific antigens in human colonic carcinomata by immunological tolerance in absorbtion techniques, *J. Exp. Med.,* 121, 439, 1965.
32. **Coligan, J. E., Henkart, P. A., Todd, C. W., and Terry, W. D.,** Heterogeneity of the carcinoembryonic antigen, *Immunochemistry,* 10, 591, 1973.
33. **Rogers, G. T., Searle, F., and Bagshawe, K. D.,** Carcinoembryonic antigen: isolation of a sub-fraction with high specific activity, *Br. J. Cancer,* 33, 357, 1976.
34. **Plow, E. G. and Edgington, T. S.,** Isolation and characterization of a homogenous isomeric species of carcinoembryonic: CEA-S, *Int. J. Cancer,* 15, 748, 1975.
35. **von Kleist, S.,** Substances immunologically related to carcinoembryonic antigen, *Ann. Immunol. (Paris),* 124C, 589, 1973.
36. **Tomita, J. T., Safford, J. W., and Hirata, A. A.,** Antibody response to different determinants of carcino-embryonic antigens (CEA), *Immunology,* 26, 291, 1974.
37. **Neville, A. M. and Cooper, E. H.,** Biochemical monitoring of cancer, *Ann. Clin. Biochem.,* 13, 283, 1976.
38. **Booth, S. N., Jamieson, G. C., King, J. P. G., Leonard, J., Oats, G. D., and Dykes, B. W.,** Carcinoembryonic antigen in the management of colorectal cancer, *Br. Med. J.,* 4, 183, 1974.
39. **Mackay, A. M., Patel, S., Carter, S., Stephens, V., Lawrence, D. J. R., Cooper, E. H., and Neville, A. M.,** Role of serial plasma carcino-embryonic antigen assays in the detection of recurrent metastatic colorectal cancer, *Br. Med. J.,* 4, 382, 1974.
40. **Booth, S. N., Lakin, G., Dykes, B. W., Burnette, D., and Bradwell, A. R.,** Cancer associated proteins in effusion fluids, *J. Clin. Path.,* 30, 537, 1977.
41. **Searle, F., Lovesey, A. C., Roberts, B. A., Rogers, G. T., and Bagshawe, K. D.,** Radioimmunoassay methods for carcino-embryonic antigen, *J. Immunol. Methods,* 4, 113, 1974.
42. **Melvin, K. E. W., Miller, H. H., and Tashjian, A. H.,** Early diagnosis of medullary carcinoma of thyroid gland by means of calcitonin assay, *N. Engl. J. Med.,* 285, 1115, 1971.
43. **Coombes, R. C., Hilliard, C., Greenberg, P. V., and McIntire, I.,** Plasma immunoreactive calcitonin in patients with non-thyroid tumors, *Lancet,* 1, 1080, 1974.
44. **Hendrick, J. C. and Franchimont, P.,** Radioimmunoassay of casein in the serum of normal subjects and patients with various malignancies, *Eur. J. Cancer,* 10, 725, 1974.
45. **Woods, R. L., Searle, F., Wilson, P., Bagshawe, K. D., and Cooper, E. H.,** Serum kappa-casein in breast cancer, *Eur. J. Cancer,* 13, 113, 1977.
46. **Russell, D. H. and Russell, S. D.,** Relative usefulness of measuring polyamines in serum, plasma and urine as biochemical markers of cancer, *Clin. Chem. (Winston-Salem, N.C.),* 21, 860, 1975.
47. **Lipton, A., Sheehan, L., Mortell, P., and Harvey, H. A.,** Urinary polyamine levels in patients with localized malignancy, *Cancer,* 38, 1344, 1976.
48. **Holes, T. J., Lees, C. L., and Bondy, P. K.,** Hydroxyproline excretion in patients with breast cancer and response to treatment, *Br. Med. J.,* 2, 164, 1975.

Chapter 8

MEDICAL GENETICS WITH PARTICULAR REFERENCE TO ENDOCRINE DISORDERS

C. E. Blank

TABLE OF CONTENTS

I. INTRODUCTION

Genetics is essentially the study of inherited differences between individuals. The units of inheritance, the "genes", are contained in the chromosomes within each cell nucleus. The presence, or absence, of a particular gene can be inferred only from its effect upon the cell or organism under investigation. For example, the presence (in double dose) of the gene for albinism is inferred because an individual lacks pigment. Chromosomes consist of deoxyribonucleic acid (DNA) and protein. The DNA fraction is responsible for the preservation, replication, and transcription of the genetic code.[1] However, the precise structure of a chromosome is not known.[2] For example, we do not know whether the DNA forms the core of the chromosome and is enclosed in a protein envelope, or vice versa. Although it might be suggested that each molecular geneticist has its own individual concept of "the gene", for most purposes the unit of inheritance may be regarded as a section of DNA situated at a particular part (the locus) of a particular chromosome, which acts in concert with a similar unit (gene) on a partner (homologous) chromosome (see Figure 1). Regulatory mechanisms initiate and control the transcription of genes producing enzymes and other polypeptides of biological significance ("structural" genes) and are of particular importance in cell and tissue differentiation. "Regulator genes" (see Figure 2) can trigger the synthesis of messenger RNAs for whole chains of enzymes.[1,4]

Man has many thousands of genes contained in 23 pairs of chromosomes, 22 pairs of autosomes, and a pair of sex chromosomes, XX in the female and XY in the male. At each locus on each member of a particular pair of chromosomes the coded information may be the same or different, although always concerned with the same metabolic step. If the information is different (genes A and a, Figure 1), the paired genes are said to be alleles and are described as being in heterozygous form. If the same form is present in each partner chromosome (gene S, Figure 1) the gene is said to be in homozygous form. Genes on the X and Y chromosomes are not paired and, in the male, are described as being in hemizygous form.

The behavior of a homologous pair of chromosomes during gamete formation (meiosis) is described in Figure 3. The most important effect of meiosis is that a gamete, either sperm or ovum, contains only one of each pair of chromosomes present in the adult. A child therefore obtains only one of a pair of genes from each parent.

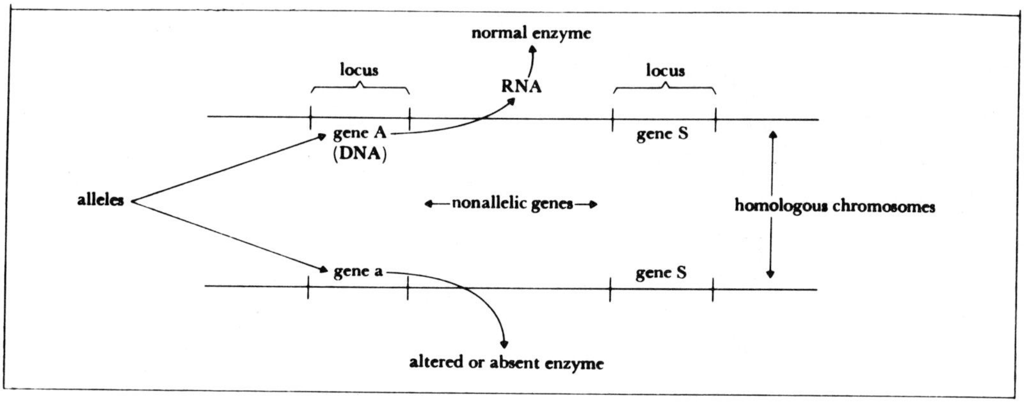

FIGURE 1. Inherited information is coded by deoxyribonucleic acid (DNA) transcribed to ribonucleic acid (RNA) and translated into protein molecules, which are often enzymes. A particular gene codes for a particular enzyme. Gene A (dominant) and gene a (recessive) are alleles. Gene S is present in homozygous form. (From Blank, C. E., *Mims Magazine*, April 1977, 75. With permission.)

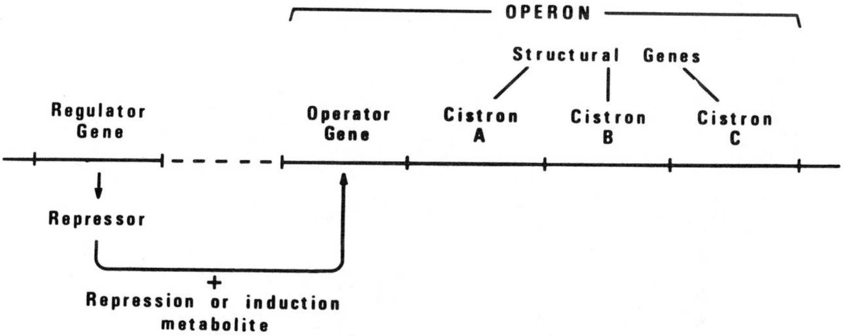

FIGURE 2. A model for regulator gene control of enzyme synthesis. The activity of structural genes (cistrons) A, B, and C is controlled by operator and regulator genes. Repressors, which can either be activated (repression) by specific metabolites or inactivated (induction), act as intermediaries between regulator and operator genes. Operator and structural genes form, together, the operon.

Disease or disorders of development in man of "genetic" origin may be divided into three main categories (see Table 1) according to the principle mechanism responsible: conditions caused by chromosome abnormality; conditions caused by the action of a single "abnormal" gene; and conditions in which inherited predisposition and environment both appear to play a part. While it is often possible to categorize the type of mechanism of inheritance present, the pathogenesis of the condition produced by abnormal gene activity is usually poorly understood. This is so in endocrine disorders of genetic origin, with the possible exception of congenital adrenal hyperplasia.

II. THE HUMAN CHROMOSOME COMPLEMENT

Modern staining methods enable the precise identification of individual pairs of chromosomes (see Figures 4 and 5); indeed, in some instances individual segments of

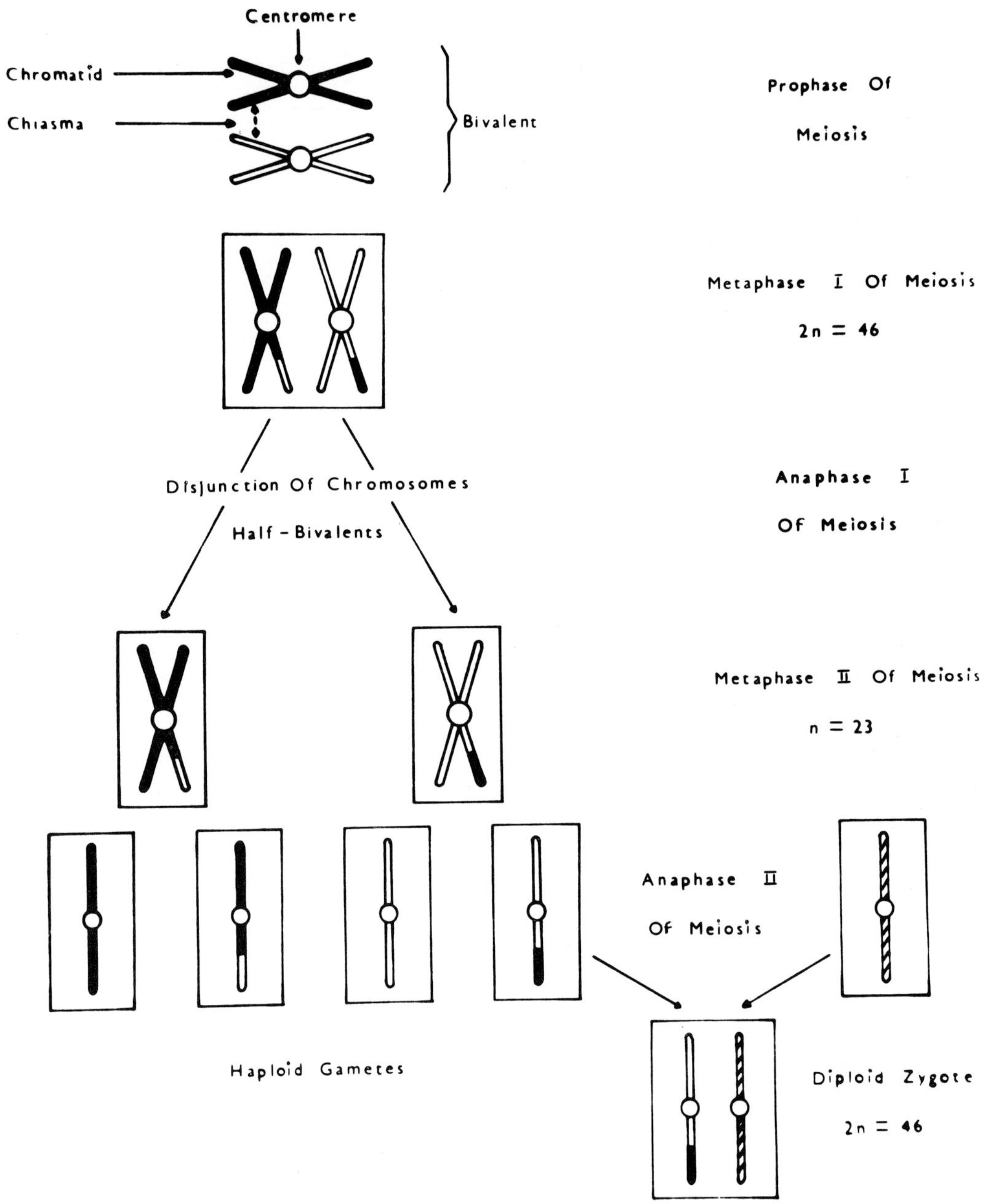

FIGURE 3. Normal meiosis (only one pair of chromosomes represented). (From Blank, C. E., *Mims Magazine*, March 1977, 69. With permission.)

chromosomes may be recognized with confidence.[6,7] Chromosome abnormality is presumed where the number of chromosomes is different from the normal or where the morphology, or "banding" pattern, of a particular chromosome is different from the normal.

A. Late-Replicating X Chromosome

One X chromosome in the female undergoes DNA replication out of phase with the rest of the chromosome complement.[8] The late-replicating chromosome can be studied

Table 1
MECHANISMS PRODUCING DISEASE OR DISORDER OF DEVELOPMENT IN MAN

	Mechanism	Mode of Action
1.	Chromosome aberration	Extra or absent genetic material Many "normal" genes in abnormal dose
2.	Single gene effect Dominant trait Recessive trait X-linked recessive trait	Particular "abnormal" gene in single dose Particular "abnormal" gene in double dose Particular "abnormal" gene in single dose on the X chromosome in the male.
3.	Multifactorial (polygenic)	Many genes with a smal effect Gene action modified by environmental factors
4.	Mainly environmental	Example: endemic goiter.

(see Figure 6) using autoradiographic techniques. A structurally abnormal X chromosome is usually the X chromosome which replicates late. Where more than two X chromosomes are present the additional X chromosomes are also late replicating.

Modern "banding" techniques are simpler and usually more informative than autoradiography and have largely replaced the latter in the identification of extra or abnormal chromosome material.

B. Sex Chromatin and Y Chromosome Fluorescence

A convenient tissue to study for sex chromatin is the buccal mucosa (see Figure 7).[8] The sex chromatin body (Barr body) is a single X chromosome in a tightly coiled (heteropyknotic) form. In a normal male a Barr body is never seen; in a normal female between 20 and 50% of nuclei show a single Barr body, the actual count depending to some extent on the staining technique and method of counting.

Individuals with a single Barr body in a proportion of buccal smear nuclei have two X chromosomes, individuals with two, three, or four Barr bodies in a proportion of nuclei have three, four, or five X chromosomes, respectively. If sex chromatin is absent then only one X chromosome is present. A large, or small, Barr body may indicate an abnormality of an X chromosome. If the proportion of cells showing a Barr body is outside normal limits, or the distribution of cells containing Barr bodies is uneven, a sex chromosome abnormality may be suspected; for example a low sex chromatin count sometimes indicates that the patient is a mixture of cell types with respect to sex chromosome complement (sex chromosome mosaicism).

A second type of sex chromatin body is the drumstick, observed in polymorphonuclear leucocytes. In a normal female more than 6 drumsticks per 500 polymorphonuclear leucocytes are observed. A normal male has very few. Like the Barr body, the drumstick is a heteropyknotic X chromosome. Drumsticks are not easy to score, even by the expert, and not as much information is to be obtained as by examination of a buccal smear. It is, however, technically easier to make a satisfactory blood smear preparation.

It is also possible to demonstrate in buccal mucosa nuclei the presence, or absence, of the Y chromosome. In interphase nuclei, or metaphase preparations, the Y chromosome takes up certain dyes preferentially, and may be made to fluoresce under ultraviolet light (see Figure 8). Two fluorescent bodies in a nucleus indicate the presence of two Y chromosomes.

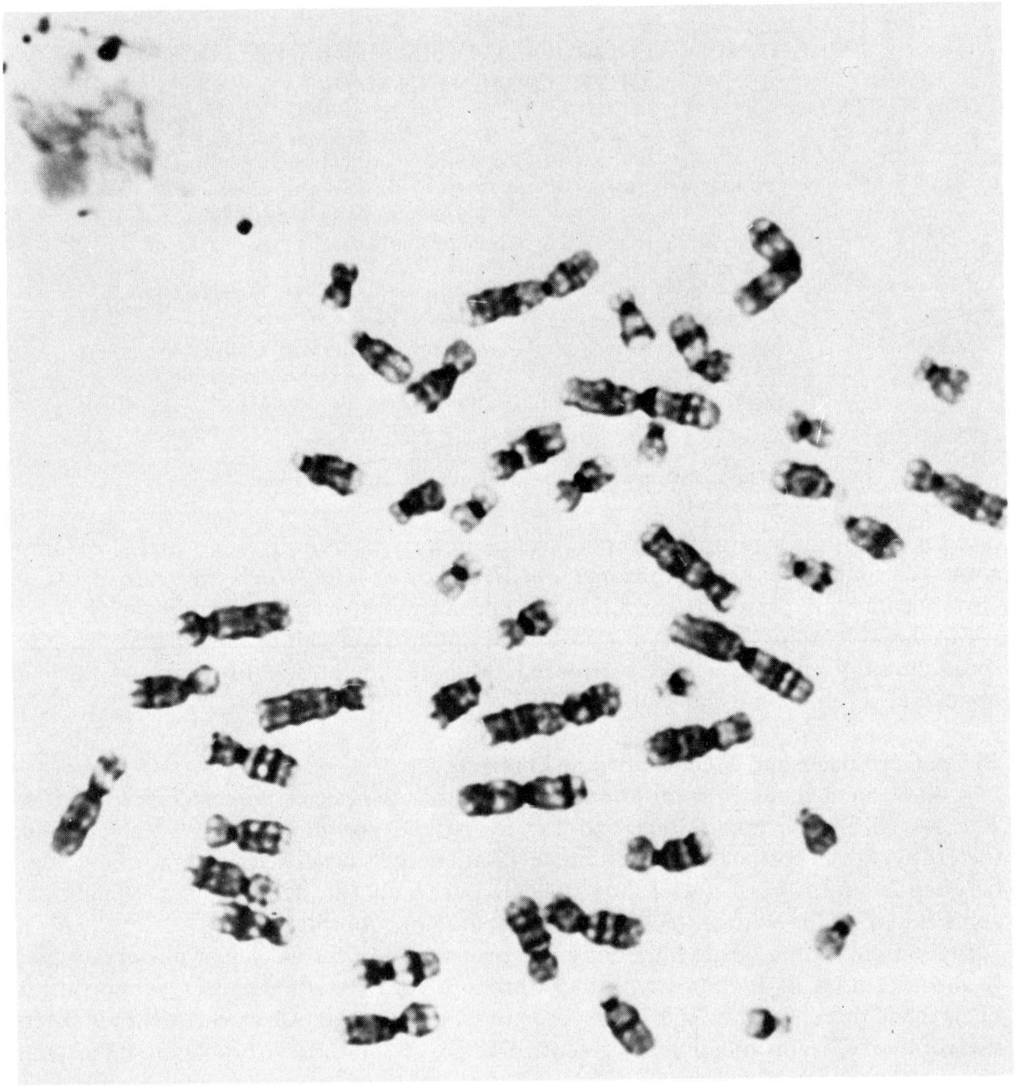

FIGURE 4. A metaphase plate from a lymphocyte culture. Pretreated and stained to show "banding" patterns. (From Blank, C. E., *Mims Magazine*, March 1977, 69. With permission.)

C. Gonadal Differentiation

It is the presence of a Y chromosome that determines the development of embryonic testes. Even where two, three, or four X chromosomes are present a single Y chromosome is sufficient to determine that the bipotential gonad shall become a testis — albeit with poorly differentiated and subfunctional tissue. On the other hand, the presence of two complete X chromosomes, without a Y chromosome, is necessary for the completion of ovarian development. The development of internal and external genitalia is secondary to the type and degree of differentiation of the gonads.

D. Lyon Hypothesis

X Chromosome activity in the mammalian female is quantitively similar to that in the male, despite the fact that the female has two X chromosomes and the male only one.[8,10] At an early state of embryonic development one of the two X chromosomes

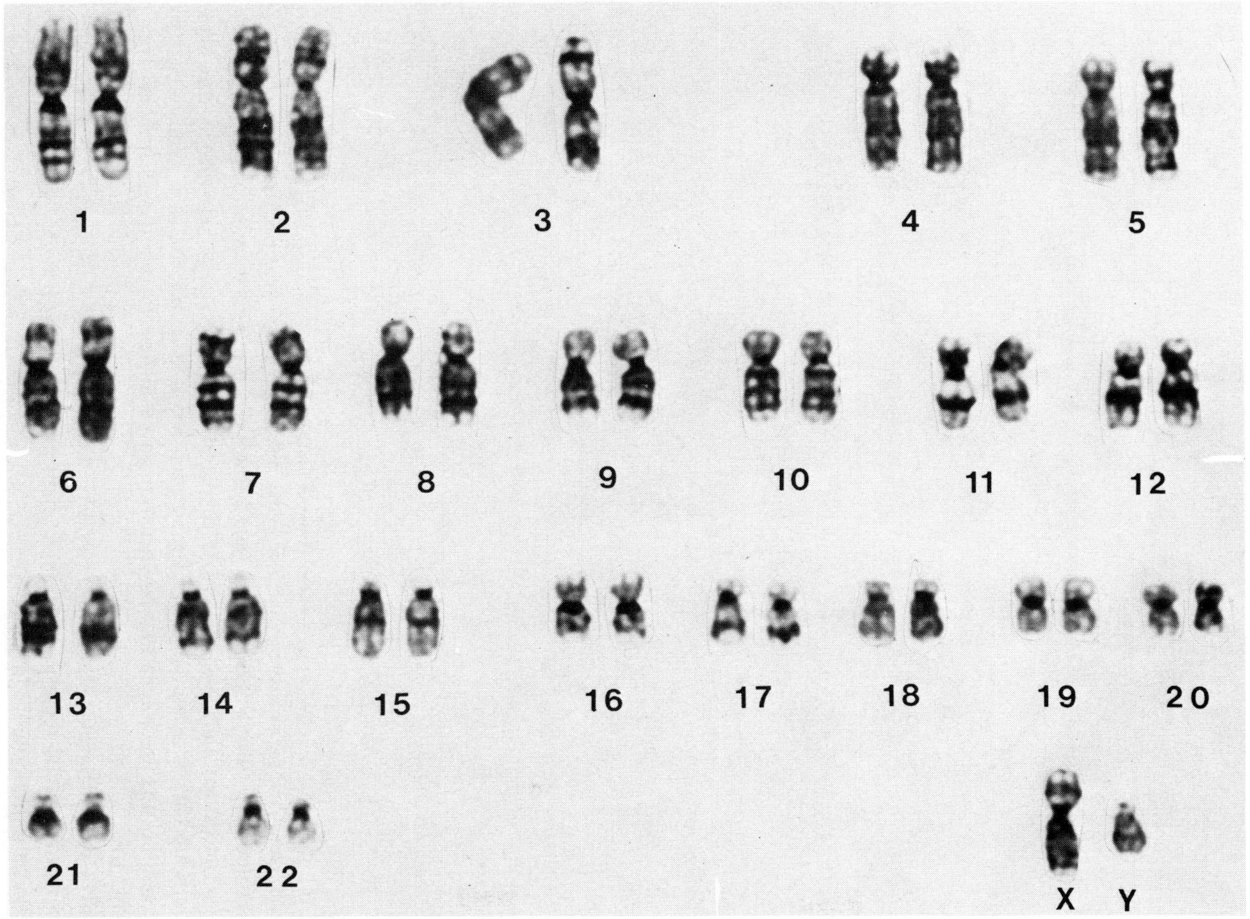

FIGURE 5. Normal male chromosome complement. Chromosomes arranged into pairs according to length of chromosome, position of centromere and banding pattern. (From Blank, C. E., *Mims Magazine*, March 1977, 69. With permission.)

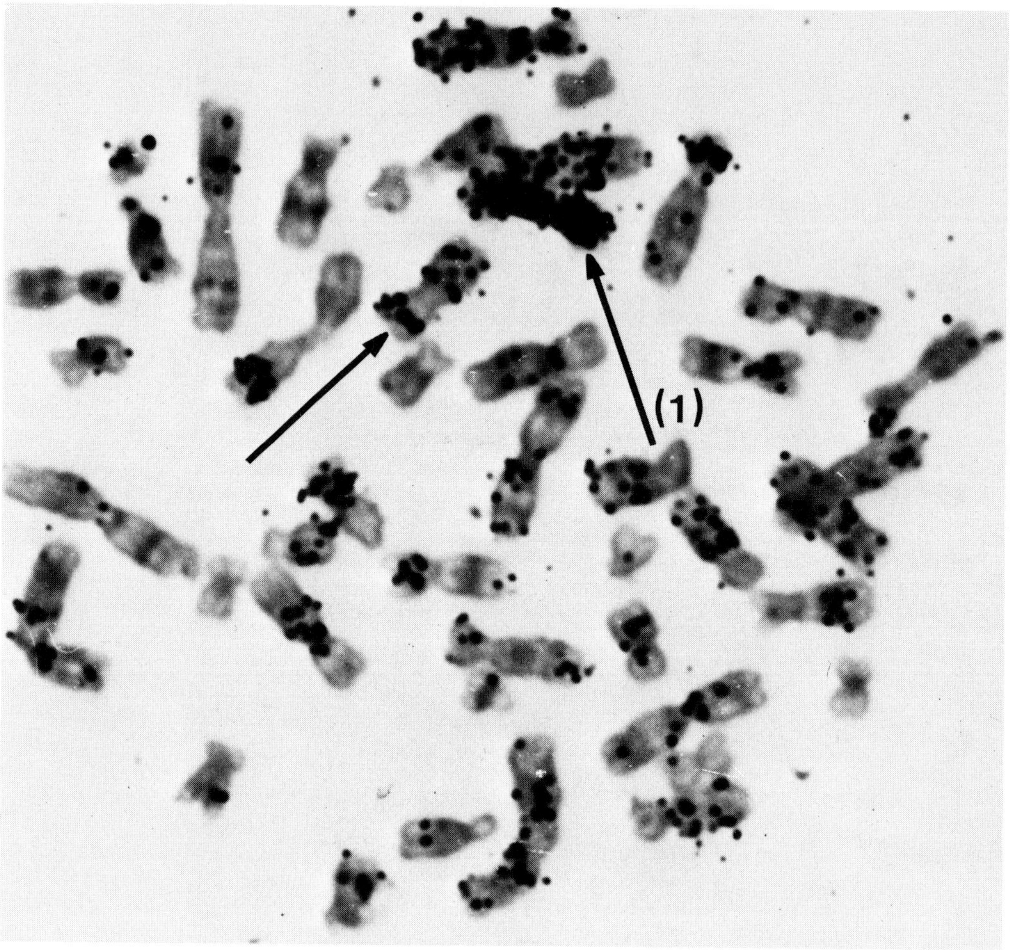

FIGURE 6. Autoradiography. Late and early replicating X chromosomes arrowed. Late replicating X indicated by (1).

in cells of the embryo is randomly inactivated (Lyon hypothesis). This has the effect of compensating for the double dose of gene products that would otherwise result. Thus the female is a functional mosaic (see Figure 9), one cell population expressing the genes of the paternal X and the other those of the maternal X. However, not all of this inactivated chromosome is nonfunctional for it is apparent that segments of both X chromosomes are necessary for normal gonadal development and indeed, for normal growth.

Gene inactivation, late labeling, and heteropyknosis are concommitant phenomena in that it is always the heteropyknotic (sex chromatin forming) X chromosome which is late labeling and genetically inactive.

E. Tissues That Might be Examined for Chromosome Complement

In clinical practice chromosome analysis is performed on the lymphocytes of the blood, the fibroblasts of the dermis and other connective tissues, the cells of the bone marrow, fetal cells derived from amniotic fluid, neoplastic tissue, and rarely, on gonadal cells undergoing meiosis. A chromosome analysis may be provided within 4 days

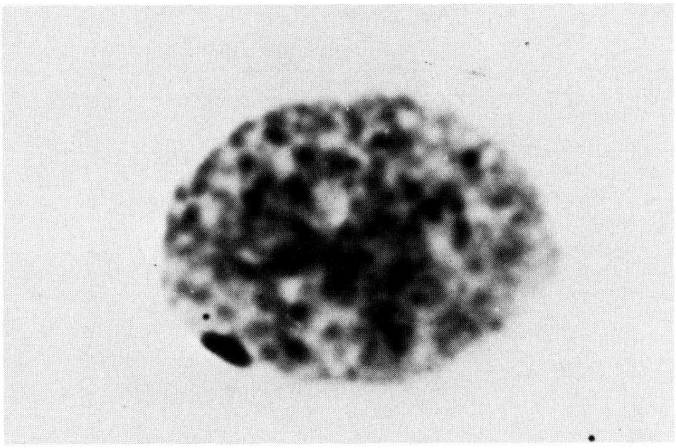

FIGURE 7. Sex chromatin in buccal mucosa. Under the nuclear membrane there is a deeply staining body about 1 μ in diameter. Interphase nucleus. (From Blank, C. E., *Mims Magazine,* March 1977, 69. With permission.)

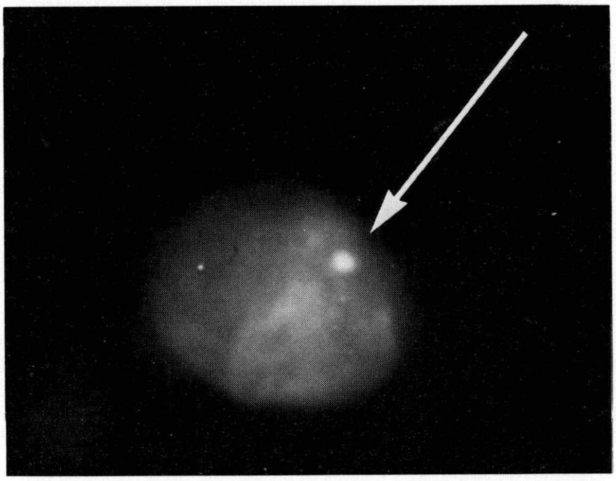

FIGURE 8. Fluorescent Y body (arrowed) under ultraviolet light in buccal mucosa. (From Blank, C. E., in *Scientific Foundations of Obstetrics and Gynaecology,* 2nd ed., Philipp, E. E., Barnes, J., and Newton, M., Eds., William Heinemann Medical Books, London, 1977, 44. With permission.)

of obtaining a specimen for lymphocyte culture, but if analysis is required immediately, the bone marrow technique can provide a result within 6 hours of obtaining a sample. A report of fetal chromosome complement usually takes 2 to 3 weeks from when the specimen of amniotic fluid is obtained.

F. Chromosome Abnormality as a Cause of Developmental Defect

Approximately 1 in 5 spontaneous abortions and more than 1 in 2 early abortions are of chromosomal origin.[11] Chromosome abnormality is the cause of at least 1 in 20

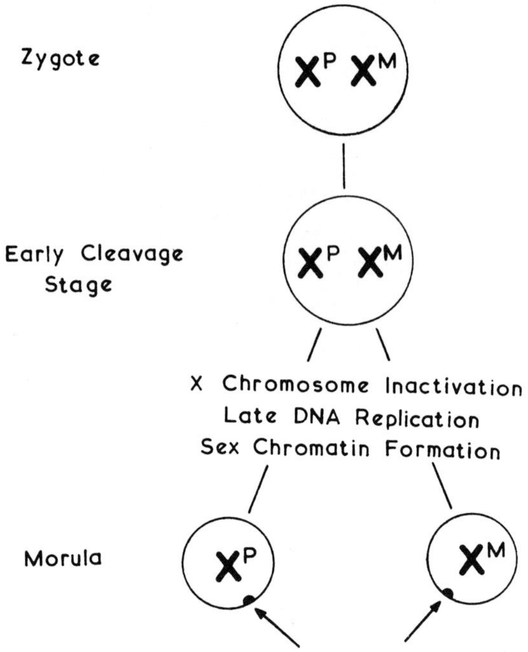

FIGURE 9. X-Chromosome inactivation during development. The paternally and maternally derived X chromosomes are represented as X^p and $X,^m$ respectively. The inactive X (arrowed) is always the late replicating and sex chromatin forming X chromosome and once "inactivated" remains so throughout succeeding cell generations.

stillbirths and about 1 in 20 neonatal deaths.[12] More than 1 in 250 liveborn children have, or will manifest by the time they reach puberty, gross defects of physical and/or mental development of chromosomal origin.[13] The main clinical syndromes associated with chromosome abnormality are indicated in Tables 2 and 3.[14] In developmental anomalies of sex, such as Klinefelter's syndrome and Turner's syndrome, gonadal dysgenesis is of major importance. Maldevelopment of the genital tract, including the gonads, is also a frequent occurrence where autosome abnormality is observed. Thyroid autoimmunity is found with increased frequency in children with mongolism and in their first degree relatives.[15] There is an increased frequency of goiter without thyroid antibodies in patients with Klinefelter's syndrome.

G. Origin of Chromosome Abnormality

Chromosome abnormality may be divided into two main types,[16] numerical anomaly and structural aberration.

1. Numerical Anomaly

Errors in the number of chromosomes present (aneuploidy) is usually the result of irregular division in parental gametogenesis. Nondisjunction (see Figure 10) results in the formation of a cell with one extra chromosome and a cell with one less. Fertilization will result in a zygote with an extra chromosome (trisomy) and one less (monosomy). Anaphase lag, where a chromosome is simply not included in either daughter nucleus, results in the loss of a chromosome. Nondisjunction or anaphase lag can occur at the first or second stage of meiosis. If irregular division occurs during early embryogenesis, two or more chromosomally distinct cell lines may be produced, the resultant condition being known as chromosome mosaicism.

Table 2
SOME AUTOSOME ABNORMALITIES ASSOCIATED WITH PARTICULAR CLINICAL FEATURES

Chromosome abnormality	Syndrome	Main clinical features
Trisomy 21	Down's (Mongolism)	Characteristic facies, mental subnormality, hypotonia, congenital heart disease (20%). Characteristic dermal ridge pattern. Those surviving infancy have a relatively normal life span.
Trisomy 18	Edwards'	Prominent occiput, micrognathia, low-set ears, flexion deformity of fingers, "rocker-bottom" feet. Characteristic dermal ridge pattern. Death in early infancy.
Trisomy 13	Patau's	Peculiar facies, cleft lip, polydactyly. Characteristic dermal ridge pattern. Death in early infancy.
Monosomy for short arm of 5	Cri-du-chat	Peculiar round moon-face, micrognathia. Cry the mewing of a kitten. Severe mental subnormality. Survival to adult life common.
Trisomy for short arm of 9	—	Characteristic facies, angulation of fingers and toes, moderate to severe mental subnormality. Characteristic dermal ridge pattern. Suvival to adult life common.

Table 3
SEX CHROMOSOME ABNORMALITY ASSOCIATED WITH DEVELOPMENTAL ANOMALY OF SEX

Clinical Syndrome	Main clinical features	Cytogenetic state usually or sometimes observed
Turner's	Small stature, primary amenorrhea, secondary sex development absent, webbing of neck, "shield" chest, "streak" gonads. Edema of feet often seen in infancy.	45, X; 46, X, isochromosome X; 45, X/46, XX mosaicism
Klinefelter's	Eunuchoid body proportions, poorly developed secondary sex characteristics, small testes, pubic hair of feminine distribution, sterility. May be educationally subnormal.	47, XXY; 47, XXXY, etc.
Hermaphroditism	Ovarian and testicular tissue present, external genitalia usually ambiguous, secondary sex development usually of female type.	Usually 46, XX; occasionally 46, XY/46, XX or 45, X/46, XY

2. Structural Aberration

A chromosome may break at one or more points. In consequence part of a chromosome may be lost (deletion) or transferred to another chromosome (translocation)

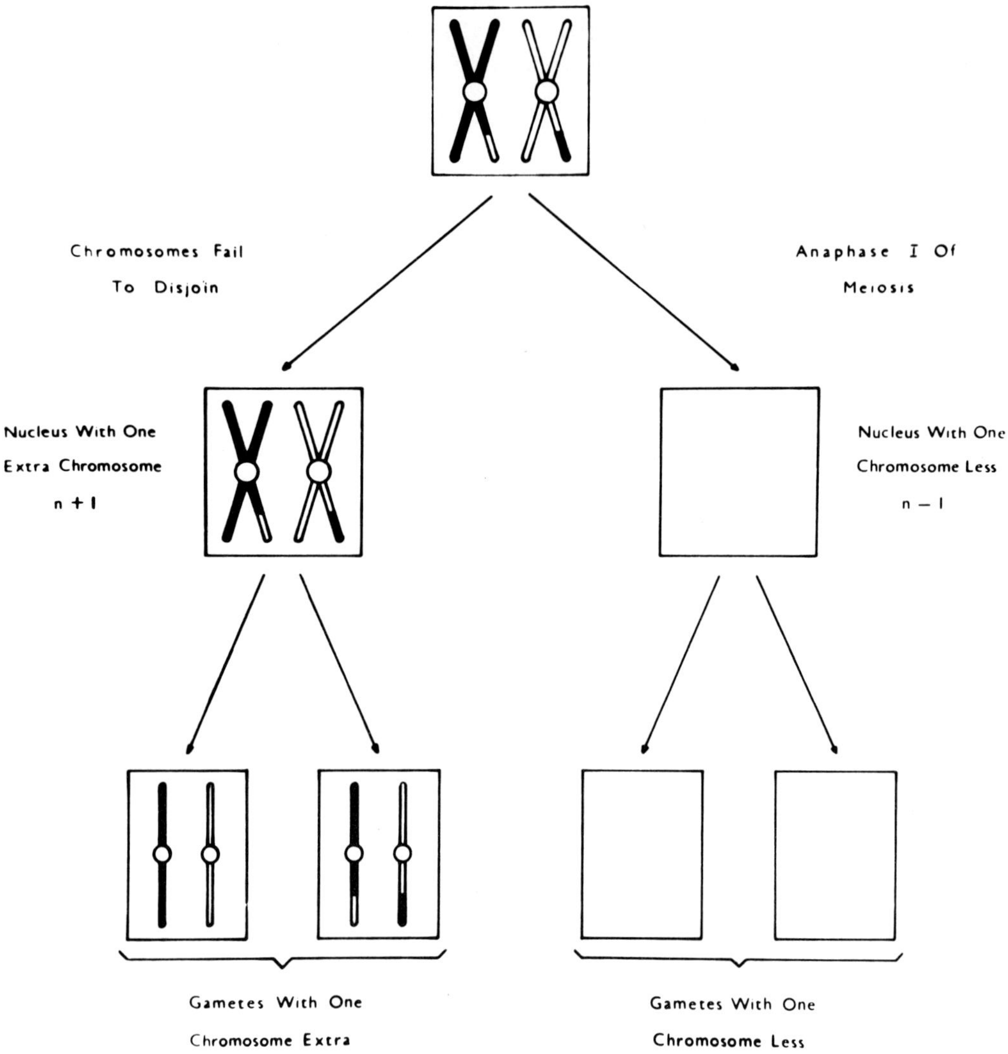

FIGURE 10. Nondisjunction: both half bivalents go to the same nucleus at anaphase I of meiosis. (From Blank, C. E., *Mims Magazine,* March 1977, 69. With permission.)

(see Figure 11). Where translocation merely rearranges the gene complement without producing an excess or deficiency of genetic material, there is usually no developmental defect, although duplication/deficiency may occur in the offspring of such a "genetically balanced" individual. Structural aberration may be produced during gamatogenesis or embryogenesis.

H. Factors Affecting the Frequency of Chromosome Abnormality

1. Maternal Age

A disproportionate number of babies with chromosome abnormality are born to older parents.[17-21] Maternal age, paternal age, and birth order are interdependent variables: the older a mother is at the birth of her child, the older the father tends to be, and the greater number of older siblings the child tends to have. Using appropriate

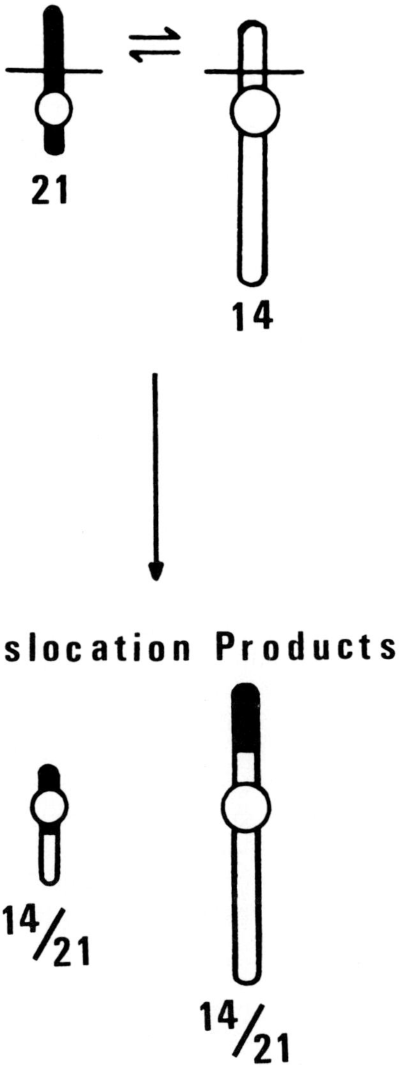

FIGURE 11. 14/21 translocation (the smaller product is usually lost in subsequent cell division). (From Blank, C. E., *Mims Magazine,* March 1977, 69. With permission.)

statistical techniques, one can study the independent effect of each of these variables on the incidence of a particular chromosome abnormality. In general, the trisomic conditions are associated with advancing maternal age (see Table 4), an exception being XYY.

An attractive explanation for this effect of maternal age is that ova are shed in the sequence in which they are laid down during embryogenesis and those produced last have fewer chiasmata. Chiasmata (see Figure 3) are important to the normal segregation of half bivalents to opposite daughter nuclei. In the absence of chiasmata, sister chromosomes might be expected to enter the same daughter nucleus frequently. Nondisjunction, leading to trisomy, might therefore be expected to occur more often in older ova.

Table 4
CHROMOSOME ABNORMALITY AND MATERNAL AGE[a]

Maternal age	Incidence of mongolism[b] among the liveborn in different maternal age groups (%)
Less than 30	0.04
30—34	0.11
35—39	0.33
40—44	1.25
45 and over	3.15

[a] Data derived from Penrose.[22]
[b] The total incidence of developmental defect of chromosomal origin among the liveborn is approximately twice the incidence of mongolism alone.

2. *Ionizing Radiation*

Ionizing radiation can produce chromosome breakage with consequent loss or gain of genetic material.[23] Large single doses of radiation, for example heavy doses of X-ray or the acute radiation from an atomic accident, are particularly likely to produce such damage. However, structural chromosome abnormality is not a frequent cause of developmental defect in man. Moreover, animal experiments on the effect of acute high dosage radiation of the testis indicate that most of the chromosome aberrations produced by high dose-rate ionizing radiation result in the death of the affected cell or its immediate descendents. However, *Drosophila* experiments on chronic low intensity radiation suggest that irradiation may also disrupt chromosome segregation.[24] Furthermore, six of nine surveys on women exposed to X-ray examination before pregnancy indicate that low dose-rate ionizing radiation may increase the frequency of trisomic offspring.[20,25] The effect appears to be substantial and is particularly marked in older mothers.

While recent trends in maternal age in Britain would be expected to reduce the frequency of trisomic states such as mongolism,[26] the increasing use in the home, industry, and medicine of equipment producing low doses of ionizing radiation may be having the opposite effect. Such use may be increasing the frequency of miscarriage, perinatal death, and mental handicap.

3. *Viral and Chemical Mutagens*

Some common viruses (such as those of measles and chickenpox), various other pathogens, and numerous chemical compounds in common usage in agriculture, medicine (for example inhalation anesthetics), industry, and the home, can produce chromosome breakage under experimental conditions.[27] Again several surveys have suggested an association between malformations of chromosomal origin and outbreaks of epidemic disease.[28,29] Nevertheless, firm evidence for viral or chemical induced developmental defect of chromosomal origin is as yet lacking.

III. SINGLE GENE DISORDERS IN MAN

A. Frequency

Although they are individually rare, with a usual frequency of less than 1 in 5000, often less than 1 in 10,000, so many conditions of single gene origin are known that, as a group, they contribute substantially to human morbidity and mortality.[30-33] About

Table 5
ENDOCRINE DISEASES WHERE SINGLE GENE INHERITANCE IS USUALLY OR SOMETIMES OBSERVED[a]

Autosomal dominant traits:	Pheochromocytoma
	Neurohypophyseal (vasopressin-sensitive) diabetes insipidis
	A type of pituitary dwarfism (isolated growth hormone deficiency)
	Hyperparathyroidism
	Pseudohypoparathyroidism[b]
	Multiple endocrine adenomatosis - peptic-ulcer complex
Autosomal recessive traits:	Goiterous cretinism[c]
	Nongoiterous cretinism
	Familial goiter with deafness (Pendred's syndrome)
	Congenital adrenal hyperplasia[c]
	Pituitary dwarfism
	Neonatal hyperparathyroidism
X-Linked recessive traits:	Congenital adrenal hyperplasia
	Nephrogenic diabetes insipidis
	Testicular feminization[d]

[a] Data mainly derived from Fialkow.[15]
[b] Sex influenced trait. An alternative explanation is X-linked dominance.
[c] Several subtypes distinguishable.
[d] Alternative explanation is sex-limited autosomal dominance.

5% of children in hospital are there because of a disorder of single gene origin, and about 10% of infant deaths in hospital have a similar cause. In excess of 1% of the adult population require medical attention because of disease of single gene origin. Endocrine disturbances where single gene inheritance is usually, or sometimes, observed are listed in Table 5. The common endocrine disorders, for example diabetes mellitus and thyrotoxicosis, are better understood in terms of "multifactorial" origin (see below).

Biochemical and clinical aberrations of single gene origin are the consequence of a change (mutation) in the DNA code at a particular locus. Studies on experimental organisms have shown that mutation may occur in a regulatory gene (see Figure 2) responsible for the control of one or more structural genes, in the promotor region of an operon, or in a structural gene itself.[1] Functional deficiency of a protein producing the clinical abnormalities of a single gene disorder can be caused by a defect in any of these three types of gene. Without detailed biochemical analysis of the affected polypeptide it is very difficult to distinguish between these three types of coding defect, for each would be expected to give rise to clinically very similar symptoms. Within any one of these three subgroups there are a host of potential alleles, adding a further pattern of variation to an already complex picture.

In man numerous alleles of structural genes are known, both benign and malign.[34] The hemoglobinopathies are a well studied group of disorders where single changes in the amino acid sequence of a protein have been shown to give rise to various changes in its functional properties. Such allelic variation would be anticipated in hormonal disorders although hormones with abnormal amino acid sequences have not yet been characterized.

Although there is no incontrovertible evidence for regulatory gene defects in man, organ agenesis, system dysgenesis, or the quantitative deficiency of structurally normal enzymes can readily be understood in terms of abnormal regulatory gene activity. It may be reasonably suggested that the various deficiencies of steroid 21-hydroxylase, the most common cause of congenital adrenal hyperplasia, may reflect various (defective) alleles of a regulatory gene.

Defects in the promotor region of an operon would be expected to produce similar effects to those produced by a defective regulatory gene. Where regulatory or operator genes control the transcription of more than one structural gene, abnormal levels of all the structural gene products would be anticipated. Thus the observation of multiple deficiencies in hormone proteins would be good evidence for such a type of defect.

B. Autosomal Dominant and Recessive Disorders

A dominant trait is the manifestation of a single gene in single dose (heterozygous form). If the condition does not impair reproductive ability, a characteristic pedigree pattern is observed (see Figure 12). When a dominant trait is incompatible with survival or reproduction is severely limited, as in achondroplasia, most cases are new mutations, the mutation occurring in a germ cell of one parent. A recessive trait is the manifestation of a single gene in double dose (homozygous form). A characteristic pedigree pattern may be observed (see Figure 13). The parents are usually quite normal clinically, although they must be presumed to be heterozygous for the gene, i.e., they are carriers of the gene. Most of the inborn errors of metabolism are recessive traits. As experience accumulates and biochemical techniques in particular become more sophisticated, the number of recessive traits grows for which the gene can be detected in heterozygous form, at least with a high probability.[34]

C. Sex-Linked Disorders

The vast majority of conditions due to single genes with major effect on the X and Y chromosome are the manifestation of genes in hemizygous form on the X chromosome (X-linked recessive traits). Mothers and sisters (see Figure 14) are often carriers of the deleterious gene. In some X-linked recessive diseases, for example Hunter's syndrome or the Lesch-Nyhan syndrome, chemical examination or detailed clinical examination can identify the carrier state in a female with virtually 100% confidence.[34,35]

Rare X-linked dominant traits occur in man, for example, vitamin D-resistant rickets. Manifestation may be more severe in the hemizygous male than in the heterozygous female. Convincing evidence of Y-linked inheritance in man is lacking, although a type of "hairy ears" may be an example.

D. Gene Linkage

With only 23 pairs of chromosomes in the chromosome complement of man, many loci will obviously be on the same chromosome pair. This association is described as gene linkage. A chromosomal map which defines the position of these loci is gradually being built up.[7,36,37] The establishment of linkage association is not of solely academic interest; if a particular deleterious gene, say for Huntington's chorea, were shown to be linked to a common "marker" gene, say at the O blood group locus, identification of marker status could be an aid to identifying, or excluding individuals at high risk of the disease. The gene for the dominant disorder dystrophia myotonica is linked to the ABH secretor locus.[38] Again, significant associations have been found between certain antigens of the histocompatibility locus-A system and juvenile diabetes (see Section IV. D).

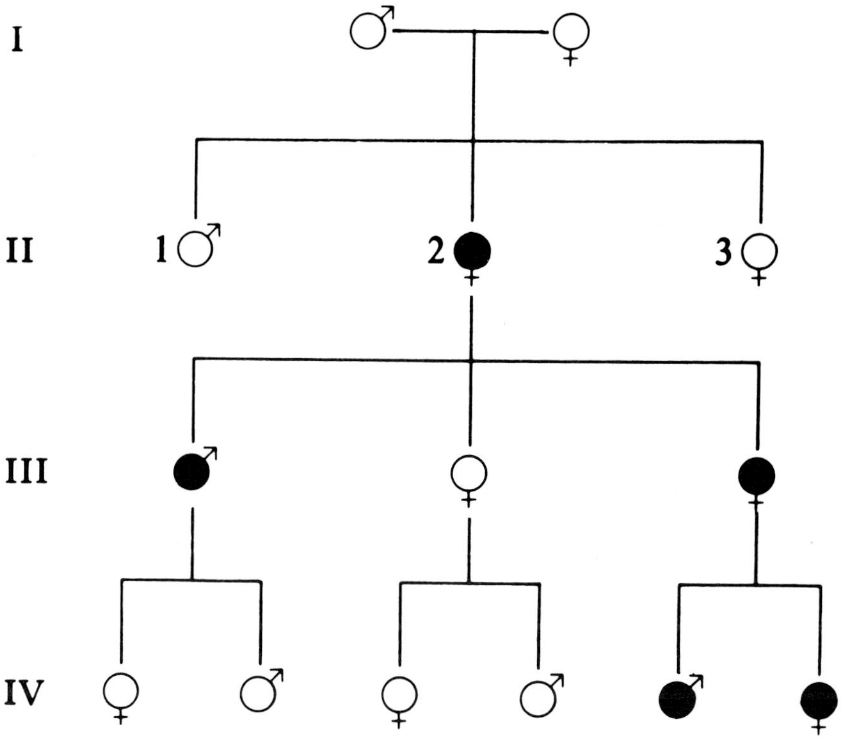

FIGURE 12. Pedigree pattern of an autosomal dominant trait. ♂ = male; ♀ = female; ● = affected. II.2 is a new mutant, mutation having occurred in a germ cell of one or other parent in the preceding generation. (From Blank, C. E., *Mims Magazine,* April 1977, 75. With permission.)

E. Factors Affecting the Frequency of Gene Mutation

In experimental organisms, many factors including ionizing radiation, ultraviolet light, various chemical agents, and changes in atmospheric pressure or temperature, have been shown to affect the rate of gene mutation.[39] Presumably these factors also influence the frequency of gene mutation in man. Considerable concern has arisen about the effect on mutation rate of ionizing radiation produced by equipment used in medicine, industry, and the home. Interest became intense when the extent of ionizing radiation attending thermonuclear explosions ("radioactive fallout") became evident. On the other hand, descendents of individuals particularly exposed to ionizing radiation, such as the survivors of Hiroshima and Nagasaki, show no statistically significant increased frequency of dominant traits attributed to new mutation.[40] One may conclude that present day practice in medicine and industry regarding equipment emitting ionizing radiation is unlikely to produce a measurable effect on, and is certainly in no danger of causing a marked increase in, the frequency of disease or disorder of development of single gene origin in man.

The frequency of some new mutations, for example, achondroplasia, Marfan's syndrome, and Apert's syndrome, rises with increasing father's age.[41] although the effect is not as marked as that of increasing mother's age in mongolism. The explanation for this paternal age effect is not clear. The phenomenon is not observed for every disorder of development referrable to a gene in heterozygous form.

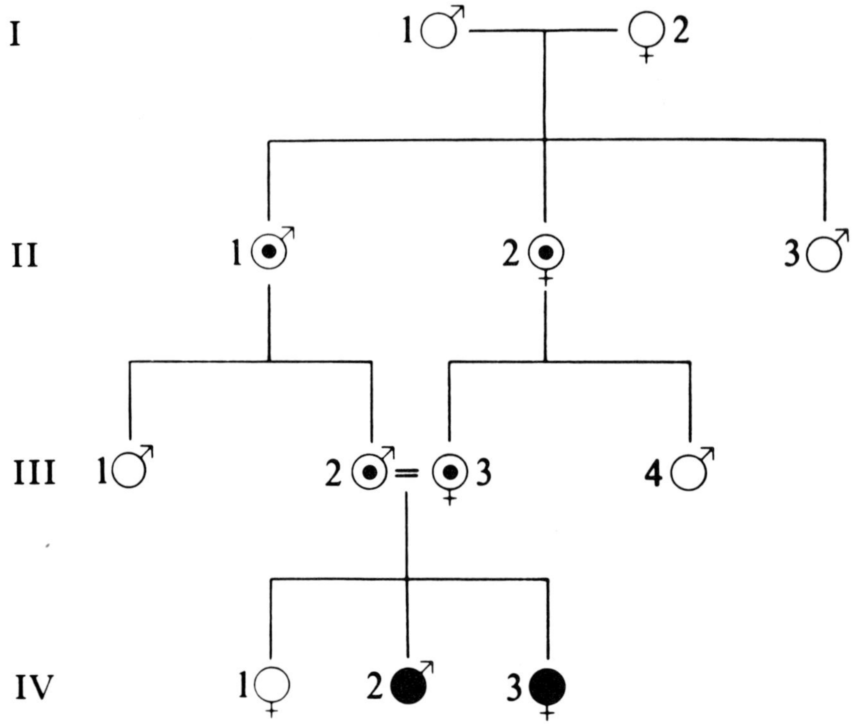

FIGURE 13. Pedigree pattern of an autosomal recessive trait. Consanguineous mating (♂ = ♀) is seen among parents of affected individuals more often than in the general population. Affected individuals are homozygous for the abnormal gene. Parents of affected individuals are obligate carriers (●). Either I.1 or I.2 must be a carrier. IV.1 has a 2 in 3 chance of being a carrier. (From Blank, C. E., *Mims Magazine*, April 1977, 75. With permission.)

IV. CONDITIONS OF MULTIFACTORIAL ORIGIN

Disease or disorder of development not known to be of single gene origin or due to chromosome abnormality may also occur in two or more members of the same family more often than can be attributed to chance. Endocrine disturbances which fit this description (Table 6) include thyroid autoimmunity, nonendemic simple goiter, most malignant thyroid tumors and diabetes mellitus (but see Section IV. B). In the absence of an obvious environmental cause inherited predisposition is often thought to play a part. In such circumstances the inherited component is believed to consist of many genes each with a small, but by itself unrecognizable, effect (polygenic inheritance).

One of the major features of medical genetics in recent years has been the development of models demonstrating how genes with a minor effect can influence development or disease.[42-45] Two such models particularly pertinent to the etiology of common disorders are outlined below. The first applies to characters, such as height, weight, skin color, intelligence, and blood pressure, which show a continuously variable range of expression (continuous variation). The second refers to conditions such as cleft lip, neural tube defect, and duodenal ulcer which are either present or absent (discontinuous variation).

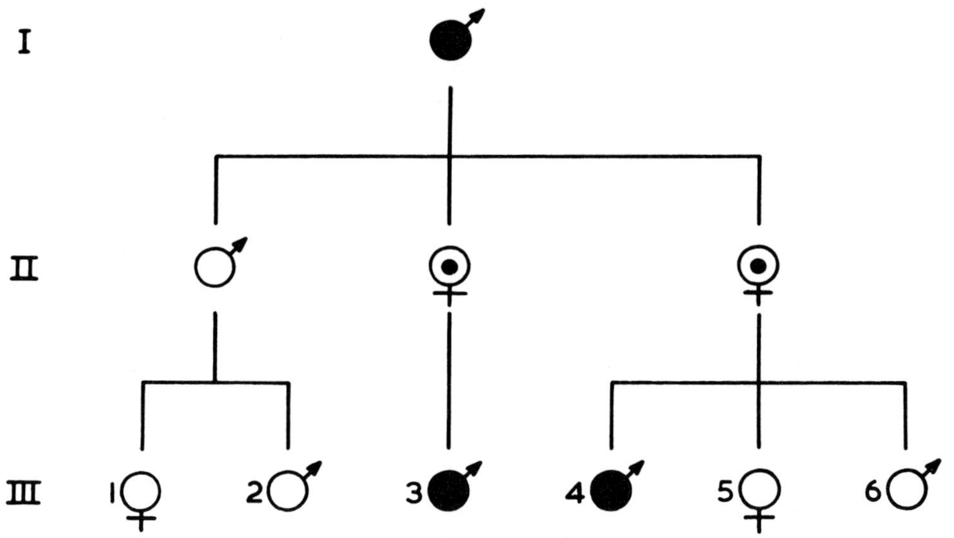

FIGURE 14. Pedigree pattern of an X-linked recessive trait. Affected males are hemizygous for the gene: mothers of affected males are heterozygous (♀). III.5 has a 1 in 2 chance of being a carrier of the gene. (From Blank, C. E., *Mims Magazine*, April 1977, 75. With permission.)

Where many genes, each with small effect are involved, environmental factors can usually be seen also to play a part (multifactorial inheritance).

A. A Model for Continuous Variation

1. The "Normal" Curve

Graded characters, such as height, weight, skin color, IQ, and blood pressure, often show all possible values between extremes, if the population studied is sufficiently large. Nevertheless, the majority of individuals in the population have values close to the average for that population. This "frequency distribution curve" is usually "bell-shaped" or "normal" (see Figure 15). A population with a frequency distribution approximating the normal curve may be conveniently described in such statistical terms as the mean (the average) and variance (a measure of spread). These statistics are used to make comparisons with frequency distributions of other populations.

2. Additive Gene Action

For most graded characters, members of a family show greater similarities than individuals taken at random from the general population. Part of the similarity may be due to the inheritance of genes with a small effect. In our model we shall assume that these genes do not show dominance or recessiveness but have an additive effect. In this model (see Figure 16) a tall man has many "tall" genes and a short man has a few — instead he has the "short" alleles. Individuals of average height have a mixture of "tall" and "short" alleles. A tall father and a tall mother contribute mainly "tall" genes to their offspring, and a short couple mainly "short" genes.

When the population character under investigation is due to many genes with an additive effect, the frequency distribution of individuals with particular gene complements (genotypes), for example particular proportions of "tall" alleles, is also normally distributed (Figure 16).

Table 6
ENDOCRINE DISORDERS WITH FAMILIAR INCIDENCE EXPLAINED IN TERMS OF "MULTIFACTORIAL" HYPOTHESIS[a]

Thyroid autoimmunity[b]
(e.g., Hashimoto's disease, Graves' disease)
Nonendemic simple goiter
Most malignant thyroid tumors
Diabetes mellitus

[a] Data derived from Fialkow[15]

[b] Other "autoimmune" diseases, e.g. Addison's disease, observed more frequently than expected by chance in relatives of patients with thyroid autoimmunity.

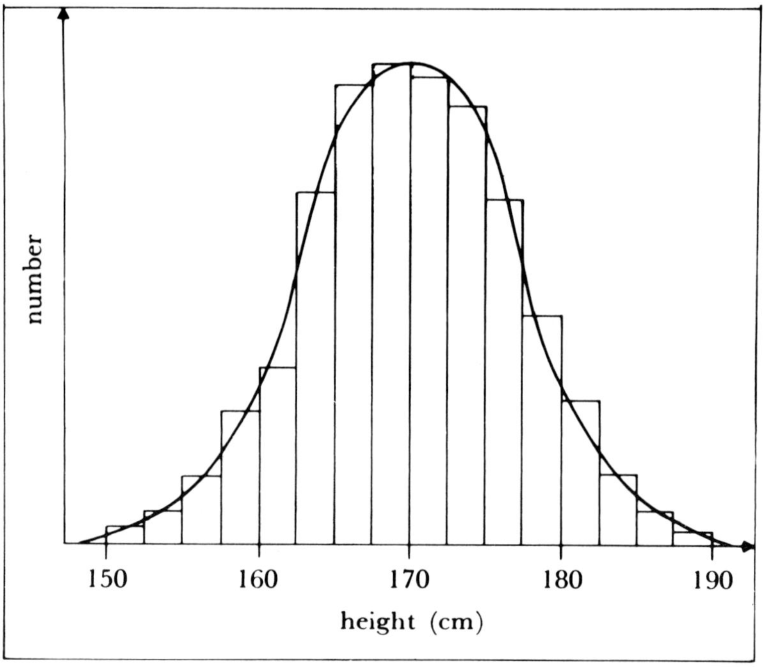

FIGURE 15. Distribution of adult male height in a population and a "normal" distribution curve fitted to the data. (From Blank, C. E., *Mims Magazine,* May 1977, 69. With permission.)

3. Interaction of Inherited Predisposition and Environment

Where inherited predisposition is believed to be polygenic, environmental factors can almost always be seen to influence the manifestation of these genes. For example, the height of a person depends on the genes inherited from his parents, but whether he realizes his inherited potential depends on many factors in his environment, including diet and exercise. Environmental influences can themselves be considered to have a normal distribution within a population. Consequently, "total liability" — inherited liability and environmental liability acting together — can be regarded as having a normal distribution.

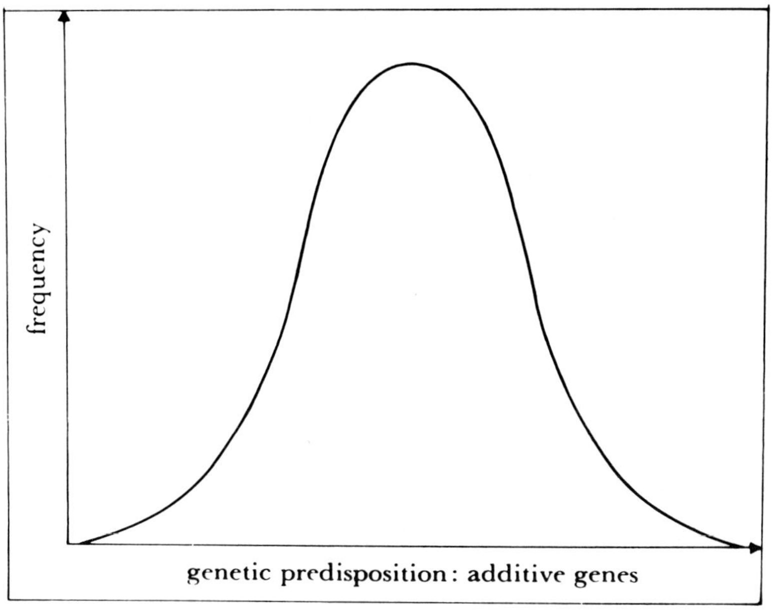

FIGURE 16. Frequency distribution of genetic predisposition where predisposition is due to many genes each having a small additive effect. An example of "polygenic" inheritance. (From Blank, C. E., *Mims Magazine,* May 1977. With permission.)

B. A Model for Discontinuous Variation

1. Liability with a "Threshold"

The familial incidence of some discontinuous traits, including many common malformations and diseases, can best be explained by a continuously distributed total liability and a "threshold" (see Figure 17).

Individuals with a total liability above the threshold show the disease or malformation, while individuals below that threshold do not. The threshold model has proved an extremely useful concept which enables us to understand many facets of disease or disorder of development previously not clear. For example, pyloric stenosis is four times commoner in the male infant than in the female; on a threshold model this can be expressed as different, although parallel, distributions of liability in the male and the female. Although inherited predisposition (in the form of many genes with an additive effect) must have the same distribution in both sexes, manifestation of these genes is obviously influenced by the hormonal environment in which they act. Again, familial incidence is also easily appreciated in terms of a threshold model. By chance some families must have more (or less) than the average concentation of liability of genetic, and perhaps environmental, origin. Such families are identified only by the occurrence of one or more affected individuals. Relatives of affected indiviuals are then at greater risk than the general population for that particular affliction — the closer the relationship to an affected individual the greater the risk.

2. Environmental Factors Modifying Gene Action

The influence of environmental factors on a condition which is believed to have a polygenic background may be indicated by correlation of the incidence or expression

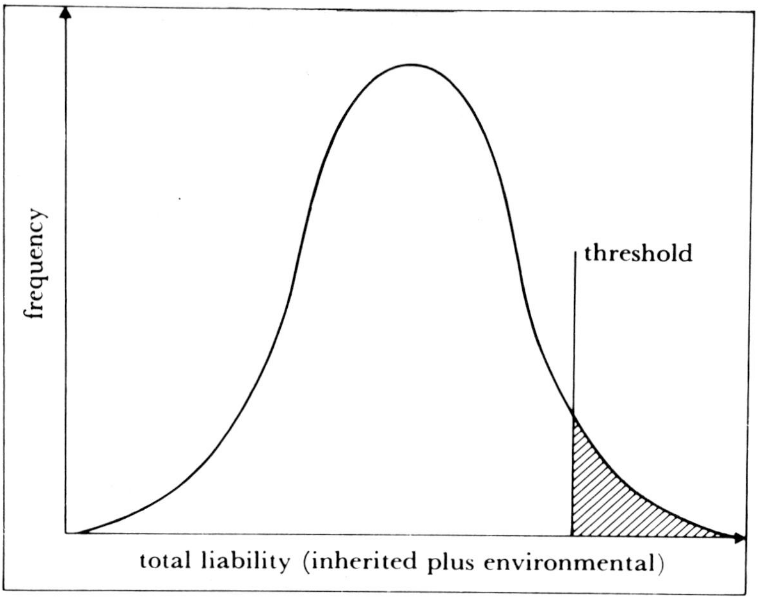

FIGURE 17. The "threshold" model. Only individuals with a total liability above the threshold will show disease or disorder of development (indicated by cross-hatched area). (From Blank, C. E., *Mims Magazine*, May 1977. With permission.)

of the defect of development or disease with sex, parental age, birth order, social class, season, year, or other environmental factor.

Of particular interest are possible "trigger" mechanisms, for example viral infection in early onset diabetes mellitus, that can produce overt manifestation of disorders involving a threshold concept; avoid the trigger and one would expect to avoid the disorder, irrespective of the "heritability" (see Section IV. C) of the disorder.

C. Measuring Heredity

What proportion of the difference between individuals, as in liability to a condition, is genetic and what proportion is environmental? The question can rarely be answered with absolute confidence. A major difficulty is that environmental influences, if they occur, are likely to be more similar among members of a family than among unrelated individuals. Genetic similarity, of course, is also stronger among relatives. Environmental influences are therefore not easily separated from inherited predisposition.

"Heritability" is usually calculated by comparing the frequency of the condition in relatives with that in the general population.[44,47] Estimates of heritability for some common diseases explicable in multifactorial terms are given in Table 7. Most statistical manipulations tend to underestimate the significance of environmental factors.

D. The Genetics of Diabetes Mellitus

Diabetes mellitus is worthy of special consideration here because of its prevalence, at 1 to 2% in Western Europe and the U.S. it is the commonest endocrine disturbance coming to the attention of the medical practitioner, and because recent work has given strong support to identifiable etiological heterogeneity and a clue as to pathogenesis.[49]

A high familial incidence and a greater concordance rate observed in identical twins

Table 7
ESTIMATES OF HERITABILITY FOR VARIOUS DISORDERS[a]

Disorder	Incidence (%)	Heritability
Asthma	4	80
Schizophrenia	1—2	80
Cleft lip ± palate	0.1	76
Pyloric stenosis (congenital)	0.3	75
Diabetes mellitus:		
early onset	0.2	75
late onset	2—3	35
Ankylosing spondylitis	0.2	70
Dislocation of hip (congenital)	0.07	70
Club foot (congenital)	0.1	68
Coronary artery disease	3	65
Hypertension (essential)	5	62
Anencephaly and spina bifida	0.5	60
Peptic ulcer	4	37
Congenital heart disease (all types)	0.5	35

[a] Data derived from Emery.[48]

(65%) compared with nonidentical twins (20%) suggest an important inherited predisposition.[49,50] Diabetes may conveniently be divided into two relatively distinct clinical subtypes according to age of onset and dependence on insulin. Those with onset as children or young adults (prevalence 0.2%) are usually dependent on insulin and those with a later age of onset are not, although this association is not absolute. Heterogeneity of etiology between early onset and late onset diabetes is suggested by the relative infrequency of occurrence of early onset and late onset diabetes in the same family and, more especially, by a difference in the concordance rate for identical twins;[52,53] for early onset diabetes the identical twin concordance rate approximates 50% and for late onset diabetes it approaches 100%.

Further support for the recognition of two main clinical and etiologically distinct subtypes of diabetes mellitus is given by the observation that certain antigens of the major histocompatibility system HLA, are associated with early onset (insulin dependent) diabetes but not with late onset (insulin independent) diabetes.[54,55] It is already clear that the antigens HLA B8, BW15, and B18 occur among early onset diabetics more frequently than expected by chance. Again there is strong circumstantial evidence that different environmental factors affect the manifestation of inherited predisposition in the two types, carbohydrate intake in late onset diabetes and viral infection in early onset diabetes.[56] A working hypothesis for early onset diabetes is outlined in Figure 18.

Although inherited predisposition in late onset diabetes is still best considered as of polygenic origin,[57] with a heritability estimate 30 to 40,[51] a major gene (or gene complex) on chromosome 6 is clearly implicated in early onset diabetes. It is of interest that the HLA B8 antigen is also seen with increased frequency in Graves' disease and in idiopathic Addison's disease, both "autoimmune" diseases.[58] In rare families,[59] where age of onset is early but the diabetes is adequately controlled by diet, the condition appears to segregate as an autosomal dominant trait.

Published data relating to the risk to the siblings or offspring of diabetics themselves developing diabetes is conflicting. However, the risk to a sibling of a juvenile diabetic

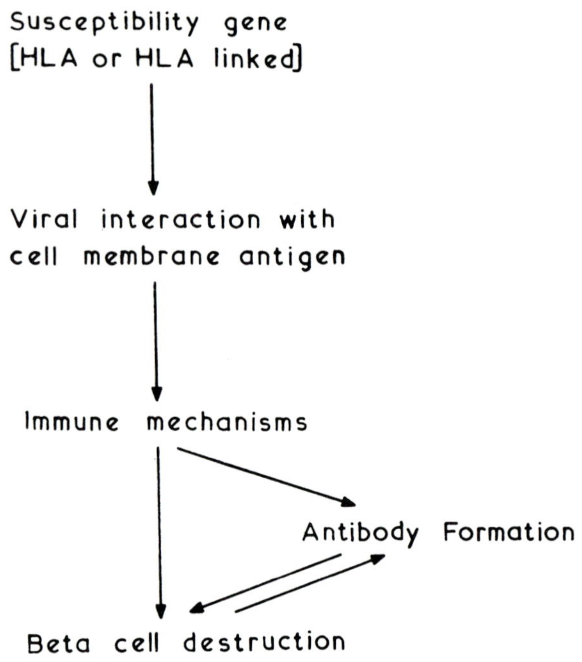

FIGURE 18. A model for the pathogenesis of early onset diabetes. (After Cudworth, A. G., *Br. J. Hosp. Med.*, 16, 207, 1976.)

of developing diabetes as a child or young adult probably approximates 1 in 12,[60] as does the risk to a parent with insulin dependent diabetes of a child developing early onset diabetes. The risk to a parent with late onset diabetes of a child developing early onset diabetes is probably less than 1 in 30. In time an appreciation of the HLA haplotypes of relatives at risk of early onset diabetes mellitus will make more precise risk estimates possible. Furthermore, HLA antigens are manifest in fibroblast culture so that analysis of fetal HLA status on cells derived from amniotic fluid, and an estimate of risk to the fetus should, eventually, be possible.[61]

Female insulin dependent diabetics have an additional problem with respect to outcome of pregnancy. Without good management perinatal death is very high. With modern management during pregnancy, and in the neonatal period, infant loss may be reduced to 10%.[62,63] However, the frequency of congenital abnormality (major malformations) in the liveborn is three to four times the normal (approximately 8%) about half of which are lethal.[64,65] The mechanism of this teratogenic effect is unknown, but the frequency of developmental defect is maximum, (eight times that expected by chance) in the children of mothers with severe vascular complications, e.g. nephropathy and/or proliferative retinopathy. There is some indication that severe limb deformities, especially reduction deformity of the legs, are particularly frequent.

V. GENETIC COUNSELING

Genetic counseling may be defined most simply as the computation and communication of a specified risk in a particular pregnancy.[66,67] The problem usually arises because the prospective parents have already experienced an unfavorable outcome to pregnancy, for example, a child with physical or mental handicap. Explanation as to the mechanism of origin — for example, birth injury, chromosomal defect, single gene effect, or multifactorial inheritance — of the particular disorder or disease, an appreciation of prognosis, an assessment of availability and adequacy of treatment and of relevent antenatal diagnostic procedures are also important aspects of management.[68-70] Where risk of recurrence is not high guarded, reassurance is much appreciated.

Although most genetic counseling is retrospective, given after an abnormal event has drawn attention to the family at risk, opportunities for prospective genetic counseling are increasing. For instance, if a woman is a diabetic (see Section IV.D), an epileptic on medication,[71] or of advanced reproductive age (see Section II.H), the greatly increased risk of unfavorable outcome to pregnancy is now well recognized.

Because a proper appreciation of prognosis and of treatment is so important the genetic counseling should usually be given by the clinician — often a pediatrician — dealing with the abnormal event initiating genetic counseling. Again, the specialist on the spot is usually in the best position to appreciate and delineate heterogeneity of origin which is of importance to risk estimate and prognosis.[72] If a second opinion is required, or if assessment is unusually complicated or difficult to obtain, a medical geneticist may be approached.

A. Special Risk Estimates

Although more than 5% of developmental defect in man can be attributed to environmental influence acting on a fetus during development,[73-79] occasions when one can confidently refer a particular congenital abnormality to a teratogen are rare.

For conditions of single gene origin, precise estimates (see Table 8) based on an understanding of mendelian segregation may be given. However, in most cases estimates are empirical, based on past experience.[72] Several admirable works are now available which deal with risk of recurrence or transmission in different groups of disease.[66,80-83] Endocrine disorders are perhaps not so well documented as many other groups of disease, e.g. muscle dystrophies or skeletal abnormalities. Where empiric risk values are not available, and the condition is believed to be multifactorial in origin, risk to first degree relatives approximates to the square root of the frequency in the general population.[43]

B. General Risk

Unfavorable outcome to pregnancy is more common than most young couples appreciate: 15% of pregnancies miscarry; about 2% of those going to term end in the birth of a dead child or a child dying within a few days of birth; and about 2% of surviving infants suffer severe physical or mental handicap. Although most couples with a history of unfavorable outcome to pregnancy are concerned about the risk of recurrence of that particular abnormal event, the general risk must be added to their special risk to give them an appreciation of overall risk in the next pregnancy.

Diabetic women on insulin (see Section IV.D), females with thyroid disease,[77,84] female epileptics receiving medication,[71] and women of advanced reproductive age (see Section II.H) have a much greater "general" risk than average. The risk of congenital abnormality in female diabetics and epileptics is between two and four times the average. It is encouraging to note that recent research indicates that, at least in experimental organisms.[85] some antiepileptic drugs are without demonstrable teratogenic effect; phenytoin and phenobarbital, commonly used medication in epilepsy, are both teratogenic in the mouse. For mothers of advancing age, much of the increased risk is of fetal chromosome abnormality. Pregnancy can be screened for fetal chromosome abnormality (see Section VI).

Table 8
RISK OF AFFECTED OFFSPRING AFTER ONE, OR TWO AFFECTED OFFSPRING

Situation	After one	After two
Autosomal dominant trait		
Affected parent	1 in 2	1 in 2
Clinically normal parents:		
Regular dominant	<1 in 100	1 in 2
Irregular dominant[a]	1 in 15	1 in 2
Autosomal recessive trait[b]	1 in 4	1 in 4
X-Linked recessive trait[c,d]	1 in 6[e]	1 in 4
Chromosome abnormality[f]		
Parents normal karyotype	1 in 70[g]	1 in 20
Parent a translocation carrier	1 in 10	1 in 5
Multifactorial, or "unknown" origin	<1 in 20	>1 in 10
Diabetes mellitus (early onset)	1 in 12	—

[a] Gene not always manifest in heterozygous form.
[b] Sometimes amenable to antenatal diagnosis (see Table 10).
[c] Clnical or laboratory examination for carrier status sometimes useful.
[d] Sometimes amenable to antenatal diagnosis. Fetus may be sexed (only males may be affected).
[e] In the absence of a positive family history.
[f] Fetal karyotype identifiable.
[g] After maternal age of 35 years risk rises rapidly.

VI. ANTENATAL DIAGNOSIS OF FETAL ABNORMALITY

In those countries where interruption of pregnancy is permissible if the risk of having a child with serious physical or mental handicap is substantial, a great deal of interest and activity has been stimulated concerning the possibility of identifying markers of fetal abnormality sufficiently early in pregnancy to permit termination if required.[86] The main antenatal diagnostic procedures currently relevant to the management of high risk situations are fetal chromosome analysis and amniotic fluid alphafetoprotein (AFP) assay.[87,88] Many inborn errors of metabolism exhibit specific enzyme deficiency in cells in tissue culture and, therefore, might be susceptible to detection by enzyme assay of fetal cells from amniotic fluid.[78] Analysis of the chemical constituents of amniotic fluid may also sometimes be expected to indicate disease of single gene origin, for example, in a pregnancy at special risk of a child with the adrenogenital syndrome. If a special risk exists of a child being born with skeletal abnormality, X-ray examination of the fetus may be helpful.[89]

Amniocentesis is transabdominal and best carried out at 15 to 16 weeks gestation, usually as an outpatient procedure. Before 15 weeks, amniocentesis is technically more difficult and sufficient quantites of amniotic fluid for reliable fetal chromosome analysis are not easily obtained. Prior to amniocentesis, the placenta is localized by ultrasonography; rhesus sensitization is prevented by administration of anti-D where the woman is rhesus negative. Amniocentesis carries a risk, probably less than 1 in 100,[90] of inducing abortion. Although (in Britain) termination is allowable up to the 28th week of pregnancy, the decision to induce abortion is usually taken much earlier. Mid-trimester abortion may conveniently be induced by administering extra-amniotic prostaglandins.[91]

The risk of a child being born with chromosome abnormality rarely exceeds 1 in 10 and is then virtually confined to situations in which one parent has a balanced translocation. Nevertheless, most couples who have had a previous child with chromosome abnormality (for example mongolism), and who have discussed antenatal diagnosis, elect to have fetal chromosome analysis in succeeding pregnancies.

Couples who have had a child with anencephaly or spina bifida cystica usually chose to have amniotic fluid AFP assay in subsequent pregnancies. Alphafetroprotein (molecular weight 60,000) is the main protein in the circulation of the early human fetus. The levels of AFP in fetal blood reach a peak of 2 to 3 mg/mℓ at the 12 to 14th week of gestation and thereafter decrease. Levels in amniotic fluid, the principal source of which is probably fetal urine, are much lower. Serum levels of up to 25 ng/mℓ occur in the normal adult. High concentrations of AFP are found in amniotic fluid where the fetus has an open neural tube defect, and are probably due to leakage of fetal cerebrospinal fluid or transduction of proteins from fetal capillaries exposed to amniotic fluid. High amniotic AFP levels almost always indicate fetal abnormality; benign causes of raised AFP may reliably be excluded. However, closed lesions, such as meningocele, may not show sufficiently high levels to indicate abnormality. Alphafetoprotein has no biological activity and is usually measured in amniotic fluid by a gel-precipitin technique (radioimmunoassay on maternal serum). In experienced hands this technique is reliable. An assay may be available a few hours after receipt of the specimen. One may expect to detect 90 to 95% of anencephaly and spina bifida cystica. However, anencephaly and spina bifida cystica are also observed at high frequencies after the birth of a child with primary congenital hydrocephaly,[92] and must, at least in part, have a common etiology. Primary hydrocephaly is not usually associated with a raised amniotic fluid AFP. The risk of a child with neural tube defect after a "normal" amniotic fluid AFP reading is calculated in Table 9 and assumes that 10% of this risk is for primary congenital hydrocephaly. Maternal serum levels of AFP also may be raised if the fetus has open neural tube abnormality, but considerable overlap is seen between in normal pregnancies and those where the fetus has neural tube abnormality (see Section VI. B).

Table 10 lists inborn errors of metabolism which have been diagnosed antenatally. Nevertheless, the reliability of a particular technique may be insufficient to encourage parents at high risk to proceed with the promise of antenatal diagnostic cover.[86] If the risk of having a child with an X-linked recessive condition is high, for example with Duchenne muscular dystrophy or hemophilia, the fetus may be sexed and the pregnancy terminated if that fetus is male. Of the more than 150 X-linked disorders only Hunter's syndrome, Fabry's disease, and the Lesch-Nyhan syndrome are specifically diagnosable antenatally.[86]

A. Screening the Pregnancies of Older Women

The incidence of almost all chromosome abnormalities is associated with maternal age (Table 4). For mothers less than 30 years old, the incidence of mongolism among the liveborn is less than 1 in 2000; between 35 and 39 years the incidence approximate 1 in 300; and above 39 years old the incidence approaches 1 in 65. Neural tube abnormality also is more frequent in older mothers, although this effect is much less marked than that in mongolism. Screening the fetuses of older mothers, by amniocentesis for fetal chromosome analysis and AFP levels, is obviously desirable.[94]

On the basis of the 1975 maternal age distribution in Britain monitoring all preganancies in women who would be 40 or more years old at delivery would be expected to reduce the frequency of liveborn mongol children by 15 to 25%; for 35 years and older, the frequency of mongolism would be reduced by approximately 40%; starting

Table 9
RISK OF RECURRENCE FOR NEURAL TUBE ABNORMALITY, ANENCEPHALY, SPINA BIFIDA CYSTICA AND PRIMARY CONGENITAL HYDROCEPHALY, AFTER NORMAL AMNIOTIC FLUID ALPHAFETOPROTEIN

Situation	Prior probability	Risk after "normal" AFP reading[a]
After one affected first degree relative	1 in 20	1 in 130
After two affected first degree relatives	1 in 8	1 in 50
After three affected first degree relatives	1 in 4	1 in 20

[a] Assuming 95% of anencephaly and/or spina bifida cystica detectable, none of primary hydrocephaly (approximately 10% of risk) detectable, and virtually no "false positives". Overall frequency of detection 85%.

Table 10
SOME EXAMPLES OF RECESSIVE DISORDERS (AUTOSOMAL AND X-LINKED) IN WHICH AN ANTENATAL DIAGNOSIS HAS BEEN MADE[a]

Disorder
Generalized gangliosidosis
Tay-Sachs disease
Sandhoff's disease
Fabry's disease
Gaucher's disease
Niemann-Pick disease
Krabbe's disease
Metachromatic leucodystrophy
Pompe's disease
Galactosemia
Maple syrup urine disease
Homocystinuria
Argininosuccinicaciduria
Propionicacidemia
Methylmalonicacidemia
Lesch-Nyhan syndrome
Hurler's and Hunter's syndromes (gargoylism)
Lysosomal acid phosphatase deficiency
Adrenogenital syndrome

[a] Data derived from Rushton.[93]

at 30 years (approximately 20% of all pregnancies in 1975), at least 60% of mongolism and more than 20% of neural tube defect would be detected.

B. Screening for Neural Tube Abnormality on Maternal Serum

In 1973, diagnosis of anencephaly was shown to be possible by assay of maternal serum AFP at 16 weeks of pregnancy.[95] A proportion of cases of both anencephaly and spina bifida cystica are now well known to be associated with serum AFP values outside the normal range at a stage in pregnancy early enough to permit termination.[88,96] The origin of the raised maternal AFP level is probably by absorption of amniotic fluid AFP through the membranes. However, the efficiency of maternal serum AFP assay in detecting different types and degrees of neural tube defect is not yet precisely defined. Although technical improvements will probably reduce the frequency of cases missed (false negatives), present assessments indicate that efficiency, particularly of detecting spina bifida cystica, is well short of 100%. Again, attempts to identify neural tube defect before the end of the first trimester seem unlikely to succeed.

Another problem in AFP serum screening is the frequency of "false positives", because of the considerable overlap of AFP values between normal pregnancies and those in which the fetus has neural tube defect. Multiple pregnancy and threatened abortion may give high AFP values. A high maternal serum AFP value is not, by itself, sufficient reason for termination but an indication that further investigation, including amniotic fluid AFP assay, is necessary.

The effect of screening by serum AFP under different conditions on the generation of "unnecessary" amniocentesis is summarized in Table 11. The ratio of "unnecessary" to "necessary" amniocenteses and the efficiency of maternal serum AFP screening in detecting neural tube defect is expected to vary with both the value taken to be a "normal" reading and the regional incidence of neural tube (anencephaly and spina bifida cystica) defect. For example, where incidence approaches 10 per 1000 births, as in South Wales, and the upper limit of normal is taken as the 95th centile, the ratio of unnecessary to necessary amniocenteses would approximate 6:1, with 70% of neural tube abnormality detected antenatally. If only those readings above the 98th centile are investigated further, the estimated ratio of unnecessary to necessary amniocentesis falls to 3:1, but the detection efficiency drops to 50%. In a region where the incidence is less than 4 per 1000 (in East Anglia and the South of England the incidence approximates 3 per 1000), even if all readings above the 95th centile are investigated, detection efficiency is calculated as only 50%, and the ratio of unnecessary to necessary amniocentesis would be greater than 24:1.

When maternal serum AFP becomes a routine aspect of obstetric management as is intended throughout Britain, the test must obviously be performed in time to allow any necessary further investigation (for example amniotic fluid AFP) and to allow termination if required — 16 to 19 weeks gestation seems to be the optimum time for maternal serum AFP assay.

C. Other Markers of Fetal Developmental Defect or Predisposition to Disease

The late (third trimester) antenatal detection of fetal disease, for example Rhesus disease, with a view to early postnatal or intrauterine treatment, is not considered here. Attention is confined to techniques that are concerned with the identification of markers of disease or disorder of development early enough in pregnancy to permit termination if required.

Epidemiological studies indicate that some disease of multifactorial origin are associated with single gene traits potentially detectable in fatal cells derived from amniotic fluid.[61,97] Ankylosing spondylitis, disseminated sclerosis, and early onset diabetes (see Section IV. D) are three such conditions — each is associated with particular antigens of the HLA system; so that the presence, or absence, of specific HLA antigens in a fetus at special risk can give an improved estimate of the susceptibility of that fetus to that disease. Again, where gene linkage (see Section III.D) is apparent, and the marker

Table 11
THE EFFECT OF SCREENING BY SERUM AFP UNDER DIFFERENT CONDITIONS ON THE GENERATION OF "UNNECESSARY" AMNIOCENTESIS[a]

Incidence of neural tube defects/1000	Upper limit of normal range (percentile)	Amniocentesis rate/1000	Detection efficiency (%)	Ratio of "unnecessary" to "necessary" amniocentesis
10	98	20	50	3:1
10	95	50	70	6:1
6	98	20	50	6:1
6	95	50	70	12:1
4	95	50	50	24:1
2	95	50	50	49:1

[a] Data derived from Brock.[88]

trait is identifiable in amniotic fluid or fetal cells, identification of the marker trait in fetuses may be useful for antenatal purposes.[98,99]

Although fetoscopy, as currently practiced,[89,100] is associated with a substantial risk of accidental abortion, it is a technique which allows direct viewing of the fetus and as such is of special value where the fetus is at high risk of morphological abnormality not otherwise detectable, for example, cleft lip. Again fetoscopy combined with sampling of fetal blood may eventually be valuable where laboratory indicators of disease susceptibility, for example, low factor VIII activity in hemophilia and increased creatine phosphokinase level in Duchenne muscular dystrophy, may be anticipated.[101] Fetal blood analysis has already been used successfully in the antenatal detection of thalasemia and sickle-cell anemia.[102,103] Fetal X-ray, fetal ultrasound scanning, and analysis of the constituents of amniotic fluid are constantly improving in ability to detect fetal abnormality, including abnormality of internal organs.[104]

Although the techniques or approaches outlined above may already be useful in appropriate situations, none has yet acquired the technical accuracy or usefulness of fetal chromosome analysis, amniotic fluid AFP assay, or maternal serum AFP assay.

REFERENCES

1. **Smith-Keary, P. F.,** *Genetic Structure and Function,* Macmillan, London, 1975.
2. **Comings,D. E.,** Chromosome organisation, in *Aspects of Genetics in Paediatrics,* Barltrop, D., Ed., Fellowship of Postgraduate Medicine, London, 1976, 17.
3. **Blank, C. E.,** Genetic counselling — conditions attributable to single genes, *Mims Magazine,* April 1977, 75.
4. **Jacob, F. and Monod, J.,** Genetic regulatory mechanisms in the synthesis of proteins, *J. Molec. Biol.,* 3, 318, 1961.
5. **Blank, C. E.,** Genetic counselling — chromosome abnormality and defects of development, *Mims Magazine,* March 1977, 69.
6. **Bobrow, M.,** New techniques in chromosome cytology, in *Chromosome Variations in Human Evolution,* Boyce, A. J., Ed., Taylor & Francis, London, 1975, 1.

7. **Baltimore Conference,** 1975, Third International Workshop on Human Gene Mapping, in *Birth Defects: Original Article Series, XII,* The National Foundation-March of Dimes, New York, 1976. 7.
8. **Mittwoch, U.,** Sex chromatin, in *The Cell in Medical Sciences,* Vol. 2, Beck, F. and Lloyd, J. B., Eds., Academic Press, London, 1974, 169.
9. **Blank, C. E.,** Chromosome abnormality and cytogenetic analysis in obstetric and gynaecological practice, in *Scientific Foundations of Obstetrics and Gynaecology,* 2nd ed., Phillipp, E. E., Barnes, J., and Newton, M., Eds., William Heinemann Medical Books, London, 1977, 44.
10. **Lyon, M. F.,** X-chromosome inactivation and developmental patterns in mammals, *Biol. Rev.,* 47, 1, 1972.
11. **Carr, D. H. and Gedeon, M.,** Population cytogenetics of human abortuses in *Population Cytogenetics: Studies in Humans,* Hook, E. B. and Porter, I. H., Eds., Academic Press, London, 1977, 1.
12. **de Grouchy, J.,** Human chromosomes and their anomalies, in *Aspects of Genetics in Paediatrics,* Barltrop, D., Ed., Fellowship of Postgraduate Medicine, London, 1976, 5.
13. **Hook, E. B. and Hamerton, J. L.,** The frequency of chromosome abnormalities detected in consecutive newborn studies — differences between studies — results by sex and by severity of phenotypic involvement, in *Population Cytogenetics: Studies in Humans,* Hook, E. B. and Porter, I. H., Eds., Academic Press, New York, 1977, 63.
14. **Valentine, G. H.,** *The Chromosome Disorders: An Introduction for Clinicians,* 3rd ed., William Heinemann Medical Books, London, 1975.
15. **Fialkow, P. J.,** The endocrine system, in *Clinical Genetics,* 2nd ed., Sorsby, A., Ed., Butterworths, London, 1973, 532.
16. **Ford, C. E.,** General mammalian cytogenetics, in *The Cell in Medical Sciences,* Vol. 2, Beck, F. and Lloyd, J. B., Eds., Academic Press, London, 1974, 53.
17. **Penrose, L. S.,** The effects of change in maternal age distribution upon the incidence of mongolism, *J. Ment. Defic. Res.,* 11, 54, 1967.
18. **Collman, R. D. and Stoller, A.,** Shift of childbirth to younger mothers and its effect on the incidence of mongolism in Victoria, Australia, 1939-1964, *J. Ment. Defic. Res.,* 13, 13, 1969.
19. **Lindsjo, A,** Down's syndrome in Sweden — an epidemiological study of a three year material, *Acta Paediatr. Scand.,* 63, 571, 1974.
20. **Alberman, E. and Creasy, M. R.,** Factors affecting chromosome abnormality in human conceptions, in *Chromosome Variations in Human Evolution,* Boyce, A J., Ed., Taylor & Francis, London, 1975, 83.
21. **Christianson, R. E.,** Down syndrome and maternal age, *Lancet,* 2, 1198, 1976.
22. **Penrose, L. S.,** Parental age and non-disjunction, in *Human Chromosome normalities,* Davidson, W. M. and Smith, D. R., Eds., Staples Press, London, 1961, 116.
22. **Penrose, L. S.,** Parental age and non-disjunction, in *Human Chromosome Abnormalities,* Davidson, W. M. and Smith, D. R., Eds., Staples Press, London, 1961, 116.
23. **Evans, H. J.,** Effects of ionizing radiation on mammalian chromosomes, in *Chromosomes and Cancer,* German, J., Ed., John Wiley & Sons, New York, 1974, 191.
25. **Uchida, I. A.,** Maternal radiation and trisomy 21, in *Population Cytogenetics: Studies in Humans,* Hook, E. B. and Porter, I. H., Eds., Academic Press, London, 1977, 285.
26. **Holloway, S. and Emery, E. H.,** Factors affecting the incidence of Down syndrome in Scotland, *J. Biosocial Sci.,* 9, 453, 1977.
27. **Evans, H. J.,** Environmental agents and chromosome damage in somatic cells in man: in vivo studies, in *Chromosome Variations in Human Evolution,* Boyce, A. J., Ed., Taylor & Francis, London, 1975, 63.
28. **Kucera, J.,** Infectious hepatitis and Down's syndrome, *Lancet,* 1, 549, 1971.
29. **Robinson, A. and Puck, T. T.,** Trisomy clusters, *Lancet,* 2, 981, 1977.
30. **Trimble, B. K. and Doughty, J. H.,** The amount of hereditary disease in human populations, *Ann. Hum. Genet.,* 38, 199, 1974.
31. **Emery, A. E. H.,** *Elements of Medical Genetics,* 4th ed., Churchill Livingstone, London, 1975, 191.
32. **Fraser, G. R.,** Disease and human genetics, in *Textbook of Human Genetics,* Fraser, G. and Mayo, O., Eds., Blackwell Scientific Publications, Oxford, 1975, 442.
33. **McKusick, V. A.,** *Mendelian Inheritance in Man: Catalogs of Autosomal Dominant, Autosomal Recessive and X-Linked Phenotypes,* 4th ed., Johns Hopkins University Press, Baltimore, 1975.
34. **Harris, H.,** *The Principles of Human Biochemical Genetics,* 2nd ed., North Holland, Amsterdam, 1975.
35. **Emery, A. E. H.,** *Elements of Medical Genetics,* 4th ed., Churchill Livingstone, London, 1975, 209.
36. **Emery, A. E. H.,** *Elements of Medical Genetics,* 4th ed., Churchill Livingstone, London, 1975, 50.
37. **Mayo, O.,** Fundamental and population genetics, in *Textbook of Human Genetics,* Fraser, G. and Mayo, O., Eds., Blackwell Scientific Publications, Oxford, 1975, 3.

38. **Renwick, J. H., Budey, S. E., Ferguson-Smith, M. A., and Izatt, M. M.,** Confirmation of linkage of the loci for myotonica dystrophy and ABH secretion, *J. Med. Genet.*, 8, 407, 1971.
39. **Smith-Keary, P. F.,** *Genetic Structure and Function,* Macmillan, London, 1975, 165.
40. **Neel, J. V. and Schull, W. J.,** *The Effect of Exposure to the Atomic Bombs on Pregnancy Termination in Hiroshima and Nagasaki,* National Academy of Sciences, Washington, D.C., 1956.
41. **Jones, K. L., Smith, D. W., Harvey, M. S., Hall, B. D. and Quan, L.,** Older paternal age and fresh gene mutation — data on additional disorders, *J. Pediat.*, 86, 84, 1975.
42. **Falconer, D. S.,** *Introduction to Quantitative Genetics,* Oliver & Boyd, Edinburgh, 1964.
43. **Edwards, J. H.,** Familial predisposition in man, *Br. Med. Bull.*, 25, 58, 1969.
44. **Smith, C.,** Quantitative inheritance, in *Textbook of Human Genetics,* Fraser, G. R. and Mayo, O., Eds., Blackwell Scientific, Oxford, 1975, 383.
45. **Carter, C. O.,** Genetics of common single malformations, *Br. Med. Bull.*, 32, 21, 1976.
46. **Blank, C. E.,** Genetic counselling — inherited conditions of multifactorial origin, *Mims Magazine,* May 1977, 69.
47. **Falconer, D. S.,** The inheritance of liability to certain diseases, estimated from the incidence among relatives, *Ann. Hum. Genet.*, 29, 51, 1965.
48. **Emery, A. E. H.,** *Elements of Medical Genetics,* 4th ed., Churchill Livingstone, London, 1975, 115.
49. **Cudworth, G.,** The aetiology of diabetes mellitus, *Br. J. Hosp. Med.*, 16, 207, 1976.
50. **White, P.,** The inheritance of diabetes, *Med. Clin. North Am.*, 49, 857, 1965.
51. **Emery, A. E. H.,** *Elements of Medical Genetics,* 4th ed., Churchill Livingstone, London, 1975, 118.
52. **Tattersall, R. B. and Pyke, D. A,** Diabetes in identical twins, *Lancet,* 2, 1120, 1972.
53. **Zonana, J. and Rimoin, D. L.,** Current concepts in genetics: inheritance of diabetes mellitus, *N. Engl. J. Med.*, 295, 603, 1976.
54. **Nerup. J., Plantz, P., Andersen, O. O., Christy, M., Lyngsøe. J., Poulsen, J. E., Ryder, L. P., Nielsen, L. S., Thomsen, M., and Svejgaard, A,** HL-A antigens and diabetes mellitus, *Lancet,* 2, 864, 1974.
55. **Cudworth, A. G. and Woodrow, J. C.,** HL-A system and diabetes mellitus, *Diabetes,* 24, 345, 1975.
56. **Gamble, D. R.,** Epidemiological and virological observation on juvenile diabetes, *Postgrad. Med. J.*, 50, 538, 1974.
57. **Simpson, N. E.,** Multifactorial inheritance — a possible hypothesis for diabetes, *Diabetes,* 13, 462, 1964.
58. **Irvine, W. J., Gray, R. S., Morriss, P. J., and Ting, A.,** Correlation of HLA and thyroid antibodies with clinical course of thyrotoxicosis treated with antithyroid drugs, *Lancet,* 2, 898, 1977.
59. **Tattersall, R. B. and Fajans, S. S.,** A difference between the inheritance of classical juvenile — onset and maturity — onset type diabetes of young people, *Diabetes,* 24, 44, 1975.
60. **Darlow, J. M., Smith, C., and Duncan, L. J. P.,** A statistical and genetical study of diabetes. III. Empiric risks to relatives, *Ann. Hum. Genet.*, 37, 157, 1973.
61. **Golup, S. H., Hanson, D. C., Sulit, H. L., Morton, D. L., Pellegrino, M. A., and Ferrone, S.,** Comparison of histocompatibility antigens on cultured human tumour cells and fibroblasts by quantitative antibody absorption and sensitivity to cell mediated cytoxicity, *J. Nat. Cancer Inst.*, 56, 167, 1976.
62. **Oakley, W.,** The evolution of the management of diabetic pregnancy, *Postgrad. Med. J.*, 45, 802, 1969.
63. **Brearley, B. F.,** The management of pregnancy in diabetes mellitus, *Practitioner,* 215, 644, 1975.
64. **Pedersen, L. M., Tygstrup I., and Pedersen J.,** Congenital malformations in newborn infants of diabetic women; correlation with maternal diabetic vascular complications, *Lancet,* 1, 1124, 1964.
65. **Soler, N. G., Walsh, C. H., and Malins, J. M.,** Congenital malformations in infants of diabetic mothers, *Q. J. Med.*, (n. s.), 45, 303, 1976.
66. **Fraser, F. C.,** Genetic counseling, *Am. J. Hum. Genet.*, 26, 636, 1974.
67. **Stevenson, A. C. and Davison, B. C. C.,** *Genetic Counselling,* 2nd ed., Wiliam Heinemann Medical Books, 1976.
68. **Murphy, E. A. and Chase, G. A.,** *Principles of Genetic Counseling,* Year Book Medical Publishing, Chicago, 1975.
69. **Antley, R. M. and Hartlage, L. C.,** Psychological responses to genetic counselling for Down's syndrome, *Clin. Genet.*, 9, 257, 1976.
70. **Riccardi, V. M.,** *The Genetic Approach to Human Disease,* Oxford University Press, New York, 1977, 195.
71. **Shapiro, S., Slone, D., Hartz, S. C, Rosenberg, L., Siskind, V., Monson, R. R, Mitchell, A. A., Heinonen, O. P, Idanpaan-Heikkila, J., Haro, S., and Saxen, L.,** Anticonvulsants and parental epilepsy in the development of birth defects, *Lancet,* 1, 272, 1976.
72. **Gustavson, K. H. and Jorulf, H.,** Recurrence risks in a consecutive series of congenitally malformed children dying in the perinatal period, *Clin. Genet.*, 9, 307, 1976.

73. **Alfrod, C. A., Stagno, S. and Reynolds, D. W.**, Toxoplasmosis: silent congenital infection, in *Infections of the Fetus and the Newborn Infant,* Krugman, S. and Gershon, A. A., Eds., A. R. Liss, New York, 1975, 133.
74. **Cooper, L. Z.**, Congenital rubella in the United States, in *Infections of the Fetus and the Newborn Infant,* Krugman, S. and Gershon, A. A., Eds., A. R. Liss, New York, 1975, 1.
75. **Marx, J. L.**, Cytomegalovirus: a major cause of birth defects, *Science,* 190, 1184, 1975
76. **Smithells, R. W.**, Environmental teratogens of man, *Br. Med. Bull.,* 32, 27, 1976.
77. **Schardein, J. L.**, Thyroid and antithyroid drugs, in *Drugs as Teratogens,* CRC Press, Cleveland, 1976, 229.
78. **Hanson, J. W., Jones, K. L. and Smith, D. W.**, Fetal alcohol syndrome, *J. Am. Med. Assoc.,* 235, 1458, 1976.
79. **Tuchmann-Duplessis, H. G.**, The effects of drugs on the embryo, in *Scientific Foundations of Obstetris and Gynaecology,* 2nd ed., Philipp, E. E., Barnes, J., and Newton, M., Eds., William Heinemann Medical Books, London, 1977, 778.
80. **Rimoin, D. L. and Schimke, R. L.**, *Genetic Disorders of the Endocrine Glands,* C. V. Mosby, Saint Louis, 1971.
81. **Sorsby, A., Ed.**, *Clinical Genetics,* 2nd ed., Butterworths, London, 1973.
82. **Bonaiti-Pell, C. and Smith, C.**, Risk tables for genetic counselling in some common congenital malformations, *J. Med. Genet.,* 11, 374, 1974.
83. **Smith, D. W.**, *Recognisable Patterns of Human Malformations,* 2nd ed., W. B. Saunders, Philadelphia, 1976.
84. **Warkany, J.**, *Congenital Malformations — Notes and Comments,* Year Book Medical Publishing, Chicago, 1971, 38.
85. **Sullivan, F. M. and McElhatton, P. R.**, A comparison of the teratogenic activity of the antiepileptic drugs carbamazepine, clonazepam, ethosuximide, phenobarbital, phenytoin and primidone in mice, *Toxicol. Appl. Pharmacol.,* 40, 365, 1977.
86. **Milunsky, A.**, Current concepts in genetics: prenatal diagnosis of genetic disorders, *N. Engl. J. Med.,* 295, 377, 1976.
87. **Laurence, K. M. and Gregory, P.**, Prenatal Diagnosis of Chromosome Disorders, *Br. Med. Bull.,* 32, 9, 1976.
88. **Brock, D. J. H.**, Prenatal diagnosis — chemical methods, *Br. Med. Bull.,* 32, 16, 1976.
89. **MacVicar, J.**, Antenatal detection of fetal abnormality — physical methods, *Br. Med. Bull.,* 32, 4, 1976.
90. **Milunsky, A.**, Risk of amniocentesis for prenatal diagnosis, *N. Engl. J. Med.,* 293, 932, 1975.
91. **Burnett, L. S., Wentz, A. C., and King, T. M.**, Techniques of pregnancy termination, Part II, *Obstet. Gynecol. Surv.,* 29, 6, 1974.
92. **Lorber, J. and De, N. C.**, Family history of congenital hydrocephalus, *Devl. Med. Child. Neurol.,* 12, 94, 1970.
93. **Rushton, D. I.**, Developmental genetics, in *Textbook of Human Genetics,* Fraser, G. and Mayo, O., Eds., Blackwell Scientific Publications, Oxford, 1975, 147.
94. **Hagard, S. and Carter, F. A.**, Preventing the birth of infants with Down's syndrome: a cost-benefit analysis, *Br. Med. J.,* I, 753, 1976.
95. **Brock, D. J. H., Bolton, A. E. and Monaghan, J. M.**, Prenatal diagnosis of anencephaly through maternal serum alphafetoprotein measurement. *Lancet,* 2, 923, 1973.
96. **Cowchock, F. S. and Jackson, L. G.**, Diagnostic use of maternal serum alpha-fetoprotein levels. *Obstet. Gynecol.,* 47, 63, 1976.
97. **Svejgaard, A., Platz, P., Ryder, L. P., Nielsen, L. S. and Thomson, M.**, HL-A and disease associations — a survey, *Transplant Rev.,* 22, 3, 1975.
98. **Schrott, H. G. and Omenn, G. S.**, Myotonic dystrophy: opportunities for prenatal prediction, *Neurology,* 25, 789, 1975.
99. **Spence, M. A., Lange, K. and Crandall, B. F.**, Computations for prenatal prediction of myotonic dystrophy, *Lancet,* 2, 1198, 1976.
100. **Scrimgeour, J. B.**, Other techniques for antenatal diagnosis, in *Antenatal Diagnosis of Genetic Disease,* Emery, A. E. H., Ed., Churchill Livingstone, Edinburgh, 1973, 40.
101. **Patrick, J. E., Perry, T. B. and Kinch, R. A. H.**, Fetoscopy and fetal blood sampling: a percutaneous approach, *Am. J. Obstet. Gynecol.,* 119, 539, 1974.
102. **Kan, Y. W., Golbus, M. S., Trecartin, R., Furbetta, M. and Cao, A.**, Prenatal diagnosis of homozygous β - thalassaemia, *Lancet,* 2, 790, 1975.
103. **Kan, Y. W., Golbus, M. S., and Trecartin, R.**, Prenatal diagnosis of sickle-cell anemia, *N. Engl. J. Med.,* 294, 1039, 1976.
104. **Bartley, J. A., Golbus, M. S., Filly, R. A., and Hall, B. D.**, Prenatal diagnosis of dysplastic kidney disease, *Clin. Genet.,* 11, 375, 1977.

Chapter 9

DISORDERS OF SEX DIFFERENTIATION

James S. Scott

TABLE OF CONTENTS

I. INTRODUCTION

Disorders of sex differentiation are much commoner than is generally realized by the lay public or even the medical profession. When they do occur they are frequently the source of great distress to the individual concerned and to the whole family. While only a very small proportion of them are amenable to specific endocrinological therapy, it is possible in most cases by sympathetic understanding combined with corrective surgical and hormonal treatment to ameliorate many of the more distressing features. While many cases have specific endocrinological features the diagnosis of most can be made on the basis of clinical, anatomical, and chromosomal findings. The endocrine features are, however, essential for diagnosis in a few cases and helpful for confirmation in others; in some they have an essential place in monitoring the effects of the therapy.

To understand the whole group of patients with disorders of sex differentiation it is important to have an understanding of the fundamental biological nature of sex. It can be defined as a species dimorphism represented at different planes by chromosomes, gonads, sex ducts, external genitalia, bodily habitus, secondary sex characteristics, and behavior or psychological attitude. The terms "chromosomal" or "gonadal" intersex are self-explanatory. Phenotypic sex refers to the apparent sex of the individual as judged by external characteristics. The term "intersex" is applied to cases in which (a) there is some contradiction between the sex manifestations or (b) the characteristics are so poorly developed as to leave doubt as to whether the individual is male or female. It is usual to include a number of situations in which the chromosomal state is not strictly one of intersexually but in which there are additional sex chromosomes.

Sex is not, as society regards it, simply a grouping of individuals into two distinct classes but rather a spectrum. This ranges from the very masculine to the very feminine. The vast majority of individuals are easily classified as male or female but in the intermediate zone of the spectrum there are some who biologically are neither male nor female. Put another way, sex rather than being a binary phenomenon is a set of characteristics with bimodal distribution. Society recognizes only the two sexes and the medical profession must go along with this simplification and ascribe intersexual individuals to whatever sex seems the most *appropriate*. It is important to appreciate that this may not be the *"true"* scientific sex in terms of chromosomes, gonads or hormones.

The majority of cases of intersex fit into a number of categories which have been given various syndrome titles when they were recognized but their etiology not clearly understood (e.g. Turner's, Klinefelter's, adrenogenital, and testicular feminization syndromes). None of these syndromes, however, is sharply demarcated and all merge into the overall spectrum. The initial development of the embryo is identical in male and female and the primitive glands and ducts are capable of developing into the male or female form. An important fact is that if there is no differentiating chromosomal or endocrine stimulus, the individual will develop as a phenotypic female. In other words, in the human the female form corresponds to neuter and masculinization involves a deviation away from that.

The most fundamental controlling feature is the second, or differentiating, sex chromosome. The normal mature ovum contributes one X chromosome to fertilization. The second and differentiating sex chromosome is contributed from the male through either an X or Y bearing spermatozoon. If the sex chromosome complement is abnormal in such a way as to produce an intersexual chromosome situation, e.g. XO or XXY, then it is likely that there will be manifestations of abnormality at all subsequent levels of sex development, i.e. gonadal, gonadal steroid, sex duct, and secondary sex characteristics. If the chromosomes are normal but the gonads abnormal then it is likely that subsequent sex manifestations will show abnormalities. It follows from these generalizations that if chromosomes and gonads are from the sexual point of view normal and compatible there are only two basic types of physical intersex which occur — *incomplete masculinization of chromosomal and gonadal males* and *partial inappropriate masculinization of chromosomal and gonadal females.*

Gynecologists and clinical or laboratory endocrinologists are mostly involved with cases having physical intersex problems, but it is important to bear in mind that while most of these cases will have some psychological problems, there is a group of individuals who are entirely normal physically but who have intersexual problems which are purely psychological. Functionally gonadal sex is controlled from the hypothalamus and pituitary and while the anatomy of these is uniform for male and female, the mode of physiology is different. In the male the production of gonadotropins from the pituitary is on a steady tonic basis whereas in the female it is on an intermittent clonic pattern. Higher centers control this phenomenon and there is evidence that intrauterine hormonal levels, to which the fetus itself contributes, are responsible for the development of centers controlling the gonadotropin releasing factor production in the hypothalamus. There are also cortical centers which control general sexual behavior and attitudes which are similarly influenced by the hormonal environment in early life. Cases of intersex can be classified into (1) chromosomal, (2) gonadal, (3) partial inappropriate masculinization of chromosomal and gonadal females, (4) incomplete masculinization of chromosomal and gonadal males, and (5) cerebral.

II. CHROMOSOMES

The human somatic cell is the possessor of two sets of 23 chromosomes, 22 autosomes plus 1 sex chromosome, one set inherited from each parental gamete, 46 in all. Each chromosome carries a multitude of genes. It has been possible since the late 1950s to analyze chromosomes by culturing cells from the body; usually lymphocytes are used since they are easy to obtain. When the cells are in the metaphase, division is arrested by colchicine, and by the use of hypotonic saline the cell is disrupted; a spread preparation allows the chromosomes to be identified. With photographic techniques the chromosomes may be *karyotyped*, which involves arranging them in sequence according to size and the position of the centromere (or junction of the arms). Morphologically the X chromosome is indistinguishable from autosomes 6 to 12 (Group C) , while the Y chromosome, which is a small acrocentric chromosome (centromere near one end), is similar in size to autosomes 21 and 22 (Group G).

A. Nuclear Chromatin (Barr) Body

Techniques are available for getting information about the sex chromosome complement of human tissues without the necessity to perform the relatively expensive and slow cell culture with karyotyping. The first of these involves counting the number of nuclear chromatin (or Barr) bodies in each cell. This body is a mass of nuclear chromatin which is seen beneath the nuclear membrane in a variable proportion of cells carrying more than one X chromosome. When Barr first observed it this was thought to be the essential tissue hallmark of femaleness but it is now clear that it is related to the number of X chromsomes present. One X chromosome only is necessary for the viability of the cell and the other one undergoes condensation and rests in a state of apparent inactivity beneath the nuclear membrane. If the cells have an excessive number of X chromosomes then the number of Barr bodies which may be seen equals the number of X chromosomes minus one. The reason that chromatin bodies are not seen in all normal XX cells is probably dependent upon the random nature of the projection. If the chromatin body happens to lie on the periphery of the nucleus as it is viewed, then it will be evident, whereas if it lies deep or superficial to the nucleus it will not stand out.

As a screening test, done usually on smears of cells taken from the internal aspect of the cheek, the Barr body analysis is a most valuable tool in making a quick assessment of the likely sex chromosome constitution in cases of poorly defined sex differentiation. In relation to the nuclear chromatin body formation the Lyon hypothesis is of some theoretical importance. This postulates that genes on the X chromosome which goes to form the chromatin body are inactive. Early in embryonic life one of the two X chromosomes in a normal female cell becomes inactive as a chromatin body and all descendants of these cells have the same X chromosome inactive. It is assumed that inactivation occurs at random, sometimes involving paternal and sometimes maternal X. Thereafter as the embryo grows there will be clusters of cells with an inactive maternal X mixed with patches of cells derived from a cell in which the paternal X has become inactive. Lyon[1] originally developed her hypothesis in relation to the fact that female mice heterozygous for a particular sex linked gene controlling skin color were patchy rather than gray. The Lyon hypothesis is of relevance in relation to possible mechanisms of development of gonadal intersex with male and female tissue present — hermaphroditism.

B. Y Chromosome Fluorescence

The Y chromosome can also be demonstrated by means of fluorescent microscopy. The terminal portion of the chromosome has a selective affinity for the fluorescent acridine derivative quinacrine dihydrochloride and it can be detected in the cultured or uncultured cells by means of this label.

C. Abnormalities Which May be Detected on Chromosome Study

It may be found that the sex chromosome complement is contrary to the phenotypic or other sex characteristic of the individual. There may also be abnormalities of the number of sex chromosomes, in the structure of the sex chromosomes (the important structural abnormalities involve isochromosomes, the result of transverse division, translocations, inversions, and deletions). Relatively recently techniques have been introduced whereby cross striations on the chromosomes can be demonstrated by special staining techniques (banding studies) and this allows more detailed characterization of each individual chromosome. In addition it may be found that the cultured cells show a variable chromosome complement, usually due to *mosaicism.* In this some error occurs at the time of a mitosis after fertilization usually with nondisjunction or loss of a chromosome, and cell strains develop with different chromosome complements. By effects of this sort it is possible for an infinite range of cell mixtures to occur thus contributing to the spectral state of sex differentiation anomalies which has been described.

Alternatively, when two chromosomal cell lines are present in the one individual it may be an example of *chimerism*. In this situation the different cell types derive from separate acts of fertilization. This has bearing on some intersexual situations and is of considerable biological interest. Sometimes an ovum may have undergone incomplete maturation before fertilization and the second polar body is not extruded. Then it is possible for an X-bearing sperm to fertilize the main ovum nucleus and a Y-bearing sperm to fertilize the second polar body. From this may develop an individual who is an XX/YY chimera and shows complex intersexual manifestations.

From study of various intersexual abnormalities seen with abnormality of the X-chromosome it has been shown that genes are present on both long and short arms necessary for the development of the functioning ovary. However, when the second X chromosome is missing there are usually certain somatic abnormalities and dwarfism (Turner's syndrome) and it can be deduced that these genes are situated on the short arm of the X chromosome.

Study of chromosomal abnormalities in abortuses has also shown that very many early abortuses possess gross chromosomal abnormality. It is now certain that very many sex chromosome anomaly conceptuses are aborted in the early weeks. Figures as high as 20% of 45, X complements have been reported in early abortuses. It has been estimated[2] that between 96% and 98% of such conceptuses have failed to be born alive; another estimate[3] is that the incidence of 45, X in spontaneous abortions is 200 times higher than in the population of extrauterine survivors.

III. EMBRYONIC SEXUAL DIFFERENTIATION

The initial development of the conceptus is asexual as has been stated. Mainly thanks to the French worker Jost we now have a reasonably clear idea of the mechanisms which result in sex differentiation. Under the control of the critical genes carried on the sex chromosomes the primitive gonad on the dorsal aspect of the coelom begins to develop either male or female form. In the male, medullary growth is predominant, while in the female cortical enlargement occurs at the expense of the medullary component. This influence is mediated through the action of chemical substances, so-called "inductors". Subsequently the gonads from their own hormone production are responsible for the development of the appropriate sex ducts and the atrophy of the inappropriate ones. This involves in the male the development of the Wolffian or mesonephric ducts with atrophy of the Müllerian or paramesonephric ducts, while in the female it is the Müllerian ducts which develop and the Wolffians atrophy. At the same time development of the external genitalia into male or female form is taking place. The reason for the female phenotype of individuals who are chromosomally or gonadally neuter may be that "in utero" they are exposed only to the sex hormones which cross the placenta from the mother and they, acting unopposed, induce the female form.

The testis "in utero" produces androgens of which testosterone is probably the most important from a very early stage, but these alone are not responsible for all the masculinizing effects. Another substance is necessary for the inhibition of the Müllerian ducts — Müllerian inhibition factor (MIF). This is not a steroid but probably a protein elaborated by the Sertoli cells of seminiferous tubules. It actively suppresses the Müllerian development at about the 8th week from conception.[4] The Leydig cells in the fetal testis are responsible for testosterone production which prevents atrophy of the Wolffian system and induces development of the epididymis, vas deferens, and seminal vesicles from it. The influence of the MIF is restricted to the side on which it is produced. Therefore if the testicle is absent on one side, Müllerian inhibition on that side will be likely to fail.

The male external genital development appears to require not only testosterone but also the enzyme 5-alpha-reductase which reduces testosterone to dihydrotestosterone.[5] The testosterone also causes the genital folds to become elevated and enclose a groove which forms ultimately the male urethra while the genital swellings lateral to the folds enlarge and form the scrotum.

IV. CHROMOSOMAL INTERSEX

A. Turner's Syndrome

Turner[6] described cases of female phenotype with sexual infantalism combined with neck webbing, retardation of growth, and bilateral cubitus valgus. It was soon afterwards found that such individuals had no ovaries, merely streaks in the site where the ovaries would have been expected, termed streak gonads. Ovarian agenesis was the description first applied but later when it was shown that these individuals lacked nuclear chromatin and it was thought that they were chromosomal males, the term *gonadal* dysgenesis was applied. When it became possible to perform chromosome karyotyping it transpired that these individuals usually had a chromosome complement of 45,X. However, many displayed various mosaic patterns, some 45,X/46,XY and some 45,X/46,XX and with all proportional gradations between the different types of cells, while others showed abnormal X chromosomes. It subsequently became clear, however, that streak gonads were present in a number of other individuals who did not show the anatomical anomalies associated with Turner's syndrome (see Section V.B).

In cases of Turner's syndrome the diagnosis is often suspected soon after birth by pediatricians because of the various anatomical abnormalities which may occur, the somewhat unusual facies which is present, and the presence of lymphatic edema of the lower limbs.

Strong support of the diagnosis is obtained from a buccal smear which is chromatin negative and it is confirmed if chromosome culture and karyotype reveals a 45, X constitution or a mosaic pattern with a high proportion of XO cells.

In the neonatal phase endocrine assessment is not of any assistance but at the time puberty is expected and fails to appear endocrine anomalies are present. The primary one involves a build-up in gonadotropin levels. The pubertal surge of gonadotropins occurs in the normal way but in the absence of a gonad capable of producing steroid hormones in response, the gonadotropin level continues to rise to abnormal heights. This is combined with insignificant circulating and excretion levels of steroid hormones produced by the ovary-estrogens and progesterone and their derivatives.

B. Klinefelter's Syndrome (or Seminiferous Tubule Dysgenesis)

From a chromosomal point of view Klinefelter's syndrome is the converse of Turner's syndrome. Instead of absence of a second differentiating sex chromosome there are two contrary differentiating sex chromosomes present, one an X and one a Y so the total chromosome complement is 47, XXY. On theoretical grounds it would be expected that the incidence of the two conditions would be approximately equal and this may be so at conception but if cases surviving into the postnatal period only are considered, Klinefelter's syndrome is very much commoner than Turner's — one or two cases per thousand. This is probably due to the fact that when a chromosome is absent there is a very high intrauterine mortality. In general, the influence of the Y chromosome tends to dominate that of the Xs present.

Cases usually present only because of infertility in marriage. About 10% of azoospermic or severely oligospermic males have this condition. Azoospermia at repeated checks is usually discovered and on examination of the phenotypic male it is found usually that he is of tall stature with a long pubis-sole measurement, the lack of production of testosterone at puberty allowing increased growth of long bones because of delayed epiphyseal fusion. There may be a degree of breast hypertrophy. The testicles are small as is the prostate and there is diminished body and facial hair. Confirmation of the diagnosis is obtained by finding a positive nuclear chromatin status, a 47, XXY chromosome complement on karyotyping and possibly testicular biopsy. There are, however, a small number of cases in which the condition presents in individuals whose chromosome complement is XY.

Endocrine features are high gonadotropin levels from puberty onwards and a subnormal plasma testosterone. In cases where the diagnosis is in particular doubt because of lack of the usual chromosomal complement the endocrine results may be helpful in giving confirmation.

C. Extra Sex Chromosome Constitution without Intersexuality (XXX and XYY)

Both of these are relatively common but have no very specific features though there is a suggestion that menstrual irregularity and amenorrhea are common in XXX females along with reduced fertility. Ovarian follicular development seems to be impaired[7] and this will be reflected in abnormal ovarian steroid patterns. The XYY syndrome was first described because of an alleged association with criminally aggressive psychopathic behavior. This is now thought to have been due to biased sampling. Endocrine reports have varied but it seems that usually the plasma testosterone and urinary androgen levels are normal; LH secretion is sometime elevated but usually gonadotropins are low.[7]

D. XX/XY Chimerism

In this very rare form of chromosomal intersex it is most unlikely that any steroid or hormonal investigations will help in the diagnosis as the endocrine situation will depend entirely upon the proportion of XX and XY cells existing in the gonadal area and this is not a feature which will show any consistency between cases.

E. Mixed Gonadal Dysgenesis

Mixed (or asymmetrical) gonadal dysgenesis is a situation in which there is a streak gonad on one side of the pelvis and a testis on the other.[8] Unilateral Müllerian development may be present and associated with partial masculinization of the external genitalia. The chromosome constitution is usually a mosaic 45,X/46,XY. Dysgenetic gonads with XY cells are very liable to malignant change and problems in classification arise when a streak gonad is found on one side and a dysgerminoma or seminoma replacing the other gonad. The Müllerian development is usually female on both sides in such cases indicating a failure of MIF production suggesting that there has been little in the way of testicular tissue present.

Endocrine features will vary according to the precise gonadal situation but gonadotropin levels may be elevated and testosterone levels intermediate between male and female ranges.

V. GONADAL INTERSEX

This term covers forms of intersex in which the chromosome complement is usually normal but there is a contradiction in the gonadal situation. The commonest type of contradiction is when both ovarian and testicular tissue are present in the same individual — ovotesticular states or *hermaphroditism,* sometimes referred to as *true hermaphroditism.*

A. Hermaphroditism (or Ovotesticular States)

The arrangement and proportions of the ovarian and testicular tissues in the hermaphrodite vary widely. Consequently genital duct and external genital development can vary widely as also can the endocrine findings. Most cases are chromatin positive and have a 46, XX chromosome complement as studied in peripheral blood cells. It seemed possible that in the gonadal region the situation might be different and that 4pan XX/XY mosaic pattern in that area accounted for the male and female gonadal tissue. However Ferguson-Smith[9] concluded that so many cases having been recorded with only XX cells, including several with multiple tissue sampling, hidden XX/XY mosaicism was unlikely to be the usual explanation. Various mosaic patterns have been recorded but these are exceptional rather than the rule. There are only a few reports of what would be the *expected* chromosome complement in ovotesticular states — XX/XY. Endocrine studies with trophic hormone stimulation may be helpful in giving a pointer towards the fact that there is a dual gonadal structure present. In some cases levels of estrogen and pregnanediol approximating to the female range may be found associated with levels of circulating testosterone above the female range or up into the male range. However these findings are not clinically diagnostic and laparotomy with biopsy and histological examination of frozen sections of gonadal tissue is necessary to provide proof.

B. Pure Gonadal Dysgenesis

This term is used to describe cases in which only streak gonads are present but the individual has none of the features of Turner's syndrome and the chromosome complement is "normal". While the phenotype is always female the chromosomes in these cases may be either 46, XY or 46, XX. These individuals are not dwarfed but fail to develop secondary sex characteristics at the age of puberty and there is amenorrhea. There is no distinction between the physical forms of the XX and XY types; there is, however, a difference in the risk with regard to gonadal malignancy, which is peculiar to the XY type.

The cause of this condition is unknown but it may be there is failure of production of the gonadal inductor substances. Endocrine findings are as in Turner's syndrome.

C. Anorchia

Congenital absence of the testis, *anorchia,* is also a form of intersexuality. These individuals show male differentiation of the internal and external genitalia but no testes are present in the postnatal phase. The fact that Müllerian duct inhibition has occurred, however, indicates that testes must have been present until about the fourth month "in utero". This development of the male internal and external genitalia differentiates the condition from XY pure gonadal dysgenesis. Deficient testosterone and high gonadotropins are the expected findings on endocrine study after the age of puberty.

D. Contrary Gonadal Development (or Sex Inversion)

Sometimes a phenotypic male with testes and normal male external genitalia is found to have a 46, XX chromosome complement. This may be regarded as a form of reversal, deviation, or inversion of sex between chromosome and gonadal level. Polani[7] reviewed 30 cases and found no evidence from banding or fluorescent studies of abnormality of the X chromosomes. The zygotes may by XXY and a Y chromosome is lost, the remaining two X chromosomes being maternal ones. Other possibilities are that the second X is paternally derived and carries some Y chromosome material, that there is a mutant abnormal masculinizing autosome which overrides the effects of the two X chromosomes, or that a strong temporary androgenic influence at the time of gonadal differentiation causes testicular production despite an XX complement. The endocrine findings are those expected of a male and it is this in association with the female chromosome complement which provides the diagnosis. The opposite type of contrary gonadal development, i.e., an XY subject with ovaries and female sex ducts and phenotype, has not been detected in man.

VI. PARTIAL INAPPROPRIATE MASCULINIZATION OF CHROMOSOMAL AND GONADAL FEMALES

A. Defects of Steroid Synthesis (Congenital Adrenal Hyperplasia or "the Adreno-Genital Syndrome")

A number of anomalies in steroid synthesis occur which are responsible for effects on the sexual development of individuals who have got a normal chromosome and gonad constitution. The outstanding endocrine effect of these enzymatic deficiencies, which are genetically inherited, is a failure in adrenal production of cortisol with a consequent failure of feedback to the hypothalamic-pituitary level which results in overproduction of adrenocorticotropic hormone (ACTH). Because of this the adrenal cortex is overstimulated and undergoes hyperplasia. This is the explanation of the anatomical description of these conditions as "congenital adrenal hyperplasia". With the hyperplasa there is increased steroid biosynthesis but this stops at the level of the enzymatic block which is present. It means, however, that very large amounts of certain steroid hormones may be produced which in normal function would only be present in small quantities as a transient step in the metabolic pathway. (The term "adrenogenital syndrome" covered a group of situations in which there was evident alteration in the genital organs and their function which the clinician was able to attribute to adrenal disorder; it included a number of cases in which the disorder in the adrenal was a neoplasm rather than an enzymatic failure.)

These enzymatic defects are inherited on recessive genes and represent one of the commonest errors of metabolism, having a gene frequency of the order of 1 in 50. They are very important in the field of intersex. The most common types present as inappropriate masculinization of females and if the condition is diagnosed it can be to a very large extent corrected by therapy. It is a situation in which the chromosome studies are only of background importance and the *precise diagnosis is based upon the endocrinological findings.*

The commonest enzyme deficiency is 21-hydroxylase and quite frequently the term "congenital adrenal hyperplasia" is used by clinicians to refer to this without specifying the enzyme. However, clearer thinking occurs if each type is referred to by its specific enzyme anomaly. While the common type is virilizing there are very rare types, such as 3-beta-hydroxysteroid dehydrogenase deficiency, which result in a failure of production of androgens and failure of the normal masculinization of the male fetus. While this is incompatible with life, it serves as a good example of how the clinical effect will vary depending on the precise step in steroid biosynthesis. Thus, within the small group of cases of inborn errors of steroid metabolism there is a complete spectrum of intersexual forms from masculinized females to unmasculinized males, but it is only the masculinized female group that present as problems of clinical management.

The biosynthetic abnormalities are considered below in the order at which they present in the pathway from cholesterol in the adrenal.

1. Cholesterol to Pregnenolone Block (Probable 20,22-Desmolase Deficiency)

This is the most fundamental and severe form and individuals suffering from it usually die at a very early age from hypoadrenalism. The cortex becomes filled with lipoid and the term "lipoid hyperplasia" has been used. The enzymatic defect is not defined with total precision but it is probably a 20, 22-desmolase deficiency. These enzyme deficiencies are related to steroid pathways in general rather than to the adrenal glands specifically and this particular one is involved in the production of androgens in the testes of male fetuses. In view of this failure, male children will appear female at birth. They can be differentiated by buccal smear for nuclear chromatin and if necessary chromosome analysis — the chromatin is of course positive and the chromosome analysis in affected males is XY. In female fetuses there is no abnormality of the sex differentiation.

2. 3-Betahydroxysteroid Dehydrogenase Deficiency

In this condition there is blockage of the conversion of pregnenolone to progesterone and there is also some inhibition of aldosterone production. The enzyme is also involved to conversion of dehydroepiandrosterone (DHA) to androstenedione. The DHA level rises but it is only mildly androgenic. In a female child the 17-oxosteroid level may be very high but there is likely to be only very mild virilization. In male children on the other hand there may be incomplete masculinization due to the failure of androstenedione production. Electrolyte disturbance with salt loss is common and is likely to lead to early death if not corrected.

The endocrine features are high circulating and secretory levels of DHA manifest in the urine analysis as an elevated 17-oxosteroid measurement. As with other forms of the condition the plasma cortisol will be low and the ACTH level high.

3. 17-Alphahydroxylase Deficiency

In this situation there is blockage of conversion of progesterone and pregnenolone to 17-hydroxyprogesterone. There is excessive production of desoxycorticosterone and corticosterone which may lead to hypertension and hypokalemia. The high mineralocorticoid activity leads to compensatory depression of aldosterone production. This enzyme is involved in gonadal steroid production and impaired isosexual development also results. The affected females have primary amenorrhea and lack of secondary sexual characteristics but are otherwise sexually normal while males are incompletely masculinized and may show gynecomastia.[10]

In addition to the findings of excess ACTH and deficient cortisol levels, the high corticosterone and low oxogenic steroid levels are diagnostic features in these cases.

4. 21-Hydroxylase Deficiency

This is the commonest form and, as stated, when the term "congenital adrenal hyperplasia" is used without qualification it can be presumed that this is the type involved. It may occur in a salt losing and a nonsalt losing form. In the salt losing type there is low production of aldosterone as well as cortisol; the abnormal metabolites may antagonize aldosterone. Frequently babies affected with this die in the neonatal period before the electrolyte disturbance can be treated. In both types there are high levels of 17-alphahydroxyprogesterone. This may be measured in the blood. From it androstenedione and testosterone can be produced in abnormal quanities, and from a few weeks of age large amounts of derivative pregnanetriol are found in the urine.

Female infants show masculinization of the external genitalia at birth. The enlarged clitoris may easily be mistaken for a penis and particularly if there is almost complete fusion of the labia minora to give an appearance of hypospadias. Despite this masculinization of the external genitalia, the internal genitalia remain normal because testicular MIF is not present and probably the relatively high concentration of testosterone required to preserve Wolffian structures is not reached. There may be a degree of skin pigmentation, probably a consequence of the high ACTH level.

If the diagnosis is suspected with the finding of an elevated 17-alphahydroxyprogesterone level in a virilized female the performance of a buccal smear may be very helpful being nuclear chromatin positive. Plasma testosterone may also be somewhat elevated but this is not diagnostic. Pregnanetriol estimation in the urine is helpful in the post-neonatal phase being specifically elevated but in newborns this metabolic pathway is not developed and diagnosis then depends upon finding high plasma 17-alphahydroxyprogesterone and showing a drop with glucocorticoid therapy. Pregnanetriol estimation and the 11-oxygenation index may be helpful in monitoring the effects of treatment. Pregnanetriol is measured in the oxogenic steroid assays.

5. 11-Betahydroxylase Deficiency

This causes a blockage of conversion of 11-desoxycortisol to cortisol and of 11-desoxycorticosterone to corticosterone. The 11-desoxycorticosterone is salt-retaining and is produced in large amounts. The precise diagnostic finding is of high levels in the urine of the tetrahydro- derivative of 11-desoxycortisol (tetrahydro-S). A degree of elevation of urinary pregnanetriol, 17-alphahydroxyprogesterone and plasma testosterone may also be found.

6. 18-Hydroxylase and 18-Dehydrogenase Deficiency

If either of these enzymes is absent there is aldosterone deficiency with high levels of excretion of corticosterone and desoxycorticosterone. Masculinization of female fetuses is not a feature. Angiotensin levels may be elevated but as in this situation the cortisol feedback is normal, there is no excessive production of ACTH.

B. Management of Steroid Synthesis Defects

There are a few cases in which the manifestations of the enzyme deficiency occur long after birth but the majority of cases present at birth. The problems of collecting specimens both of urine and blood in the early neonatal period are considerable.

Another problem with diagnostic tests on urine in early life is that the usual steroid pathways are only becoming established. After the initial phase, however, normal oxosteroid excretion is less than 2 mg/24 hr until puberty approaches. In the absence of 24-hr urinary collections the ratio of steroids derived from before and after the metabolic step of 21-hydroxylation can be used to diagnose the 21-hydroxylation defect. Normally this ratio of 11-desoxysteroids to 11-oxysteroids is 0.4, but in affected cases this should rise towards unity as the 11-desoxy fraction is contributed to by the pregnanetriol. In difficult cases ACTH stimulation may be employed to facilitate identification of the specific enzymatic defect in urinary metabolism; if this is done after cortisone therapy has been started this should be replaced temporarily with an equivalent dose of dexamethasone which does not confuse the pattern of steroid excretion. In a few cases when the occurrence of 21-hydroxylase deficiency is suspected because of its presentation with younger siblings, the diagnosis has been made antenatally from examination of liquor amnii specimens obtained by transabdominal amniocentesis.[11] In such circumstances it is also possible that abnormally high levels of maternal urinary estriol may give a clue, these being attributable to the high levels of dehydroepiandrosterone coming to the placenta from the affected fetus.

In all suspected cases the electrolyte situation should be checked. With 21-hydroxylase deficiency, serum potassium tends to rise as does the blood urea; this is followed by a fall in the bicarbonate and finally in the serum sodium. These changes may develop rapidly and monitoring by ECG may be helpful. Such checks should also be done in any newborn male infant that is systemically ill even if there are no signs of intersexuality. The condition is inherited as a genetic recessive one and detection of carriers may be achieved. Differential assessment of the steroid production in response to ACTH or metyrapone is the method of approach.

The treatment is to give hydrocortisone to replace the natural cortisol and thus suppress the excessive ACTH production by the pituitary. The amount required is about 150% of the physiological needs. A guide to the dosage is 0.66 mg/kg of body weight per day in 6-hourly divided dosage with a larger dosage at night to effect ACTH suppression until the morning. However this requires to be monitored on the basis of effect and either the urinary or blood steroid situation may be used for this purpose. Growth should also be carefully monitored. In the salt losing type fluorocortisone 50 to 100 μg per day is also required with intravenous electrolytes if a crisis develops. Plastic surgery should be arranged as necessary to external genitalia that are virilized.

Failure to diagnose the condition is most likely when it presents in the male. In the common form accelerated skeletal maturation occurs with early epiphyseal fusion and resultant dwarfism. Also precocious puberty may develop with excessive libido and aggressive behavior but ultimately there may be inhibition of gonadotropin production with sterility. Cortisone therapy will usually control these undesirable effects.

In some cases even with proper treatment ovulation fails to occur at puberty despite good control and satisfactory gonadotropin levels. It seems in these cases that prolonged or excessive androgen influence on the hypothalamus has resulted in the development of an acyclic male pattern of gonadotropin release rather than the cyclic femle pattern.[12]

C. Masculinization of Females Induced by Exogenous Hormones

Synthetic steroid preparations with a potential to virilize may, if given to the mother, result in virilization of the fetus. It has been reported with a variety of testosterone preparations and in association with nortestosterone-derived progestogenic steroids which have in the past been used in the treatment of a tendency to abortion. There are no features specific to this condition on endocrine assessment; the diagnosis must be based on careful retrospective history of maternal drug ingestion.

D. Masculinization from Maternal Tumors

Very rarely it transpires that a virilizing maternal tumor, usually of the ovary, occurs in association with pregnancy and virilizes the fetus. Again there are no specific endocrine findings in the fetus but maternal studies may reveal abnormal androgenic steroid metabolites of a variety of types.

VII. FAILURE OF COMPLETE MASCULINIZATION OF CHROMOSOMAL AND GONADAL MALES

A. Testicular Feminization (or Androgen Insensitivity) Syndrome

In many ways the most remarkable of the specific syndromes of abnormal sex differentiation is the testicular feminization syndrome. In this condition the individuals are chromosomally male (46, XY) and chromatin negative. They have testicles, usually within the abdomen, but are born with a frankly female phenotype. Amenorrhea is the rule for there is a short blind vagina and no Müllerian development. It has become appreciated that a major feature is that the tissues are insensitive to androgens and hence the term "androgen insensitivity syndrome" has come to be used. The study of this rare syndrome has led to an understanding of many basic facets of the endocrinology of sex differentiation.[13]

Cases are rarely diagnosed before puberty; prior to this they appear to be entirely normal girls. At puberty spontaneous female breast development occurs, sometimes even to excessive degrees. The voice is feminine, but pubic and axillary hair is usually absent or scant, though this is not invariable. The external genitalia are normal female without any clitoral hypertrophy. The testes while usually in the abdomen may be in the inguinal region and are histologically similar to undescended testes in otherwise normal males. Although chromosomally and gonadally males, these individuals are usually psychologically completely feminine and well adapted to their female role. The condition is familial with an apparent X linked recessive inheritance. Carrier states may exist in females with diminished axillary and pubic hair and a history of late menarche.

The diagnosis can usually be made clinically by nuclear chromatin smear which is negative and by determining the XY chromosome constitution. The steroid findings are specific when considered in association with the physical state. Plasma testosterone level is in the normal male range; furthermore exogenous testosterone may be given without producing a virilizing effect. The plasma testosterone levels rise further on administration of human chorionic gonadotropin. Tissue incubation studies using labeled precursors demonstrated that androstenedione and dihydroepiandrosterone can be produced. These precursors can be converted to testosterone. The fact that Müllerian inhibition takes place as in a normal male indicates that MIF production is normal.

With the appreciation that despite the presence of normal male testosterone levels none of the expected effects occurred, interest focused on the mechanism of peripheral action of testosterone. This varies to some extent with tissue and age but frequently conversion of the circulating testosterone to 5-alphadihydrotestosterone by the enzyme 5-alphareductase is involved. In certain incomplete forms of the syndrome 5-alphareductase deficiency exists and therefore no 5-alphadihydrotestosterone is formed peripherally (see later). However in the fully developed androgen insensitivity syndrome this is not the case.

In general biological terms the syndrome can be regarded as the antithesis of 21-hydroxylase deficiency in which there is a central abnormality of steroid production which causes inappropriate masculinization, whereas in the testicular feminization syndrome there is a peripheral action failure which results in failure of masculinization.

The breast development which occurs at puberty and may even be excessive is still not fully explained. It appears probable that the failure of action of testosterone to some extent extends to failure of the feedback inhibitory mechanism and high levels of luteinizing hormone production result in an increase in the testicular production of estrogen. At the same time it is possible that peripheral conversion of androgens to estrogen by aromatization of androstenedione and testosterone may take place on an increased scale.[14]

B. Incomplete Forms of the Androgen Insensitivity Syndrome

Very rare types of the condition exist in which the androgen insensitivity is incomplete while in others the feminizing component is absent. These have been studied in detail by Wilson et al.[15] and Walsh et al.[14] and there appear to be two incomplete forms, types 1 and 2. Type 1 is inherited on an X-linked basis as in the complete form and there may be defective virilization of the urogenital sinus and external genitalia with hypospadias and bifid scrotum. In addition there may be Wolffian duct differentiation defects, testicular abnormality such as cryptorchidism, and incomplete male secondary sex characteristic development at puberty with a degree of gynecomastia. There is, however, always complete Mullerian duct inhibition indicating normal MIF activity. The endocrine situation in these type 1 cases appears to be similar to that in the full syndrome but the peripheral insensitivity defect is not complete and there is a variable degree of partial masculinization.[16] 5-Alphareductase is present and the end organ failure is evidently beyond this stage in the pathway.

The mode of inheritance of type 2 is autosomal recessive, and Wolffian duct derivatives (epididymis, vas deferens, and seminal vesicles) are present as in the normal male but the tissues derived from the urogenital sinus and external genitalia fail to masculinize. There is in these cases a local deficiency of 5-alphareductase with failure of dihydrotestosterone formation. It appears that the androgen feedback to the hypothalamus operates normally so there is no elevation in LH secretion and these cases do not show breast enlargement at puberty.

C. Defective Androgen Production Syndromes

A few very rare steroid enzymatic deficiencies have been recorded that result in failure of testosterone production and some of these have been considered in relation to the congenital adrenal hyperplasia, for example 21,22-desmolase deficiency, 3-betahydroxysteroid-dehydrogenase deficiency and 17-alphahydroxylase deficiency. In addition 17,20-desmolase and 17-oxosteroid reductase deficiency may have similar effects with regard to testosterone production.[15,17] Clinical manifestations may range from partial to complete failure of masculinization depending on the quantitative abnormality in testosterone production and biological effects of the precursor steroids which accumulate at the site of the metabolic block. In 17-oxosteroid reductase deficiency there is gynecomastia due to build up of estrone and estradiol levels. With 17,20-desmolase deficiency deficient testosterone levels can be expected to be associated with raised levels of 17-hydroxypregnenolone and 17-hydroxyprogesterone. With 17-oxosteroid reductase there is a low testosterone level combined with an elevated plasma androstenedione and estrone level. The LH level is elevated as is the 17-oxosteroid excretion. The elevated 17-oxosteroid level and 17-hydroxyprogesterone do not suppress with dexamethasone.[17]

D. Defective Müllerian Regression Syndrome

There are a number of reports of 46, XY individuals showing persistent Müllerian duct structures sometimes in the form of an inguinal hernia containing a uterus.[15,18]

This condition is apparently inherited as an autosomal recessive or is X linked. The picture is what would be expected if there is defective MIF production "in utero" but there is no direct way of measuring this.

VIII. CEREBRAL INTERSEX

In this category are cases in which there is no physical abnormality of sex differentiation but there is a psychological abnormality. In one form the individual has a conviction of belonging to the sex contrary to the chromosomal, gonadal, endocrinological, and phenotypic sex — *transsexuality.* When there is a desire to wear the clothes of the opposite sex the term *transvestitism* is used and when the sex drive is directed towards members of the same phenotypic sex *homosexuality* is the term applied. These conditions are not commonly considered with physical errors of sex differentiation as they usually only present at psychiatric clinics. Occasionally some appear in gynecological clinics requesting operations which will alter their physical sexual features towards that of the opposite sex. (In this connection it should be appreciated that there is no such thing as a "sex change operation"; all that can be done is a very limited amount of plastic surgery which is easier to perform towards the female than towards the male because of the technical difficulty in constructing an approximation to a male phallus in a phenotypic female.)

It has in the past been widely assumed that these psychological forms were not related to the endocrine status. In some cases this is probably true but there is now evidence that in males with low heterosexual drive the testosterone level is lower than in active heterosexual males.[19] Also some information obtained in the study of physical forms of intersex and related animal experimentation does indicate ways that hormonal factors may play a part in cases which are apparently purely psychological. In the animal world in general the same principle applies as in the human on the physical plane, namely that for the male pattern to emerge androgens are necessary to change the phenotypic sex from the neuter or female pattern. It appears from evidence on XY pure gonadal dysgenesis and the testicular feminization syndrome that the XY chromosomal constitution does not carry any genetic factor specifically responsible for masculine psychology and behavior. Some other variable factors are needed to convert the chromosomal and genetic constitution into psychological sexuality. The evidence is strong that the mediators are hormonal. It is probable that there is a critical time in the course of cerebral differentiation when if there is an abnormal hormone present, as for example from maternal ingestion, maternal tumor, or blockage of the steroid pathway in some form, the cerebral imprint may be contrary to the chromosomal and gonadal sex of the individual. The gonadotropin releasing center which is activated may be the tonic rather than the clonic one if androgens are circulating in a female fetus at the appropriate time. Also it seems likely that at higher cortical levels a similar androgenic imprint may produce inappropriate masculinization of behavior. This has been seen in individuals with 21-hydroxylase deficiency. Conversely in the testicular feminization syndrome despite there being XY chromosomes and testicles with ample testosterone production, from a psychological point of view the individual remains completely feminine psychologically and this is presumably one manifestation of the androgen insensitivity state.

Animal experiments with the anti-androgen preparation cyproterone acetate which apparently competes with androgens at the end organ level have reproduced all the manifestations of the testicular feminization syndrome. Typical female sexual behavior was shown in male animals exposed to cyproterone acetate in the second half of gestation and in the early weeks after delivery.[20] It therefore seems possible that if some similar type of substance circulates at the time for normal male cerebral differentiation it could block this occurrence.

Other possibilities are that androgen or estrogen receptors may be variably present or absent in an inappropriate way or their ratio disturbed. Also the abnormality may be a physical one of the tanycyte layer of the ependyma and the third ventricle or the hypothalamus.[21]

These comments are only hinting at the possible role that endocrine factors may have in cerebral sex differentiation. There is, however, no precise way in which steroid or other endocrine hormone measurement can be used to make a specific diagnosis.

IX. POINTS ON GENERAL MANAGEMENT OF INTERSEX PROBLEMS

There are no rules for management of errors of sex differentiation. Virtually never can these be completely corrected. Full investigation however is appropriate in all cases as only if the situation is defined as precisely as possible can maximum help be given. It is important to know if gonadal tissue contrary to the phenotypic sex is present, as in cases of hermaphroditism, for it will frequently be necessary to remove this either because of the likelihood of unwanted hormonal influences at puberty or the risk of malignancy. Prior to any laparotomy full studies should have been carried out by all other possible techniques and a clear line of action should be established between the endocrinologist and the surgeon as to what should be done in the event of each possible finding. It is important that at the time of operation frozen histological section facilities should be available in order to be able to be certain immediately of the precise nature of any gonadal tissue of doubtful naked eye appearance.

Sex change never occurs but occasionally it becomes clear that the sex registration given at birth is inappropriate for the individual and in these circumstances reregistration by the Registrar General can be performed, though there are many problems about this. It should be in the forefront of the clinician's mind that nothing should be done to convert the individual to what is the theoretical sex as judged by chromosomes, gonads, or hormones, as this may be entirely inappropriate for any prospect of the individual achieving a reasonable life. In the testicular feminization syndrome, for example, all the basic sex parameters — chromosomes, gonads, and hormones — are male, yet female integration is usually good and there is no realistic possibility of fulfilling a male role.

REFERENCES

1. **Lyon, M. F.,** Genetics; gene action in the X-chromosome of the mouse, *Nature,* 190, 372, 1961.
2. **Hecht, F. and Macfarlane, J. P.,** Mosaicism in Turner's syndrome reflects the lethality of XO, *Lancet,* 2, 1197, 1969.
3. **Polani, P. E.,** The incidence of chromosomal malformations, *Proc. Roy. Soc. Med.,* 63, 50, 1970.
4. **Blanchard, M. and Josso, N.,** Source of the anti-Müllerian hormone synthesized by the fetal testis: Müllerian-inhibiting activity of fetal bovine Sertoli cells in tissue culture, *Pediatr. Res.,* 8, 968, 1974.
5. **Wilson, J. D. and Walker, J. D.,** The conversion of testosterone to 5α-androstan-17β-ol-3-one (dihydrotestosterone) by skin slices of man, *J. Clin. Invest.,* 48, 371, 1969.
6. **Turner, H. H.,** A syndrome of infantilism, congenital webbed neck, and cubitus valgus, *Endocrinology,* 23, 566, 1938.
7. **Polani, P. E.,** Errors of sex determination and sex chromosome anomalies, in *Gender Differences, Their Ontogeny and Significance,* Ounsted, C. and Taylor, D. C., Eds., Churchill-Livingstone, Edinburgh and London, 1972, 13.
8. **Sohval, A. R.,** "Mixed" gonadal dysgenesis: a variety of hermaphroditism, *Am. J. of Hum. Genet.,* 15, 155, 1963.
9. **Ferguson-Smith, M. A.,** X-Y Chromosomal interchange in the aetiology of true hermaphroditism and of XX Klinefelter's syndrome, *Lancet,* 2, 475, 1966.
10. **Hall, R., Anderson, J., Smart, G. A., and Besser, M.,** *Fundamentals of Clinical Endocrinology,* (2nd ed.), Pitman Medical Publishing, London, 1974.
11. **Jeffcoate, T. N. A., Fliegner, J. R. H., Russell, S. H., Davis, J. C., and Wade, A. P.,** Diagnosis of the adrenogenital syndrome before birth, *Lancet,* 2, 553, 1965.
12. **Lev-Ran, A.,** Isosexual development of women with late-treated congenital adrenal hyperplasia, *Obstet. Gynecol.,* 46, 313, 1975.
13. **Simmer, H. H., Pion, R. J., and Dignam, W. J.,** *Testicular Feminisation: Endocrine Function of Feminising Testes; Comparison with Normal Testes,* Charles C Thomas, Springfield, Illinois, 1965.
14. **Walsh, P. C., Madden, J. D., Harrod, M. J., Goldstein, J. L., MacDonald, P. C., and Wilson, J. D.,** Familial incomplete male pseudohermaphroditism, type 2: decreased dihydrotestosterone formation in pseudovaginal perineoscrotal hypospadias, *N. Eng. J. Med.,* 291, 944, 1974.
15. **Wilson, J. D., Harrod, M. J., Goldstein, J. L., Hemsell, D. L., and MacDonald, P. C.,** Familial incomplete male pseudohermaphroditism, type 1: evidence for androgen resistance and variable clinical manifestations in a family with the Reifenstein syndrome. *N. Engl. J. Med.,* 290, 1097, 1974.

16. **Barragry, J. M., Makin, H. L. J., Morris, D. V., Trafford, D. J. H., and Mason, A. S.,** Male pseudohermaphroditism due to partial end-organ insensitivity to androgens, *Clin. Endocrinol. (Oxford),* 7, 137, 1977.
17. **Givens, J. R., Wiser, W. L., Summitt, R. L., Kerber, I. J., Andersen, R. N., Pittaway, D. E., and Fish, S. A.,** Familial male pseudohermaphroditism without gynecomastia due to deficient testicular 17-ketosteroid reductase activity, *N. Engl. J. Med.,* 291, 938, 1974.
18. **Brook, C. G. D., Wagner, H., Zachmann, M., Prader, A., Armendares, S., Frenk, S., Aleman, P., Najjar, S. S., Slim, M. S., Genton, N., and Bozic, C.,** Familial occurrence of persistent Müllerian structures in otherwise normal males, *Br. Med. J.,* 1, 771, 1973.
19. **Cooper, A. J., Ismail, A. A. A., Smith, C. G., and Loraine, J. A.,** Androgen function in "psychogenic" and "constitutional" types of impotence, *Br. Med. J.,* 3, 17, 1970.
20. **Neumann, F., Berswordt-Wallrabe, R. von, Elger, W., Steinbeck, H., Hahn, J. D., and Kramer, M.,** Aspects of androgen-dependent events as studied by antiandrogens, *Rec. Prog. in Horm. Res.,* 26, 337, 1970.
21. **Hamilton, W. and Walker, D. M.,** Gender: Quaesto quid Juris?, *Med. Sci. Law,* 15, 79, 1975.

INDEX

A

B

C

D

E

F

G

H

I

J

K

L

M

N

O

P

Q

R

S

T

U

V

W

X

Y

Z